Methods in Molecular Biology

Series Editor
John M. Walker
School of Life and Medical Sciences
University of Hertfordshire
Hatfield, Hertfordshire, AL10 9AB, UK

For further volumes:
http://www.springernature.com/series/7651

Colorectal Cancer

Methods and Protocols

Edited by

Jean-François Beaulieu

Laboratory of Intestinal Physiopathology, Department of Anatomy and Cell Biology, Faculty of Medicine and Health Science, Université de Sherbrooke, Sherbrooke, QC, Canada

Humana Press

Editor
Jean-François Beaulieu
Laboratory of Intestinal Physiopathology
Department of Anatomy and Cell Biology
Faculty of Medicine and Health Science
Université de Sherbrooke
Sherbrooke, QC, Canada

ISSN 1064-3745 ISSN 1940-6029 (electronic)
Methods in Molecular Biology
ISBN 978-1-4939-7764-2 ISBN 978-1-4939-7765-9 (eBook)
https://doi.org/10.1007/978-1-4939-7765-9

Library of Congress Control Number: 2018936904

Printed on acid-free paper

This Humana Press imprint is published by the registered company Springer Science+Business Media, LLC part of Springer Nature.
The registered company address is: 233 Spring Street, New York, NY 10013, U.S.A.

Dedication

I would like to thank my former mentors, Raymond Calvert, Daniel Ménard, Robert Tanguay, and Andrea Quaroni, who initiated me to the world of cell and molecular biology and its applications to the field of intestinal physiopathology.

Jean-François Beaulieu

Preface

Colorectal cancer is a complex disease and still one of the leading causes of cancer-related deaths worldwide. A better understanding of the molecular basis underlying colorectal cancer progression, from adenomas to metastasis, is crucial to establishing new noninvasive efficient tests for the detection of early lesions as well as for advancing the development of new therapeutic approaches for preventing advanced disease.

This edition of the book *Colorectal Cancer: Methods and Protocols* covers the most recent developments in the study of the mechanisms, diagnostics, screening methods, and therapeutics of colorectal cancer. The chapters were written by the scientists who established and or adapted these procedures and assays in the field of intestinal physiopathology. The first part (Chaps. 1–10) examines current approaches and techniques in use for the discovery of the molecular mechanisms underlying colorectal cancer development and progression. The second part (Chaps. 11–17) is devoted to the development of innovative tools for the diagnosis and detection of cancer lesions at early stages using cell and molecular biology approaches. Finally, the third part (Chaps. 18–22) presents recent advances in the treatment of colorectal tumors and approaches for the identification of novel therapeutic molecules. It is hoped that this book will be of great use to scientists in the field of colorectal cancer.

I would like to thank all the contributors for making this book possible.

Sherbrooke, QC, Canada *Jean-François Beaulieu*

Contents

Dedication . . . . *v*
Preface . . . . *vii*
Contributors . . . . *xi*

Part I Molecular Basis of Colorectal Cancer

1 Cell Line Models of Molecular Subtypes of Colorectal Cancer 3
Jennifer K. Mooi, Ian Y. Luk, and John M. Mariadason

2 Dissecting Oncogenic RTK Pathways in Colorectal Cancer Initiation and Progression 27
Stephen McManus, Walid Chababi, Dominique Arsenault, Claire M. Dubois, and Caroline Saucier

3 Identification of Response Elements on Promoters Using Site-Directed Mutagenesis and Chromatin Immunoprecipitation 43
Salah Boudjadi, Julie C. Carrier, and Jean-François Beaulieu

4 Identification and Functional Analysis of Gene Regulatory Sequences Interacting with Colorectal Tumor Suppressors 57
Katja Dahlgaard and Jesper Thorvald Troelsen

5 Methods for In Vivo Functional Studies of Chromatin-Modifying Enzymes in Early Steps of Colon Carcinogenesis 79
Martine Chevillard-Briet and Fabrice Escaffit

6 The Colorectal Cancer Microenvironment: Strategies for Studying the Role of Cancer-Associated Fibroblasts 87
Rahul Bhome, Massimiliano Mellone, Katherine Emo, Gareth J. Thomas, A. Emre Sayan, and Alex H. Mirnezami

7 Methods for Assessing Apoptosis and Anoikis in Normal Intestine/Colon and Colorectal Cancer 99
Pierre H. Vachon

8 Molecular Analysis of the Microbiome in Colorectal Cancer 139
Fiona Clegg, Susan H. Berry, Richard Hansen, and Georgina L. Hold

9 Proteomics Analysis of Colorectal Cancer Cells 155
Anaïs Chauvin and François-Michel Boisvert

10 Autophagic Flux Assessment in Colorectal Cancer Cells 167
Annie Lauzier and Steve Jean

Part II New Developments in Colorectal Cancer Diagnostics and Screening

11 Classification of Colorectal Cancer in Molecular Subtypes by Immunohistochemistry 179
Sanne ten Hoorn, Anne Trinh, Joan de Jong, Lianne Koens, and Louis Vermeulen

12 Stool DNA Integrity Method for Colorectal Cancer Detection 193
Claudia Rengucci, Giulia De Maio, Maura Menghi, and Daniele Calistri

13 RT-qPCR for Fecal Mature MicroRNA Quantification and Validation......... 203
Farid E. Ahmed, Nancy C. Ahmed, Mostafa M. Gouda, Paul W. Vos, and Chris Bonnerup

14 A Stool Multitarget mRNA Assay for the Detection of Colorectal Neoplasms... 217
Elizabeth Herring, Shigeru Kanaoka, Eric Tremblay, and Jean-François Beaulieu

15 Colorectal Cancer Detection Using Targeted LC-MS Metabolic Profiling 229
Danijel Djukovic, Jiangjiang Zhang, and Daniel Raftery

16 Proteomic Profiling for Colorectal Cancer Biomarker Discovery............. 241
Paula Álvarez-Chaver, Loretta De Chiara, and Vicenta Soledad Martínez-Zorzano

17 Tumor-Derived Microparticles to Monitor Colorectal Cancer Evolution....... 271
Diane Mege, Laurence Panicot-Dubois, and Christophe Dubois

PART III RECENT ADVANCES IN COLORECTAL CANCER THERAPEUTICS

18 Molecular Testing for the Treatment of Advanced Colorectal Cancer: An Overview 281
Patrick S. Lin and Thomas J. Semrad

19 Testing Cell-Based Immunotherapy for Colorectal Cancer 299
Jong Soon Kang, Yeo Dae Yoon, Myeong Youl Lee, Chang Woo Lee, Suk Jong Lee, and Sang-Bae Han

20 Patient-Derived Xenograft Models of Colorectal Cancer: Procedures for Engraftment and Propagation 307
Danielle M. Burgenske, David J. Monsma, and Jeffrey P. MacKeigan

21 Use of Organoids to Characterize Signaling Pathways in Cancer Initiation 315
Christina Oatway, Calley L. Hirsch, and Alex Gregorieff

22 Identification of Novel Molecules Targeting Cancer Stem Cells............... 333
Yannick D. Benoit

Index *349*

Contributors

FARID E. AHMED • *GEM Tox Labs, Institute for Research in Biotechnology, Greenville, NC, USA*
NANCY C. AHMED • *GEM Tox Labs, Institute for Research in Biotechnology, Greenville, NC, USA*
PAULA ÁLVAREZ-CHAVER • *Proteomics Unit, Structural Determination, Proteomics and Genomics Service, CACTI, University of Vigo, Vigo, Spain*
DOMINIQUE ARSENAULT • *Department of Pediatrics, Faculty of Medicine and Health Science, Université de Sherbrooke, Sherbrooke, QC, Canada; Department of Immunology Division, Faculty of Medicine and Health Science, Université de Sherbrooke, Sherbrooke, QC, Canada*
JEAN-FRANÇOIS BEAULIEU • *Laboratory of Intestinal Physiopathology, Department of Anatomy and Cell Biology, Faculty of Medicine and Health Sciences, Université de Sherbrooke, Sherbrooke, QC, Canada*
YANNICK D. BENOIT • *Department of Cellular and Molecular Medicine, University of Ottawa, Ottawa, ON, Canada*
SUSAN H. BERRY • *Gastrointestinal Research Group, School of Medicine, Medical Sciences and Nutrition, Institute of Medical Sciences, University of Aberdeen, Aberdeen, UK*
RAHUL BHOME • *Cancer Research UK Centre, University of Southampton Cancer Sciences Division, Southampton University Hospital NHS Trust, Southampton, UK; University Department of Surgery, Southampton University Hospital NHS Trust, Southampton, UK*
FRANÇOIS-MICHEL BOISVERT • *Department of Anatomy and Cell Biology, Faculty of Medicine and Health Sciences, Université de Sherbrooke, Sherbrooke, QC, Canada*
CHRIS BONNERUP • *Department of Physics, East Carolina University, Greenville, NC, USA*
SALAH BOUDJADI • *Cancer Molecular Pathology Section, Laboratory of Pathology, National Cancer Institute, Bethesda, MD, USA*
DANIELLE M. BURGENSKE • *Center for Cancer Cell Biology, Van Andel Research Institute, Grand Rapids, MI, USA*
DANIELE CALISTRI • *Istituto Scientifico Romagnolo per lo Studio e la Cura dei Tumori (IRST) IRCCS, Meldola, Forlì-Cesena, Italy*
JULIE C. CARRIER • *Department of Medicine, Faculty of Medicine and Health Science, Université de Sherbrooke, Sherbrooke, QC, Canada*
WALID CHABABI • *Department of Anatomy and Cell Biology, Faculty of Medicine and Health Science, Université de Sherbrooke, Sherbrooke, QC, Canada*
ANAÏS CHAUVIN • *Department of Anatomy and Cell Biology, Faculty of Medicine and Health Sciences, Université de Sherbrooke, Sherbrooke, QC, Canada*
MARTINE CHEVILLARD-BRIET • *Laboratoire de Biologie Cellulaire et Moléculaire du Contrôle de la Prolifération (LBCMCP), Centre de Biologie Intégrative (CBI), Université de Toulouse, CNRS, UPS, Toulouse, France*
LORETTA DE CHIARA • *Department of Biochemistry, Genetics and Immunology, Faculty of Biology, University of Vigo, Vigo, Spain*
FIONA CLEGG • *Gastrointestinal Research Group, School of Medicine, Medical Sciences and Nutrition, Institute of Medical Sciences, University of Aberdeen, Aberdeen, UK*
KATJA DAHLGAARD • *Department of Science and Environment, Roskilde University, Roskilde, Denmark*

DANIJEL DJUKOVIC • *Department of Anesthesiology and Pain Medicine, University of Washington, Seattle, WA, USA*

CHRISTOPHE DUBOIS • *Aix Marseille University, INSERM UMR-S1076, C2VN, Marseille, France*

CLAIRE M. DUBOIS • *Department of Pediatrics, Faculty of Medicine and Health Science, Université de Sherbrooke, Sherbrooke, QC, Canada; Department of Immunology Division, Faculty of Medicine and Health Science, Université de Sherbrooke, Sherbrooke, QC, Canada*

KATHERINE EMO • *Cancer Research UK Centre, University of Southampton Cancer Sciences Division, Southampton University Hospital NHS Trust, Southampton, UK*

FABRICE ESCAFFIT • *Laboratoire de Biologie Cellulaire et Moléculaire du Contrôle de la Prolifé ration (LBCMCP), Centre de Biologie Intégrative (CBI), Université de Toulouse, CNRS, UPS, Toulouse, France*

MOSTAFA M. GOUDA • *Department of Nutrition and Food Science, National Research Center, Cairo, Egypt*

ALEX GREGORIEFF • *Lunenfeld-Tanenbaum Research Institute, Sinai Health System, Toronto, Canada; Department of Pathology, McGill University, Montreal, Canada; Cancer Research Program of the Research Institute of McGill University Health Centre, Montreal, Canada*

SANG-BAE HAN • *College of Pharmacy, Chungbuk National University, Cheongju, Chungbuk, Republic of Korea*

RICHARD HANSEN • *Department of Paediatric Gastroenterology, Royal Hospital for Children, Glasgow, UK*

ELIZABETH HERRING • *Laboratory of Intestinal Physiopathology, Department of Anatomy and Cell Biology, Faculty of Medicine and Health Sciences, Université de Sherbrooke, Sherbrooke, QC, Canada*

CALLEY L. HIRSCH • *Lunenfeld-Tanenbaum Research Institute, Sinai Health System, Toronto, Canada*

GEORGINA L. HOLD • *Gastrointestinal Research Group, School of Medicine, Medical Sciences and Nutrition, Institute of Medical Sciences, University of Aberdeen, Aberdeen, UK*

SANNE TEN HOORN • *Laboratory for Experimental Oncology and Radiobiology (LEXOR), Center for Experimental and Molecular Medicine (CEMM), Academic Medical Center and Cancer Center Amsterdam, Amsterdam, The Netherlands*

STEVE JEAN • *Department of Anatomy and Cell Biology, Faculty of Medicine and Health Sciences, Université de Sherbrooke, Sherbrooke, QC, Canada*

JOAN DE JONG • *Laboratory for Experimental Oncology and Radiobiology (LEXOR), Center for Experimental and Molecular Medicine (CEMM), Academic Medical Center and Cancer Center Amsterdam, Amsterdam, The Netherlands*

SHIGERU KANAOKA • *Department of Gastroenterology, Hamamatsu Medical Center, Hamamatsu, Japan*

JONG SOON KANG • *Korea Research Institute of Bioscience and Biotechnology, Cheongju, Chungbuk, Republic of Korea*

LIANNE KOENS • *Department of Pathology, Academic Medical Center, Amsterdam, The Netherlands*

ANNIE LAUZIER • *Department of Anatomy and Cell Biology, Faculty of Medicine and Health Sciences, Université de Sherbrooke, Sherbrooke, QC, Canada*

CHANG WOO LEE • *Korea Research Institute of Bioscience and Biotechnology, Cheongju, Chungbuk, Republic of Korea*

MYEONG YOUL LEE • *Korea Research Institute of Bioscience and Biotechnology, Cheongju, Chungbuk, Republic of Korea*
SUK JONG LEE • *College of Pharmacy, Chungbuk National University, Cheongju, Chungbuk, Republic of Korea*
PATRICK S. LIN • *Division of Hematology/Oncology, Department of Internal Medicine, University of California Davis Comprehensive Cancer Center, Sacramento, CA, USA*
IAN Y. LUK • *Olivia Newton-John Cancer Research Institute, Melbourne, VIC, Australia*
JEFFREY P. MACKEIGAN • *Center for Cancer Cell Biology, Van Andel Research Institute, Grand Rapids, MI, USA; College of Human Medicine, Michigan State University, Grand Rapids, MI, USA*
GIULIA DE MAIO • *Istituto Scientifico Romagnolo per lo Studio e la Cura dei Tumori (IRST) IRCCS, Meldola, Forlì-Cesena, Italy*
JOHN M. MARIADASON • *Olivia Newton-John Cancer Research Institute, Melbourne, VIC, Australia*
VICENTA SOLEDAD MARTÍNEZ-ZORZANO • *Department of Biochemistry, Genetics and Immunology, Faculty of Biology, University of Vigo, Vigo, Spain*
STEPHEN MCMANUS • *Department of Anatomy and Cell Biology, Faculty of Medicine and Health Science, Université de Sherbrooke, Sherbrooke, QC, Canada*
DIANE MEGE • *Aix Marseille University, INSERM UMR-S1076, C2VN, Marseille, France*
MASSIMILIANO MELLONE • *Cancer Research UK Centre, University of Southampton Cancer Sciences Division, Southampton University Hospital NHS Trust, Southampton, UK*
MAURA MENGHI • *Diatech Pharmacogenetics, Jesi, Ancona, Italy*
ALEX H. MIRNEZAMI • *Cancer Research UK Centre, University of Southampton Cancer Sciences Division, Southampton University Hospital NHS Trust, Southampton, UK; University Department of Surgery, Southampton University Hospital NHS Trust, Southampton, UK*
DAVID J. MONSMA • *Center for Cancer Cell Biology, Van Andel Research Institute, Grand Rapids, MI, USA; College of Human Medicine, Michigan State University, Grand Rapids, MI, USA*
JENNIFER K. MOOI • *Olivia Newton-John Cancer Research Institute, Melbourne, VIC, Australia*
CHRISTINA OATWAY • *Lunenfeld-Tanenbaum Research Institute, Sinai Health System, Toronto, Canada*
LAURENCE PANICOT-DUBOIS • *Aix Marseille University, INSERM UMR-S1076, C2VN, Marseille, France*
DANIEL RAFTERY • *Department of Anesthesiology and Pain Medicine, University of Washington, Seattle, WA, USA*
CLAUDIA RENGUCCI • *Istituto Scientifico Romagnolo per lo Studio e la Cura dei Tumori (IRST) IRCCS, Meldola, Forlì-Cesena, Italy*
CAROLINE SAUCIER • *Department of Anatomy and Cell Biology, Faculty of Medicine and Health Science, Université de Sherbrooke, Sherbrooke, QC, Canada*
A. EMRE SAYAN • *Cancer Research UK Centre, University of Southampton Cancer Sciences Division, Southampton University Hospital NHS Trust, Southampton, UK*
THOMAS J. SEMRAD • *Division of Hematology/Oncology, Department of Internal Medicine, University of California Davis Comprehensive Cancer Center, Sacramento, CA, USA; Gene Upshaw Memorial Tahoe Forest Cancer Center, Truckee, CA, USA*
GARETH J. THOMAS • *Cancer Research UK Centre, University of Southampton Cancer Sciences Division, Southampton University Hospital NHS Trust, Southampton, UK*

Eric Tremblay • *Laboratory of Intestinal Physiopathology, Department of Anatomy and Cell Biology, Faculty of Medicine and Health Sciences, Université de Sherbrooke, Sherbrooke, QC, Canada*

Anne Trinh • *Li Ka Shing Centre, Cancer Research UK Cambridge Institute, University of Cambridge, Cambridge, UK; Department of Medical Oncology, Dana-Farber Cancer Institute, Boston, MA, USA*

Jesper Thorvald Troelsen • *Department of Science and Environment, Roskilde University, Roskilde, Denmark*

Pierre H. Vachon • *Département d'anatomie et de biologie cellulaire, Faculté de médecine et des sciences de la santé, Université de Sherbrooke, Sherbrooke, QC, Canada*

Louis Vermeulen • *Laboratory for Experimental Oncology and Radiobiology (LEXOR), Center for Experimental and Molecular Medicine (CEMM), Academic Medical Center and Cancer Center Amsterdam, Amsterdam, The Netherlands*

Paul W. Vos • *Department of Biostatistics, East Carolina University, Greenville, NC, USA*

Yeo Dae Yoon • *Korea Research Institute of Bioscience and Biotechnology, Cheongju, Chungbuk, Republic of Korea*

Jiangjiang Zhang • *Department of Anesthesiology and Pain Medicine, University of Washington, Seattle, WA, USA*

Part I

Molecular Basis of Colorectal Cancer

Check for updates

Chapter 1

Cell Line Models of Molecular Subtypes of Colorectal Cancer

Jennifer K. Mooi, Ian Y. Luk, and John M. Mariadason

Abstract

Colorectal cancer (CRC) is a genetically diverse disease necessitating the need for well-characterized and reproducible models to enable its accurate investigation. Recent genomic analyses have confirmed that CRC cell lines accurately retain the key genetic alterations and represent the major molecular subtypes of primary CRC, underscoring their value as powerful preclinical models. In this chapter we detail the important issues to consider when using CRC cell lines, the techniques used for their appropriate molecular classification, and the methods by which they are cultured in vitro and as subcutaneous xenografts in immune-compromised mice. A panel of commonly available CRC cell lines that have been characterized for key molecular subtypes is also provided as a resource for investigators to select appropriate models to address specific research questions.

Key words Colorectal cancer cells, Molecular subtype, DNA profiling, Chromosomal instability, Microsatellite instability, CpG island methylator phenotype, Signaling pathways

1 Introduction

Colorectal cancers (CRC) are broadly classified according to the global genomic or epigenomic aberrations they harbor. Approximately 80% of sporadic CRCs have chromosomal instability (CIN) characterized by whole or partial chromosomal duplication or deletion, while the remainder have microsatellite instability (MSI), underpinned by inactivation of DNA mismatch repair genes [1, 2]. In addition, approximately 20% of CRCs harbor the CpG island methylator phenotype (CIMP), characterized by increased rates of DNA promoter methylation [3]. CIMP is also highly associated with MSI CRC. In both CIN and MSI CRCs, the underlying genetic instability drives disease progression through the sequential deregulation of five key signaling pathways: Wnt, MAPK, p53, TGFβ, and PI3K [4–6].

Jennifer K. Mooi and Ian Y. Luk contributed equally to this work.

Jean-François Beaulieu (ed.), *Colorectal Cancer: Methods and Protocols*, Methods in Molecular Biology, vol. 1765, https://doi.org/10.1007/978-1-4939-7765-9_1, © Springer Science+Business Media, LLC, part of Springer Nature 2018

The molecular subtype and mutation spectrum of CRCs impact significantly on patient prognosis and response to therapy. For example, MSI tumors have significantly lower rates of relapse after early stage resection, while in the metastatic setting, tumors harboring *KRAS* mutations are largely refractory to EGFR-targeted therapies [7, 8].

More recently, global gene expression profiling has been used to classify CRCs into one of four consensus molecular subtypes (CMS 1–4) [9]. Prognostic associations of CMS have been described, and associations with treatment are still being investigated. The established molecular classifiers (CIN, MSI, and CIMP) are enriched within particular CMS groups, such as CMS1, which is enriched for MSI and CIMP CRCs. Comparatively, the CMS2 subgroup is enriched for CRCs with high expression of Wnt target genes, CMS3 is enriched for *KRAS* mutant tumors, and CMS4 is enriched for tumors with high stromal content and TGFβ signaling.

Comprehensive characterization of the genetic aberrations, or determining the CMS of a CRC cell line, requires high-throughput genomic approaches and gene expression profiling respectively. These specialized methods are beyond the scope of this chapter. Instead, this chapter will describe the key quality control measures to consider prior to using CRC cell lines, specifically cell line authentication and mycoplasma screening. The chapter then details the methods for MSI and CIMP classification which can be used by investigators needing to characterize new CRC cell lines, patient-derived xenografts, or to confirm the molecular subtypes of existing cell lines. Finally we detail methods for culturing CRC cell lines in vitro and as subcutaneous xenografts in immune-compromised mice.

As a resource, we provide a list of commonly used and well characterized CRC cell lines to aid investigators in selecting appropriate models to address specific research questions (Appendix 1).

2 Materials

2.1 Short Tandem Repeat (STR) Profiling

1. Reagents for isolation of genomic DNA from cells (including various commercially available kits) (*see* **Note 1**).
2. STR profiling Kit. Various commercial kits are available, such as the GenePrint™10 system (Promega, USA).

2.2 Mycoplasma Testing

For PCR and agarose gel electrophoresis

1. *Taq* DNA Polymerase PCR kit (*Taq* Polymerase, dNTP mixture, $MgCl_2$ and PCR buffer).
2. Sense primer GPO-3 (10 μM) (5′-GGGAGCAAACAGGATTA GATACCCT-3′) [10].
3. Antisense primer MGSO (10 μM) (5′-TGCACCATCTGTCA CTCTGTTAACCTC-3′) [10].

4. Agarose.
5. 50× Tris-Acetate-EDTA (TAE) Buffer: Prepare by adding 242 g Tris base to 57.1 mL glacial acetic acid, and 100 mL of 500 mM EDTA (pH 8.0) solution, and bring the volume up to 1 L.
6. SYBR Safe DNA Gel Stain (Life Technologies).
7. 1 kb Plus DNA Ladder.

2.3 Cell Culture

All materials need to be sterile and used only in a tissue culture flow hood in order to prevent biological contamination.

1. Base Culture Medium: A number of different culture media are available. Almost all CRC cell lines grow well in Dulbecco's Modified Eagle Medium: Nutrient Mixture F-12 (DMEM F-12), RPMI-1640, DMEM (1×) or MEM (Gibco, USA). Occasionally, a cell line may require a specific culture medium. It is therefore best to check with the cell line supplier regarding the most appropriate culture medium for each cell line. When comparing effects across multiple cell lines it is best to use a single culture medium. We have used DMEM-F12 when performing experiments in which drug effects on multiple CRC cell lines are compared [11–13].
2. To prepare complete culture medium, supplement 500 mL of base cell culture medium with the following: 50 mL of fetal bovine serum (FBS) (various suppliers), 5 mL of GlutaMAX 100× supplement (Gibco, USA), 5 mL of Penicillin–Streptomycin antibiotic (10,000 units/mL), and 5 mL of HEPES buffer 1M. (When confident with aseptic technique, the use of antibiotics may be omitted.)
3. Trypsin solution (various suppliers, e.g., TrypLE Express Enzyme, Gibco, USA).
4. Dulbecco's phosphate-buffered saline (DPBS).

2.4 Formalin-Fixed Paraffin-Embedded (FFPE) Cell Blocks

1. Plasma, undiluted (bovine, goat, rabbit, or human) (sources—*see* **Note 2**).
2. Thrombin, topical (bovine), 1000 IU/mL concentration.
3. Long thin wooden stick (e.g., single ended cotton bud on a 15 cm wooden stick).
4. 10% neutral buffered formalin.
5. 80% ethanol.
6. Dulbecco's phosphate-buffered saline (DPBS).

2.5 Xenografts

1. Corning Matrigel matrix.
2. Complete culture medium (*see* Subheading point 2.3.2), without antibiotics.
3. Trypan Blue.

2.6 MSI Analysis

1. For Immunohistochemistry (IHC), primary antibodies for human MLH1, PMS2, MSH2, MSH6 and the relevant secondary antibodies and detection system reagents (*see* **Note 3**).
2. Reagents for isolation of genomic DNA from cells (including various commercially available kits) (*see* **Note 1**).
3. Reagents for PCR and fragment analysis of MSI markers, available as MSI Analysis System Version 1.2 (Promega, USA).

2.7 CIMP Analysis

1. Reagents for isolation of genomic DNA from cells (including various commercially available kits) (*see* **Note 1**).
2. Reagents for bisulfite treatment of gDNA (available in various commercially available kits such as the EpiTect Bisulfite kit, Qiagen).
3. Probes and primers as per Table 1.
4. Methylated DNA reference.
5. Nuclease-free water.
6. Reagents for methylation-specific PCR: Taq DNA polymerase, dNTP mix (dATP, dCTP, dGTP, dUTP), $MgCl_2$, Tween 20, gelatin. These reagents are also available as components of the Epitech MethyLight PCR kit, Qiagen).

3 Methods

3.1 Short Tandem Repeat (STR) Profiling of CRC Cell Lines

Prior to commencing work with cell lines it is important to authenticate that the cell line being used is indeed the correct line. Misidentification of cell lines can occur through human error, by simple mislabeling, or cross-contamination of two or more independent lines.

The authenticity of a cell line can be determined by STR profiling, and is now a requirement of many journals prior to publication. The importance of cell line authentication is underscored by the revelation that some CRC cell lines (such as HT-29 and WiDR) that were previously considered independent are in fact the same cell line.

STR's are short sequences of DNA, typically 2–5 base pairs in length, that are repeated multiple times in a row on a DNA strand [14]. STR profiling exploits the polymorphic (variable) nature of specific STRs located throughout the human genome to generate a unique genetic profile for a given sample with a very low probability of producing a random match.

3.1.1 Genomic DNA Isolation

1. Various methods can be used to isolate gDNA from colon cancer cell lines including well-optimized and validated protocols in the form of commercially available kits. We recommend isolating gDNA using a commercially available kit, as per the manufacturer's instructions (*see* **Note 1**).

Table 1
Probes and primers for MethyLight CIMP classification assay

Gene	Forward primer	Reverse primer	Probe
CACNA1G	TTTTTTCGTTTCGCGTTTAGGT	CTCGAAACGACTTCGCCG	6FAM-AAATAACGCCGAATCCGACAACCGA-BHQ
IGF2	GAGCGGTTTCGGTGTCGTTA	CCAACTCGATTTAAACCGACG	6FAM-CCCTCTACCGTCGCGAACCCGA-BHQ
NEUROG1	CGTGTAGCGTTCGGGTATTTGTA	CGATAATTACGAACACACTCCGAAT	6FAM-CGATAACGACCTCCCGCGAACATAAA-BHQ-1
RUNX3	CGTTCGATGGTGGACGTGT	GACGAACAACGTCTTATTACAACGC	6FAM-CGCACGAACTCGCCTACGTAATCCG-BHQ-1
SOCS1	GCGTCGAGTTCGTGGGTATTT	CCGAAACCATCTTCACGCTAA	6FAM-ACAATTCCGCTAACGACTATCGCGCA-BHQ-1
ALU[a]	GGTTAGGTATAGTGGTTTATATTTGTAATTTTAGTA	ATTAACTAAACTAATCTTAAACTCCTAACCTCA	6FAM-CCTACCTTAACCTCCC-MGBNFQ

[a]The *ALU* reaction is a non-methylation-dependent reaction used as a control for normalizing concentrations of input bisulfite-converted DNA

2. From cultured cell lines, collect up to 10^6 cells in a microcentrifuge tube.
3. Centrifuge the cell suspension at 300 × *g* for 5 min at 4 °C to form a cell pellet and aspirate the supernatant.
4. Proceed as per manufacturer's instructions.

3.1.2 STR Profiling

1. Perform STR profiling as per the manufacturer's instructions using the reagents provided in the STR profiling kit. We have used the GenePrint™10 System (Promega, USA) which provides reagents for the coamplification of ten human loci (*TH01, TPOX, vWA, Amelogenin, CSF1PO, D16S539, D7S820, D13S317, D5S818, and D21S11*). Collective assessment of these loci prov ides a genetic profile with a very low random match probability (estimated 1 in 10^9).
2. Detection of the amplified fragments can be performed using a number of genetic analyzers, including the Applied Biosystems 3500 or 3500 × L Genetic Analyzer with POP-4™ Polymer (*see* **Note 4**).

3.1.3 Interpreting STR Results

1. An example electropherogram of STR profiling performed on the SW480 CRC cell line is provided in Fig. 1. Examination of the *TH01* locus in the top panel reveals a single peak and the number eight. This means that SW480 is homozygous at both alleles of *TH01* and has eight repeats on each chromosome. In comparison, the *CSF1PO* locus in the middle panel has two peaks, one labeled 13 and one labeled 14. This corresponds to a heterozygous locus in which one allele has 13 repeats and the other has 14.
2. To confirm authenticity, a minimum 80% match across the panel of allele markers is recommended. Reference STR profiles of CRC cell lines can be obtained from databases such as ExPASy Bioinformatics Resource Portal Cellosaurus Database (http://web.expasy.org/cellosaurus) or the relevant source institutions. Reference STR profiles of some commonly used CRC cell lines are provided in Appendix 1.

3.2 Mycoplasma Testing of Cell Lines by PCR

A further important consideration when using cell lines is to ensure they are free of biological contamination. This includes contamination with bacteria, molds, yeasts, and mycoplasma. While bacterial, mold, and yeast contaminations can be detected by visual inspection of the culture medium, the smaller size of mycoplasmas make them much harder to detect. Mycoplasmas are small bacterial organisms (0.15–0.3 μm) that lack a cell wall and have a flexible membrane that allows them to adhere to the host cell surface [15]. They are able to bind and invade into a host eukaryotic cell using specialised tip organelles. Once inside the cell, they multiply

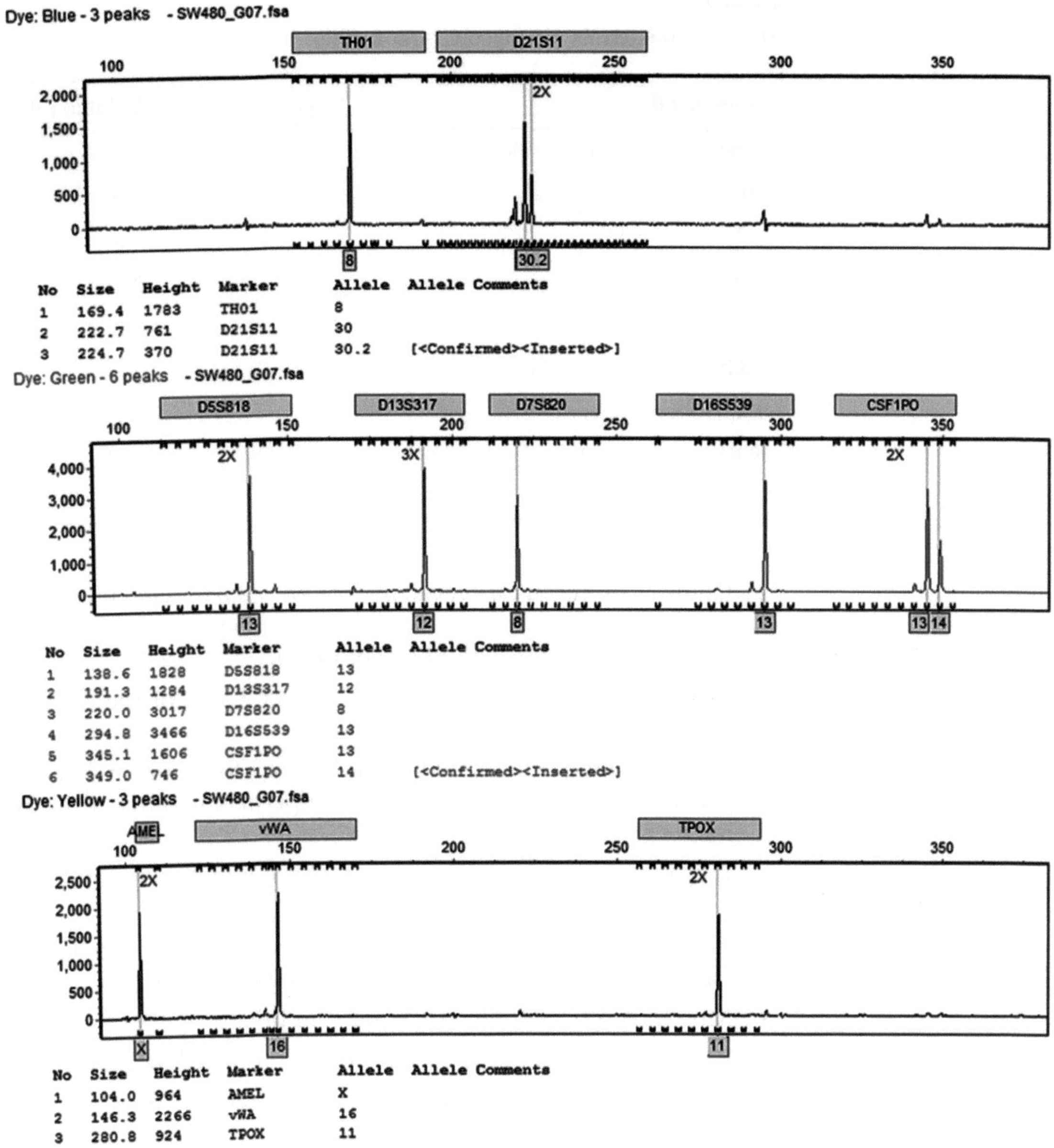

Fig. 1 STR profiling electropherogram of the SW480 colorectal cancer cell line

and compete with the host for biosynthetic precursors and nutrients and can alter cell physiology. Mycoplasma contamination, which may occur during routine cell culture, can be detected using a number of methods including fluorescent staining (e.g., Hoechst staining), ELISA, immunostaining, autoradiography, microbiological assays, or PCR. It is strongly recommended that cell cultures are periodically tested for this contamination. Here we describe a method for detecting mycoplasma contamination by PCR.

Table 2
Reaction mastermix for mycoplasma testing

Component	Volume (μL)
Supernatant (from cell line)	1
10× PCR buffer	2.5
dNTPs (10 mM)	0.5
$MgCl_2$ (50 mM)	0.75
GPO-3 primer (10 μM)	0.5
MGSO primer (10 μM)	0.5
Taq DNA polymerase	0.1
Nuclease free H_2O	19.2
Total reaction volume	*25*

1. Culture colorectal cancer cell line for 48–72 h in regular culture medium without antibiotics. Do not perform any media changes during this period (*see* **Note 5**).
2. At the end of the culture period, collect 1 mL of the culture medium in a microcentrifuge tube.
3. Centrifuge the culture medium at 300 × *g* for 5 min at 4 °C to pellet cell debris. Transfer the supernatant into a fresh microcentrifuge tube.
4. Prepare PCR master mix using the components listed in Table 2.
5. Add 24 μL of PCR mastermix and 1 μL of cell culture supernatant to each PCR tube for a 25 μL reaction (*see* **Note 6**).
6. Mix the reaction in the tubes and spin briefly.
7. Perform PCR using the cycling conditions listed in Table 3.
8. Prepare 2 L of 1× TAE buffer by adding 40 mL of 50× TAE to 1.6 L of MilliQ water.
9. Weigh out 2 g of agarose and add to a conical flask with 100 mL of 1× TAE to create a 2% agarose gel.
10. To dissolve the agarose, heat the mixture in a microwave until completely dissolved (*see* **Note 7**).
11. Add 10 μL of SYBR Safe DNA gel stain to the agarose mix and pour the gel mixture into a sealed gel moulding tank.
12. Place a well-moulding comb into the gel mix appropriate for the number of samples, and allow the gel to set for approximately 30 min.

Table 3
Cycling conditions for mycoplasma testing

Step	Temperature (°C)	Time
Denaturing, 1 cycle	95	5 min
Cycling, 36 cycles		
Denature	94	30 s
Anneal	55	30 s
Elongation	72	1 min
Elongation, 1 cycle	72	10 min
Hold, 1 cycle	4	∞

13. Once set, carefully remove the well-comb from the gel and place the gel into the electrophoresis tank.
14. Pour 1× TAE buffer to completely submerge the gel.
15. Run 10 μL of the PCR-amplified product on the 2% agarose gel at 100 V for 1.5 h. Run an appropriate volume of 1 kb DNA ladder in one well.
16. Visualize and image the gel under UV light. Detection of a 270 bp PCR product indicates a cell line is positive for mycoplasma contamination.

3.3 Growth and Subculture of CRC cell Lines In Vitro

CRC cell lines are maintained and passaged using standard cell culture techniques. The majority of CRC cell lines grow as adherent monolayers (e.g., HCT116, SW948, and SW1116), while some grow as semiadherent cultures (e.g., Colo-201, Colo-205, and Colo-320) or in suspension (e.g., SNU175 and SNUC1). It is important to be aware of the in vitro growth characteristics of the cell line you are working with to carry out the appropriate cell culture technique. The following is a general protocol for the subculture of CRC cell lines.

Carry out all procedures using proper aseptic technique in a laminar flow cabinet. Pre-warm the culture medium, trypsin, and DPBS to 37 °C prior to commencing.

1. For adherent cell lines, aspirate the old culture medium when cells reach approximately 80% confluence. For semiadherent cell lines, collect the medium containing the nonadherent population with a pipet and transfer to a fresh falcon tube.
2. Add 5 mL of pre-warmed sterile PBS per 25 cm^2 of culture flask to wash the adherent cells on the flask and to remove any residual culture medium.
3. Aspirate the PBS.

4. Add 1 mL of trypsin per 25 cm^2 of culture flask and incubate at 37 °C for approximately 5 min with intermittent tapping of the side of the flask to induce cell detachment (*see* **Note 8**).
5. Once the cells have detached, quickly neutralize the trypsin by adding an equal volume of fresh FBS-containing culture medium to the cell suspension, gently resuspend the cells by pipeting and transfer to a fresh tube. For semiadherent cell lines, add the detached adherent cell population to the non-adherent population collected previously.
6. Centrifuge at 300 × *g* at 4 °C for 5 min to pellet the cells.
7. Remove the supernatant and resuspend the cell pellet in an appropriate volume of fresh medium.
8. At this point cell number can be quantified using either a haemocytometer or an automated cell counter (e.g., Bio-Rad TC10), and an appropriate number of cells seeded into flasks, plates, or dishes as required for experimentation. Trypan Blue staining can be used to enumerate dead versus viable cells (*see* **Note 9**).
9. For routine maintenance of the cell line, cells should be diluted 1:5 to 1:10 in fresh medium (depending on the growth characteristics of the cell line) and seeded into a new flask.
10. For suspension cell lines no detachment procedure is necessary. Simply carry out steps 6–9 above to passage cells or change culture medium.

3.4 Creation of Formalin-Fixed Paraffin-Embedded Cell Blocks from CRC Cell Lines Cultured In Vitro

Formalin-fixed paraffin-embedded (FFPE) blocks of CRC cell lines grown in vitro can be created for subsequent histopathological, immunohistochemical and fluorescence-based analyses.

1. Culture the CRC cell line using the in vitro culture technique described in Subheading 3.3 to approximately 80% confluence in a 175 cm^2 tissue culture flask, to obtain approximately 10^7 cells (*see* **Note 10**).
2. Remove the culture medium, and wash the cells in cold DPBS. Aspirate the DPBS.
3. Add 10 mL of cold DPBS and remove the monolayer of cells from the culture flask by scraping gently with small angled rubber scraper.
4. Transfer the cell suspension into a 15 mL tube.
5. Centrifuge the cell suspension at 4 °C, at 300 × *g*, for 5 min.
6. Remove the supernatant, and resuspend the cell pellet in 10 mL of fresh DPBS and centrifuge again as above.
7. Remove the supernatant to leave the cell pellet at the bottom of the tube. Add 150 μL of plasma and 150 μL of thrombin (*see* **Note 11**) onto the pellet and use a thin wooden stick to gently

resuspend. Leave the end of the wooden stick in the centre of pellet and allow the clot to form around it by incubating for 5–10 min at room temperature.

8. Once the clot has formed, gently lift the clot out of the tube using the wooden stick. The cell pellet should have clotted and be attached to the end of the stick.
9. Gently dab the cell clot on a piece of filter paper to remove any excess liquid.
10. Use a scalpel blade to transfer the cell clot off the end of the stick and into a histology cartridge, lined with porous membranes to protect the cell clot (*see* **Note 12**). Fix in 10% formalin for 24–48 h (*see* **Note 13**).
11. Process and embed the sample into a formalin block using standard histology procedures.

3.5 Growth of CRC Cell Lines as Xenografts

1. Grow CRC cells to approximately 80% confluence in a 175 cm^2 tissue culture flask and detach by trypsinization as described in Subheading 3.3.
2. Determine cell number as described in Subheading 3.3 and calculate the volume of cell suspension required for 2×10^6 viable cells (*see* **Note 9**).
3. Transfer the volume of cell suspension containing 2×10^6 cells into a sterile microcentrifuge tube.
4. Centrifuge cells at $300 \times g$ for 5 min at 4 °C to form a cell pellet.
5. Resuspend the cell pellet in 75 μL of antibiotic-free complete culture medium.
6. To the resuspended cells, add 75 μL of matrigel matrix making sure the mixture is homogenous to create a cell-matrigel mixture (*see* **Note 14**).
7. Inject the cell-matrigel mixture subcutaneously into the flanks of Balb/*c nu/nu* immunodeficient mice (*see* **Notes 15** and **16**).
8. Monitor the animals for any visible signs of distress as per Institute Review Board/Animal Ethics Committee guidelines.
9. Monitor tumor growth at regular intervals (every day or every second day) by measurement of the length and the width of the tumor and computation of tumor volume according to the formula $(4/3 \times \text{PI}\ ((\text{tumor width} + \text{tumor length})/4)^3)$. Once tumors have reached the maximum size approved by the Institute Review Board/Animal Ethics Committee, animals should be humanely euthanized. If required, tumors can be extracted and either snap frozen or fixed in 10% buffered formalin for further analysis.

3.6 Microsatellite Instability (MSI) Analysis in CRC Cell Lines

The MSI status of a cell line can be determined in multiple ways. In this chapter we will describe two commonly used methods:

1. Detecting loss of expression of the mismatch repair proteins (MLH1, PMS2, MSH2 and MSH6) by immunohistochemistry (IHC).
2. Assessment of alteration in length of specific microsatellite sequences in the genome by PCR and fragment analysis (commonly referred to as Microsatellite Testing) (*see* **Note 17**).

3.6.1 Loss of Expression of Mismatch Repair Proteins by Immunohistochemistry

Microsatellite instability is caused by loss of function of one or more of the mismatch repair proteins MLH1, PMS2, MSH2 and MSH6. The MSI status of a CRC cell line can be determined by immunohistochemical assessment of expression of all four MMR proteins, or if resources are limited, just MLH1 and MSH2 (*see* **Note 18**). This can be performed on FFPE sections of colon cancer cell lines prepared as cell blocks (per Subheading 3.4) or grown as xenografts.

1. Cut the required number of 4 μm-thick sections of a CRC cell line from FFPE blocks, and mount on electrostatic glass slides.
2. Carry out standard IHC staining for each MMR protein (*see* **Note 18**).
3. Optimal IHC staining protocols including antigen retrieval method, primary antibody concentration, incubation times and secondary antibody-detection system will need to be optimized by the end-user for each primary antibody used.
4. Interpretation of IHC staining results: staining is interpreted as either the presence or absence of nuclear staining of each MMR protein in tumor cells. Loss of any one of the four MMR proteins is considered evidence for microsatellite instability (MMR-deficient), while positive staining in all four proteins (or two if only MLH1 and MSH2 are tested) is considered evidence of a microsatellite stable (MMR-proficient) cell line (*see* **Note 19**) (Fig. 2).

3.6.2 Microsatellite Testing

Loss of MMR proteins result in failure to correct DNA replication errors. These errors occur at high frequency in repetitive DNA sequences (microsatellites) due to "slippage" of the polymerase in these regions, hence the term microsatellite instability. A number of nonpolymorphic microsatellites have been identified in the human genome and detection of alterations in the length of these microsatellites by their PCR amplification followed by fragment analysis provides a reliable means of identifying microsatellite instability in CRC cell lines or tumors.

1. Isolate genomic DNA from CRC cell lines. Various methods can be used to isolate gDNA from CRC cell lines including

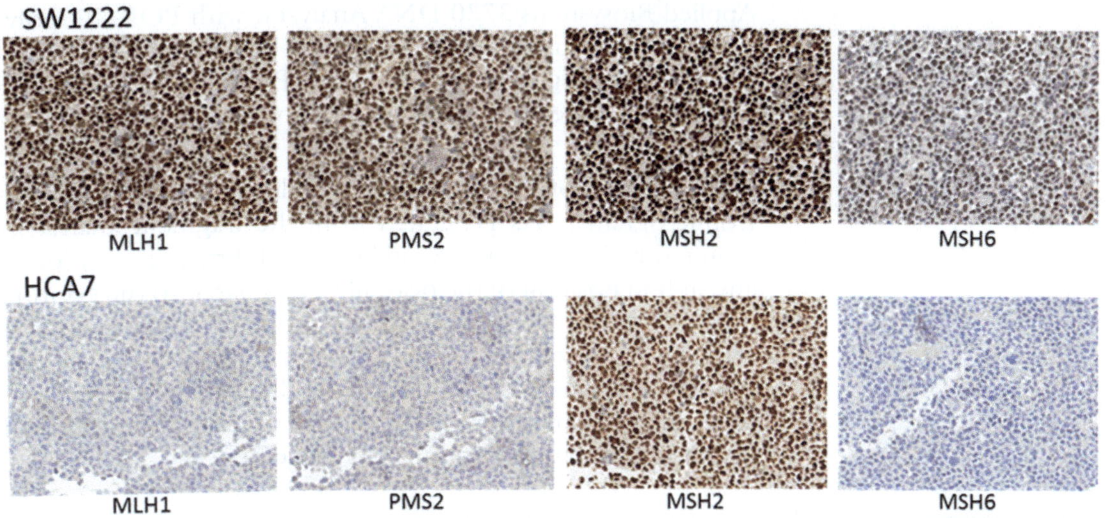

Fig. 2 IHC for MMR proteins on SW1222 and HCA7 cells (in cell block sections). In SW1222, all four MMR proteins are expressed indicating microsatellite stable status. In HCA7, expression of MLH1, PMS2, and MSH6 is lost, indicating microsatellite instability (*see* **Note 19**)

well-optimized and validated protocols in the form of commercially available kits. We recommend isolating gDNA using a commercially available kit, as per the manufacturer's instructions (*see* **Note 1**).

2. PCR amplification of a panel of microsatellite markers. The commercially available kit, MSI Analysis System Version 1.2 (Promega, USA) [16] provides all of the reagents required for this analysis. The kit contains reagents to perform a multiplex PCR assay of five validated mononucleotide markers (*BAT-25*, *BAT-26*, *NR-21*, *NR-24*, and *MONO-27*) (*see* **Note 20**). The MSI Analysis System allows for multiplexing of PCR products of the panel of markers in a single sample using probes conjugated to individual fluorophores. Perform PCR amplification of cell line gDNA using the reagents provided according to the manufacturer's instructions. We have provided additional guidance from our experience of using this protocol in **Notes 21–23**. The user manual for the MSI Analysis System Version 1.2 can be found at www.promega.com.
3. Detection of amplified PCR products (fragment analysis). This step requires resolution of the fluorophore-labeled PCR products by capillary electrophoresis and detection of amplified fragments of various lengths using an appropriate instrument. The detailed instrument-specific protocol for spectral calibration required for recognition of the multiplexed fluorescent fragments is available in the User Manual for the MSI Analysis System Version 1.2 (www.promega.com). We have used the

Applied Biosystems 3730 DNA Analyzer, with POP-7™ polymer and a 36 cm capillary array for resolution and detection of PCR products generated using the Promega MSI Analysis System. *See* **Notes 24** and **25** for additional guidance regarding this step.

4. Interpretation of microsatellite instability. Inspection of electropherogram peaks generated from the fragment analysis is required to interpret microsatellite instability. For each locus, any shift in position of the peak allele compared to the position in the reference electropherograms provided in the manual is regarded as instability. *Instability at two or more of the five markers is diagnostic of MSI* (*see* **Note 26**). Analysis of electropherograms from samples of known MSI status can be helpful in the interpretation of results (*see* **Note 23**).

3.7 Assessment of CpG Island Methylator Phenotype (CIMP) in CRC Cell Lines

There are a number of methods available for assessing the CIMP status of CRC tumors and cell lines [17–21]. All of these methods involve bisulfite treatment of gDNA which converts unmethylated cytosine residues to uracil, while methylated cytosine remains unaffected. Thus bisulfite-treated gDNA reveals methylation-specific information on DNA sequences which can be analyzed by a number of downstream assays following PCR amplification. In addition, the methylation status of different panels of marker genes can be used to assess CIMP status [3, 22–24] (*see* **Note 27**). Here, we describe a method that can be used for assessing CIMP status of CRC cell line samples using the MethyLight assay, a multiplex PCR assay which simultaneously detects the methylation status of five CIMP marker genes (*CACNA1G, IGF2, NEUROG1, RUNX3,* and *SOCS1*) as described by Weisenberger *et al.* [17, 18].

3.7.1 Isolation of Genomic DNA from CRC Cell Lines

Various methods can be used to isolate gDNA from CRC cell lines including well-optimized and validated protocols in the form of commercially available kits. We recommend isolating gDNA using a commercially available kit, as per the manufacturer's instructions (*see* **Note 1**).

3.7.2 Bisulfite Conversion of Extracted gDNA

Various commercially available kits can be used for this step, such as the EpiTect Bisulfite kit (Qiagen). We recommend performing bisulfite conversion using the reagents provided in one of these commercially available kits by following the manufacturer's instructions.

3.7.3 MethyLight PCR Assay

The MethyLight assay uses "methylation-specific" primers to only amplify loci that are methylated. Primers are specifically designed to be complementary only to unconverted (methylated) cytosines on bisulfite-treated gDNA. A methylation-prone CpG dinucleotide is also usually placed at the 3′-end of the primer to improve sensitivity.

Table 4
Reaction mastermix for methylation-specific PCR

Component	Final concentration
$MgCl_2$	3.5 mM
Tween-20	0.01%
Gelatin	0.05%
Taq polymerase	0.1 U
Primers (forward and reverse)	300 nM each
Probes	100 nM each
dNTPs	200 μM
Template bisulfite-converted DNA[a]	≤100 ng/reaction
Nuclease-free H_2O	[b]

Include a reaction for methylated DNA reference (positive control)
[a]Template DNA concentrations are adjusted and optimized by end-user
[b]Make up to final reaction volume

This method is highly sensitive and specific for interrogating CpG-rich loci with high methylation density such as the CIMP-high markers listed above.

1. Add the components for the PCR reaction mix to the desired final reaction volume (25–50 μL) as per Table 4.
2. Probes and primer sequences for the CIMP MethyLight assay have been previously validated and are listed in Table 1 (Materials) [22]. The first five markers (*CACNA1G, IGF2, NEUROG1, RUNX3,* and *SOCS1*) form the panel for CIMP classification. The *ALU* marker is a non-methylation-dependent reaction used as a control for normalizing the concentrations of input bisulfite-converted DNA.
3. Include a fully methylated DNA reference sample in the PCR reactions to serve as a positive control and for computing the percentage methylation of your sample (*see* **Note 28**). A negative control reaction (nuclease-free water) should also be included.
4. Perform PCR using the cycling conditions provided in Table 5.

3.7.4 Data Analysis and Interpretation

1. The percent methylation rate (PMR) of each locus is calculated as follows:

$$\text{PMR} = 100 \times (\text{Ct CIMP marker}/\text{Ct ALU})_{\text{sample}}/(\text{Ct CIMP marker}/\text{Ct ALU})_{\text{methylated DNA reference}}.$$

Table 5
Cycling conditions for methylation PCR analysis

Step	Temperature	Time
Initial PCR activation	95 °C	5 min
2-step cycling:		
Denaturation	95 °C	15 s
Annealing/extension	60 °C	60 s
Number of cycles	40–50[a]	

[a]No. of cycles depends on amount of template DNA, user to optimize

Ct: cycle threshold.

Sample: test sample.

Methylated DNA reference (*see* **Note 28**).

CIMP marker: *CACNA1G, IGF2, NEUROG1, RUNX3*, or *SOCS1*.

2. A CIMP marker is considered methylated if the PMR is ≥10. Cell line samples with methylation in ≥3 of these five markers are classified as CIMP-high, those with two or fewer methylated markers are considered CIMP-low, and those unmethylated at all five markers are considered CIMP-negative.

4 Notes

1. A number of kits suitable for extraction of genomic DNA (gDNA) from cell lines can be used. It is also possible to isolate gDNA from cell line xenografts that have been freshly frozen or formalin-fixed and paraffin-embedded (FFPE). In the case of extracting gDNA from FFPE material, commercially available kits specific for this purpose need to be used. We recommend isolating gDNA from in vitro cultured cells whenever possible as this produces the highest quality of gDNA.
2. We use human plasma obtained via a hospital blood bank. However, plasma from any animal species would be suitable and can be purchased from a number of biomedical research suppliers. Make sure plasma, not serum, is used. The coagulation factors in plasma are required to interact with thrombin to form the cell clot.
3. Primary antibody targeting *human* MMR proteins should be used.
4. POP-4 polymer is a separation matrix for performing DNA sequencing and fragment analysis applications.

5. Cells need to be cultured for this time period in order for any mycoplasma contamination that may be present to reach detectable levels in the culture medium. During this period, we recommend culturing cells in antibiotic-free medium to avoid masking of any low level contamination.
6. If possible include 1 μL of supernatant from a known mycoplasma-positive sample as a positive control and 1 μL of H_2O as a negative control.
7. Usually 1 min of heating is required per 100 mL of agarose/ TAE mixture. Microwave in intervals to prevent overflow. If the agarose has not dissolved, continue microwaving until the agarose is completely dissolved.
8. Incubation time for each cell line will vary as some CRC cell lines are more adherent than others.
9. Trypan Blue selectively stains dead cells and can be used to determine the percentage of viable cells in the cell suspension. When using Trypan Blue, add 10 μL of Trypan Blue to 10 μL of cell suspension (1:1 ratio), mix well by resuspending with a micropipette. Use this mixture on the counting slide.
10. User can modify the number of cells used to generate the cell pellet for cell block creation. Larger numbers of cells can be used if a larger-sized cell pellet is desired for the paraffin block. We find that a minimum of 2×10^7 cells is required to produce an average-sized pellet that is easy for handling and embedding into a standard paraffin block. For accurate comparison between cell lines, we recommend adding fresh medium to the culture approximately 8 h prior to collection.
11. When working with a large cell pellet, a longer incubation period or more thrombin and plasma may be required to induce clotting. If a clot has not formed after 15 min, add a further 150 μL of thrombin and 150 μL of plasma to the cell pellet.
12. We use two porous sponge sheets cut to size, to line the histology cartridge. The cell clot is then placed in between the sponge sheets which protects the clot in the cartridge. An alternative to the sponge sheets is porous cigarette rolling paper (purchased from any tobacconist). Place the cell clot in the centre of the cigarette paper and fold the paper around the clot, then place in histology cartridge.
13. Do not leave cell clot in formalin for longer than 48 h. If necessary, after 24–48 h remove the sample from formalin and store in 80% ethanol before processing and paraffin embedding. If working with a small cell pellet, staining the fixed pellet with eosin prior to embedding may help to improve

the visibility of the cell pellet when embedded into a paraffin block.

14. Ensure all procedures or samples containing matrigel are performed on ice as matrigel will solidify when it begins to warm. It also helps to use pipette tips which have been cooled.
15. We use a 29G × ½" needle with a 0.5 ml syringe. Ensure that needle and syringes are cooled (or on ice) prior to use to prevent the matrigel from solidifying.
16. Be sure to rid the needle and syringe of all air bubbles prior to injecting.
17. Fragment analysis of microsatellite markers will not reveal which MMR gene/proteins are deficient, whereas IHC analysis for the individual MMR proteins (MLH1, PMS2, MSH2 and MSH6) will identify which of these are lost resulting in microsatellite instability.
18. The MMR proteins function as heterodimers, with MLH1 partnering with PMS2, and MSH2 partnering with MSH6 for stability. If only two proteins are to be tested, then assessment of MLH1 and MSH2 expression provides the best sensitivity and specificity, as these proteins are required for stabilizing their corresponding partner protein. Comparatively, loss of PMS2 or MSH6 can be compensated for by other minor proteins, such as MSH3, MLH3 or PMS1. IHC testing for loss of MLH1 and MSH2 provides 92% sensitivity and 100% specificity for detecting MSI, compared to assessment of MSI status by fragment analysis [25]. To increase sensitivity, IHC for all four MMR proteins should be performed.
19. Due to the dimerization of MMR proteins, loss of staining of both major and minor proteins in a dimer pair commonly occurs, e.g., MLH1 and PMS2 or MSH2 and MSH6. Thus the concurrent loss of expression of these protein pairs provides added confidence in calling a cell line as MSI. However in the case of isolated loss of a minor protein such as PMS2, the major protein MLH1 may remain intact due to redundancy in binding to other minor proteins, although in some cases this can still result in microsatellite instability [26]. Confirmatory microsatellite testing by fragment analysis is recommended in such cases. In our experience, CRC cell lines with microsatellite instability typically demonstrate loss of more than two MMR proteins on IHC testing. The loss of additional MMR proteins may reflect secondary mutations subsequent to development of MSI.

20. An alternative to assessment of the microsatellite markers in the Promega MSI Analysis system is a different panel of microsatellite markers, the "Bethesda panel," which were recommended by the National Cancer Institute in 1997. The Bethesda panel consists of two mononucleotide markers *BAT-25, BAT-26* (which are also part of the Promega panel) and three dinucleotide markers, *D2S123, D5S346,* and *D17S250* [27]. The exclusive use of mononucleotide markers in the Promega panel has been reported to provide high sensitivity and specificity of MSI detection (almost 100% for both). Furthermore, the monomorphic nature of these markers (i.e., almost all individuals are homozygous for the common allele of the given marker) simplifies data interpretation [16, 28].
21. Accurate quantification of template DNA is important when using the MSI Analysis System. DNA isolated from cell lines cultured in vitro or from fresh frozen xenograft material can be quantified by NanoDrop spectrophotometry. For quantification of DNA isolated from FFPE material we recommend using the Qubit fluorescence-based assay, as NanoDrop is less accurate in this setting [29, 30].
22. Promega recommends using 1–2 ng of genomic DNA as template in the PCR reactions. We find that the user may need to adjust the amount of template DNA due to variations in DNA quality related to individual DNA isolation methods and sample properties, especially when dealing with low concentrations. If working with a large number of samples, we suggest optimization of the assays using various amounts of DNA template (1, 2, 5, 10 ng) from a small number of samples prior to commencing.
23. Assay controls: For the amplification step, the Promega MSI Analysis System kit provides a positive amplification control. Nuclease-free water can be used as a negative amplification control. To facilitate data analysis, we suggest including cell line samples of known microsatellite status (stable and unstable) to serve as analysis controls (*see* Appendix 1).
24. Matrix standards: Spectral calibration for the fluorescent dyes used in the MSI Analysis System is required for each genetic analyzer machine in order to evaluate the multiplexed fluorescent fragments. Matrix standards used for spectral calibration are specific to the genetic analyzer machine and can be purchased from Promega (PowerPlex Matrix Standards, Promega). It is important to consult Promega if unsure about which matrix standards to use.

25. The Promega MSI Analysis System was developed and optimized for use with Applied Biosystem's Genetic Analyzers using POP-4™ polymer, however amplification products can also be detected using instruments with POP-7™ polymer. Promega has a published protocol for this which can be found online (http://manualzz.com/doc/6951420/use-of-the-msi-analysis-system-with-the-applied).
26. The *Penta C/ Penta D* loci which are included in the Promega assay are not required for interpretation of MSI status of CRC cell line samples, as there is typically no paired normal DNA sample. These markers are useful only when using this assay for analysis of samples with paired tumor and normal DNA to confirm correct pairing of tumor and normal samples.
27. Various panels of CpG gene loci can be used to define CIMP-high status. These include the original "Issa panel" of five markers: *MINT1, MINT2, MINT31, CDKN2A (p16)*, and *MLH1* [3], and another panel of five markers (*CACNA1G, IGF2, NEUROG1, RUNX3*, and *SOCS1*) described by Weisenberger et al. (also referred to as the "Laird Panel") [22]. Subsequent studies have further extended the latter panel to eight markers (*CACNA1G, IGF2, NEUROG1, RUNX3, SOCS1, CDKN2A, CRABP1*, and *MLH1*) or 16 markers: (*CACNA1G, IGF2, NEUROG1, RUNX3, SOCS1, CDKN2A, CRABP1, MLH1, CHFR, HIC1, IGFBP3, MGMT, MINT1, MINT31, MLH1, CDKN2A/ARF (p14)*, and *WRN* [23, 31].
28. A methylated DNA reference sample is human DNA that has been completely methylated by in vitro treatment using *SssI methylase,* and bisulfite-converted. Amplification of this reference template in the MethyLight assay allows the extent of methylation of each locus in your test samples to be expressed as a percentage of this fully methylated reference (percent methylation rate, PMR). This methylated DNA reference sample can be purchased separately from Qiagen (EpiTech control DNA, methylated #59655, Qiagen).

Appendix 1

Reference STR profiles and properties of 30 commonly used CRC cell lines

CRC cell line name	In vitro growth	STR (short tandem repeats) profiles of cell lines at 10 loci										MSI/MSS status	CIMP status
		AMEL	CSF1PO	D5S818	D7S820	D13S317	D16S539	D21S11	TH01	TPOX	vWA		
CACO2	Adherent	X	11	12, 13	11, 12	11, 13, 14	12, 13	30	6	9, 11	16, 18	MSS	Neg/low
COLO201[a]	Semiadherent	X	11, 12	10, 13	9, 10	10	12, 13	30.2, 33.2	8, 9	11	15	MSS	High
COLO205[a]	Semiadherent	X	11, 12	10, 13	9, 10	10, 12	12, 13	30.2, 33.2	8, 9	11	15	MSS	High
COLO320	Semiadherent	X	11	12	9, 12	11	11, 12	33.2	9	8, 9	15, 18	MSS	Neg/low
DLD1	Adherent	X, Y	11, 12	13	10, 12	8, 11	12, 13	29, 32.2	7, 9.3	8, 11	18, 19	MSI	High
HCA7	Adherent	X	11, 14	8, 12	11, 12	9	10, 11	26, 28.2	6, 7	8, 10	14, 16	MSI	High
HCT116	Adherent	X, Y	7, 10	10, 11	11, 12	10, 12	11, 13	29, 30	8, 9	8, 9	17, 22	MSI	High
HCT15[b]	Adherent	X, Y	12	13	10, 12	8, 11	12, 13	29, 32.2	7, 9.3	8, 11	18, 19	MSI	High
HCT8[b]	Adherent	X, Y	12	13	10, 12	8, 11	12, 13	29, 32.2	7, 9.3	8, 11	18, 19	MSI	High
HT115	Adherent	X	7, 12	12	11, 12	13	10	30, 32.2	6, 9	8	18	MSS	Neg/low
HT29[c]	Adherent	X	11, 12	11, 12	10	11, 12	11, 12	29, 30	6, 9	8, 9	17, 19	MSS	High
KM12	Adherent	X	10, 12	10, 17	8, 9	12, 15	11	27	9.3	11, 12	17	MSI	High
LIM1215	Adherent	X, Y	10	9, 12	9	8, 12	8, 12	29, 31	9.3, 10	8	16	MSI	Neg/low
LIM1899	Adherent	X, Y	10, 11	11, 14	8, 9	9, 12	10, 11, 12	29	6, 9.3	9, 11	18, 19	MSI	Neg/low
LIM2405	Adherent	X, Y	14, 15	12, 13	7, 8	8, 11	14, 15	29, 30	9.3	8	14, 18	MSI	High
LIM2537	Adherent	X	9	10	8, 11	8, 14	12	28, 29, 30	6	8, 9	14, 17	MSI	High
LIM2551	Semiadherent	X, Y	9, 10, 11	12, 16	9, 11	8, 11	11	27, 28, 33.2	6, 9.3	8, 11	17, 19	MSI	Neg/low
LS174T[d]	Adherent	X	10, 13, 14	11, 15, 16	10.3, 11	10	11, 13	29, 31	6, 7	8, 9	15, 17, 18	MSI	Neg/low
LS180[d]	Adherent	X	10, 13	10, 15	9.3, 11	10	11, 13	29, 31	6, 7	8, 9	15, 18	MSI	Neg/low
RKO	Adherent	X	8, 10	11, 13, 15	8, 10	8, 11	12, 13	27, 30	6, 10	11	15, 16, 17, 22	MSI	High
SNU175	Suspension	X	10, 12	11	11	9, 12	9, 12	30, 32.2	7, 9	8, 11	14, 17	MSI	Neg/low

(continued)

CRC cell line name	In vitro growth	STR (short tandem repeats) profiles of cell lines at 10 loci										MSI/MSS status	CIMP status
		AMEL	CSF1PO	D5S818	D7S820	D13S317	D16S539	D21S11	TH01	TPOX	vWA		
SNUC1	Suspension	X	12	10	10, 11	9, 11	9, 11	30	7, 9	11, 12	16, 18	MSS	Neg/low
SW1116	Adherent	X, Y	10, 11	11, 12	12	11, 14	9, 12	28, 29	6	8, 11	14, 19	MSS	Neg/low
SW1222	Adherent	X, Y	11	9	10, 12	9, 13	9, 10	29	7	10	18	MSS	Neg/low
SW403	Adherent	X	10, 13	11	8, 9	13	10, 12	28, 29	6	8, 9	14, 18	MSS	Neg/low
SW480[e]	Adherent	X	13, 14	13	8	12	13	30, 30.2	8	11	16	MSS	Neg/low
SW620[e]	Adherent	X	13, 14	13	8, 9	12	9, 13	30, 30.2	8	11	16	MSS	Neg/low
SW948	Adherent	X	12	11	9, 11	10, 11	11, 12	25.2, 29	6, 9.3	8, 11	16, 18	MSS	Neg/low
T84	Adherent	X	10	12	8, 10	9	10, 11	31	6, 9	8, 11	17, 18	MSS	Neg/low
WIDR[c]	Adherent	X	11, 12	11, 12	10	11, 12	11, 12	29, 30	6, 9	8, 9	17, 19	MSS	High

Reference STR profiles were obtained from ExPASy Bioinformatics Resource Portal Cellosaurus Database, and data on LIM cell lines were obtained from the source institute (Olivia Newton-John Cancer Research Institute)

[a,b,c,d,e]Cell lines derived from the same individual are marked by same symbols

References

1. Shibata D, Peinado MA, Ionov Y et al (1994) Genomic instability in repeated sequences is an early somatic event in colorectal tumorigenesis that persists after transformation. Nat Genet 6 (3):273–281
2. Lengauer C, Kinzler KW, Vogelstein B (1997) Genetic instability in colorectal cancers. Nature 386(6625):623–627
3. Issa J-P (2004) CpG island methylator phenotype in cancer. Nat Rev Cancer 4(12):988–993
4. Bellam N, Pasche B (2010) TGF-β signaling alterations and colon cancer. In: Pasche B (ed) Cancer genetics. Springer, Boston, MA, pp 85–103. https://doi.org/10.1007/978-1-4419-6033-7_5
5. Cathomas G (2014) PIK3CA in colorectal cancer. Front Oncol 4:35. https://doi.org/10.3389/fonc.2014.00035
6. Colussi D, Brandi G, Bazzoli F et al (2013) Molecular pathways involved in colorectal cancer: implications for disease behavior and prevention. Int J Mol Sci 14(8):16365–16385. https://doi.org/10.3390/ijms140816365
7. Barras D (2015) BRAF mutation in colorectal cancer: an update. Biomark Cancer 7(Suppl 1):9–12. https://doi.org/10.4137/bic.s25248
8. Morkel M, Riemer P, Bläker H et al (2015) Similar but different: distinct roles for KRAS and BRAF oncogenes in colorectal cancer development and therapy resistance. Oncotarget 6(25):20785–20800
9. Guinney J, Dienstmann R, Wang X et al (2015) The consensus molecular subtypes of colorectal cancer. Nat Med 21(11):1350–1356. https://doi.org/10.1038/nm.3967
10. Young L, Sung J, Stacey G et al (2010) Detection of mycoplasma in cell cultures. Nat Protoc 5(5):929–934
11. Tögel L, Nightingale R, Chueh AC et al (2016) Dual targeting of bromodomain and extra-terminal domain proteins, and WNT or MAPK signaling, inhibits c-MYC expression and proliferation of colorectal cancer cells. Mol Cancer Ther 15(6):1217
12. Shin J, Carr A, Corner GA et al (2014) The intestinal epithelial cell differentiation marker intestinal alkaline phosphatase (ALPi) is selectively induced by histone deacetylase inhibitors (HDACi) in colon cancer cells in a kruppel-like factor 5 (KLF5)-dependent manner. J Biol Chem 289(36):25306–25316. https://doi.org/10.1074/jbc.M114.557546
13. Wilson AJ, Chueh AC, Tögel L et al (2010) A coordinated Sp1/Sp3-mediated transcriptional response involving immediate-early gene induction is linked to HDAC inhibitor-induced apoptosis in colon cancer cells. Cancer Res 70(2):609–620. https://doi.org/10.1158/0008-5472.CAN-09-2327
14. Butler JM (2007) Short tandem repeat typing technologies used in human identity testing. BioTechniques 43(4):ii–iv
15. Nikfarjam L, Farzaneh P (2012) Prevention and detection of mycoplasma contamination in cell culture. Cell J 13(4):203–212
16. Bacher JW, Flanagan LA, Smalley RL et al (2004) Development of a fluorescent multiplex assay for detection of MSI-high tumors. Dis Markers 20(4–5):237–250
17. Eads CA, Danenberg KD, Kawakami K et al (2000) MethyLight: a high-throughput assay to measure DNA methylation. Nucleic Acids Res 28(8):E32
18. Weisenberger DJ, Campan M, Long TI et al (2005) Analysis of repetitive element DNA methylation by MethyLight. Nucleic Acids Res 33(21):6823–6836. https://doi.org/10.1093/nar/gki987
19. Gu H, Bock C, Mikkelsen TS et al (2010) Genome-scale DNA methylation mapping of clinical samples at single-nucleotide resolution. Nat Methods 7(2):133–136. https://doi.org/10.1038/nmeth.1414
20. Wojdacz TK, Dobrovic A (2007) Methylation-sensitive high resolution melting (MS-HRM): a new approach for sensitive and high-throughput assessment of methylation. Nucleic Acids Res 35(6):e41. https://doi.org/10.1093/nar/gkm013
21. Jasmine F, Rahaman R, Roy S et al (2012) Interpretation of genome-wide infinium methylation data from ligated DNA in formalin-fixed, paraffin-embedded paired tumor and normal tissue. BMC Res Notes 5:117. https://doi.org/10.1186/1756-0500-5-117
22. Weisenberger DJ, Siegmund KD, Campan M et al (2006) CpG island methylator phenotype underlies sporadic microsatellite instability and is tightly associated with BRAF mutation in colorectal cancer. Nat Genet 38(7):787–793. https://doi.org/10.1038/ng1834
23. Nosho K, Irahara N, Shima K et al (2008) Comprehensive biostatistical analysis of CpG island methylator phenotype in colorectal cancer using a large population-based sample. PLoS One 3(11):e3698. https://doi.org/10.1371/journal.pone.0003698
24. Ogino S, Kawasaki T, Brahmandam M et al (2006) Precision and performance

characteristics of bisulfite conversion and real-time PCR (MethyLight) for quantitative DNA methylation analysis. J Mol Diagn 8 (2):209–217. https://doi.org/10.2353/jmoldx.2006.050135

25. Lindor NM, Burgart LJ, Leontovich O et al (2002) Immunohistochemistry versus microsatellite instability testing in phenotyping colorectal tumors. J Clin Oncol 20(4):1043–1048. https://doi.org/10.1200/JCO.2002.20.4.1043
26. Shi C, Washington K (2012) Molecular testing in colorectal cancer: diagnosis of lynch syndrome and personalized cancer medicine. Am J Clin Pathol 137(6):847–859. https://doi.org/10.1309/AJCPI83DINULUJNI
27. Berg KD, Glaser CL, Thompson RE et al (2000) Detection of microsatellite instability by fluorescence multiplex polymerase chain reaction. J Mol Diagn 2(1):20–28
28. Murphy KM, Zhang S, Geiger T et al (2006) Comparison of the microsatellite instability analysis system and the Bethesda panel for the determination of microsatellite instability in colorectal cancers. J Mol Diagn 8 (3):305–311. https://doi.org/10.2353/jmoldx.2006.050092
29. Sah S, Chen L, Houghton J et al (2013) Functional DNA quantification guides accurate next-generation sequencing mutation detection in formalin-fixed, paraffin-embedded tumor biopsies. Genome Med 5(8):77. https://doi.org/10.1186/gm481
30. Simbolo M, Gottardi M, Corbo V et al (2013) DNA qualification workflow for next generation sequencing of histopathological samples. PLoS One 8(6):e62692. https://doi.org/10.1371/journal.pone.0062692
31. Ogino S, Kawasaki T, Kirkner GJ et al (2007) Evaluation of markers for CpG island methylator phenotype (CIMP) in colorectal cancer by a large population-based sample. J Mol Diagn 9 (3):305–314. https://doi.org/10.2353/jmoldx.2007.060170

Chapter 2

Dissecting Oncogenic RTK Pathways in Colorectal Cancer Initiation and Progression

Stephen McManus, Walid Chababi, Dominique Arsenault, Claire M. Dubois, and Caroline Saucier

Abstract

Colorectal cancer (CRC) is a progressive disorder associated with an accumulation of multiple heterogeneous genetic alterations in intestinal epithelial cells (IEC). However, when these cells undergo neoplastic transformation and become cancerous and metastatic, they invariably acquire hallmarks conferring them the ability to hyperproliferate, escape growth-inhibitory and death-inducing cues, and promote angiogenesis as well as epithelial-to-mesenchymal transformation (EMT), fostering their invasive dissemination from primary tumor into distant tissues. Compelling clinical and experimental evidence suggest that aberrant engagement of cell surface growth factor receptor tyrosine kinase (RTK) signaling, like that of the hepatocyte growth factor (HGF)/MET receptor, underlies CRC metastatic progression by promoting these cancer hallmarks. To date, though, the use of RTK-targeting agents has been viewed as a promising approach for the treatment of metastatic CRC, clinical success has been modest.

Our vision is that the prospect of designing RTK-based, improved and innovative CRC therapies and prognostic markers likely rests on a comprehensive understanding of the biological processes and underlying regulatory molecular mechanisms by which deregulation of RTK signaling governs IEC's neoplastic transformation and their transition from noninvasive to metastatic and malignant cells. Herein, we describe our scheme for defining the full scope of oncogenic MET-driven cancer biological processes, in cellulo and in vivo, as well as the individual contribution of MET-binding effectors in a nontransformed IEC model, the IEC-6 cell line.

Key words Receptor tyrosine kinase, Hepatocyte growth factor (HGF), MET receptor, Intestinal epithelial cells, GRB2, SHC, EMT, Angiogenesis, Tumorigenesis, Metastasis

1 Introduction

Pathogenesis of colorectal cancer (CRC) involves a series of well-defined stages known as the adenoma–carcinoma sequence [1, 2]. This is initiated by hyperplasia and neoplastic transformation of intestinal epithelial cells (IEC) within the colon or the rectum that become dysplastic, resulting in the formation of aberrant crypt foci and then benign tumors (adenomas). Invariably, a subset of adenomas progresses to form in situ carcinomas, and eventually

Jean-François Beaulieu (ed.), *Colorectal Cancer: Methods and Protocols*, Methods in Molecular Biology, vol. 1765, https://doi.org/10.1007/978-1-4939-7765-9_2,

invasive and metastatic tumors, if they are not surgically removed [3]. As normal IECs evolve to become malignant CRC cells they acquire hallmarks enabling them to grow aberrantly, to disregard normal growth-inhibitory and death signals, to sustain angiogenesis and to invade tissue [4]. Incidentally, these are biological attributes coordinated primarily by growth factor receptor tyrosine kinases (RTK) in normal cells. Not surprisingly, compelling lines of clinical and experimental evidence entail a causal role for aberrant activation of RTK signaling in the initiation and metastatic progression of CRC, including that of the hepatocyte growth factor (HGF)/MET receptor (Reviewed in [5]).

Expressed mainly in epithelial cells, MET is activated in a paracrine manner by its unique ligand, HGF, which is produced by mesenchymal cells. Once activated, MET engages multiple signaling pathways regulating cell proliferation, survival, migration, invasion, and angiogenesis, which coordinate epithelial cell morphogenesis and tissue repair (Reviewed in [6, 7]). Deregulation of the HGF-MET axis in CRC involves the overexpression of *MET* and *HGF* genes resulting in autocrine/paracrine-mediated or ligand-independent constitutive activation of MET. This is often seen early at the adenoma stage, but in nearly all invasive carcinomas and metastases. Notably, elevated MET protein levels in primary CRC tissues have been linked with tumor invasion and lymph node metastasis, whereas increased coexpression of the *HGF* and *MET* genes is predictive of advanced disease stage and poor survival. Furthermore, *MET* gene amplification, which occurs in approximately 10% of liver metastases, may account for primary and acquired resistance to anti-EGFR (epidermal growth factor receptor) therapies in a subset of CRC patients harboring KRAS wild-type (WT) tumors [8]. Thus, aberrant HGF-MET signaling is acknowledged as a driver of CRC metastatic progression, providing the rationale for anti-MET therapies for this cancer. However, results from recent clinical trials combining MET inhibitors with agents targeting the either epidermal or vascular growth factor RTKs (EGFR or VEGFR) for patients with metastatic CRC have been limited, showing little correlation between treatment and survival [9–11]. Notably, no robust association between MET levels in tumors and clinical responses has been observed [9–11]. Thus, a comprehensive understanding of MET-driven oncogenic biological processes and the underlying molecular pathways in CRC-relevant cell models is required for the identification of molecular targets representing biomarkers for predicting those CRC patients who are most likely to benefit from anti-MET therapies.

Biological relevance of signaling proteins recruited to RTKs is typically investigated by approaches relying on their overexpression or silencing in cells. Limitations of such strategies are that normal regulatory mechanisms provided by receptor–effector interaction investigated may be ineffective, and that these RTK-binding effectors are also interacting with other types of receptors and nonreceptor signaling proteins. To define the individual functional contribution of MET-binding signaling proteins in neoplastic transformation of IECs, we exploit instead variant forms of the oncogenic MET, TRP-MET, engineered to directly bind to a single signaling protein of choice, and consequently activating in isolation its downstream signal transduction pathways [12–17]. The receptor MET was first isolated as the product of a carcinogen-induced chromosomal rearrangement, fusing a leucine zipper dimerization domain of the translocated promoter region (TPR) to the MET kinase domain and C-terminus [7]. The resulting MET oncoprotein is cytoplasmic and constitutively activated by dimerization in the absence of ligand. For creating docking-specific TPR-MET variants, we have exploited a unique characteristic of MET; that its downstream signaling and biological activities rely on the phosphorylation of two tyrosine (Tyr) residues in the MET C-terminal tail (Tyr-482/486 in TPR-MET or Tyr-1349/1356 in MET) [12]. When phosphorylated, these Tyr residues form direct binding sites for the adaptor proteins GAB1 (GRB2-associated binder-1), GRB2 (growth factor receptor-bound protein-2), and SHC (Src-homology collagen) (review in [7]). These proteins are devoid of catalytic activity but contain multiple protein–protein interaction motifs and domains; allowing them to assemble protein complexes to RTKs that relay diverse signaling pathways and biological responses directly linked to the initiation and progression of cancer [12, 13]. The engineered GRB2 and SHC specific docking TPR-MET variants consist of a TPR-MET mutants in which the multisubstrate binding region is replaced with a motif selective for the recruitment of a single signaling protein found in other RTKs [12].

In this chapter, we present the pipeline that we have developed for defining critical cancer biological processes regulated by oncogenic MET activation, as well as the specific role of the recruitment of the GRB2 and SHC adaptor proteins in a nontransformed IEC model (IEC-6 cell line) [18, 19]. Through the series of cell-based biological assays described herein, we show that it is possible to appraise in a quantitative manner which cancerous features critical for the initiation and malignant progression of CRC cancers are conferred to IEC-6 cells upon the oncogenic activation of MET or of its downstream pathways. Notably, the in vivo cancer assays that we depict allow defining whether the cancer features driven by oncogenic engagement of RTK pathways in cellulo translate into tumorigenic and metastatic attributes in vivo.

2 Materials

2.1 Cell Lines and Culture

1. Normal-derived rat intestinal epithelial crypt immortalized cell line (IEC-6) is from Dr. A. Quaroni (Cornell University, Ithaca, NY) [20] and are available from the American Type Culture Collection (ATCC) (*see* **Note 1**).
2. Human embryonic kidney (HEK) 293T cells are from the ATCC.
3. Complete DMEM: Dulbecco's modified Eagle's medium supplemented with 10% fetal bovine serum (FBS) and 50 μg/mL of gentamicin.
4. 0.25% trypsin–EDTA.

2.2 Generation of Stable IEC-6 Cell Populations

1. TPR-MET pLXSN cDNA and variants encoding the GRB2- and SHC-binding TPR-MET were provided by Dr. M. Park (McGill University, Montreal, QC) (*see* **Note 2**).
2. Plasmids encoding the viral packaging Gag-Pol protein (pVPack-GP) and vesicular stomatitis virus G envelope glycoprotein (pVPack-VSV-G).
3. Lipofectamine 2000 transfection reagent.
4. DMEM supplemented with 10% heat-inactivated FBS.
5. Polyvinylidene fluoride (PVDF) membrane syringe filters.
6. 4 μg/mL polybrene (hexadimethrine bromide) in DMEM.
7. 400 μg/mL neomycin (G418).
8. Phase contrast microscope equipped with a digital camera.

2.3 In Cellulo Biological Assays

1. Hemacytometer or an automated cell counter.
2. 100% methanol at −20 °C.
3. 0.6% crystal violet staining solution prepared in 100% methanol.
4. 0.3 and 0.6% solutions of Noble agar in DMEM supplemented with 10% FBS.
5. 1 mg/mL *methylthiazol tetrazolium or* 3-(4,5-dimethyl-2-thiazolyl)-2,5-diphenyl-2H-tetrazolium bromide (MTT) solution.
6. 10 mg/mL poly-(2-hydroxyethyl methacrylate) (PolyHEMA) in 100% ethanol. Dissolve polyHEMA powder overnight at room temperature (or by heating at 60 °C for 5–6 h).
7. XTT solution, 0.5 mg/mL 2,3-bis-(2-methoxy-4-nitro-5-sulfophenyl)-2*H*-tetrazolium-5-carboxanilide and 3.75 μg/mL phenazine methosulfate (PMS) in Opti-MEM.
8. Twenty-four (24) Transwell chambers with 8.0 μm pore polycarbonate membrane insert.

9. 20 μg/mL type I collagen, in 0.02 N acetic acid for coating (or 2 mg/mL for gels).
10. CellTrace Calcein Green AM (acetoxymethyl ester).
11. Low-power magnification microscope equipped with a digital imaging system.
12. Confocal laser scanning microscope.
13. ImageJ software [21].
14. Prism (GraphPad software, Inc).

2.4 In Vivo Assays

1. Female athymic CD1 nude mice, 4–5 week-old (Charles River).
2. Serum-reduced Matrigel (Becton Dickinson Labware).
3. 30 G1/2 inch syringe needles.
4. Vernier caliper.
5. Anesthetic solution: 10 mg/mL acepromazine, 20 mg/mL xylazine, and 100 mg/mL ketamine.

3 Method

3.1 IEC-6 Cell Culture

1. Cells are maintained in complete DMEM at 37 °C in a humidified 5% carbon dioxide atmosphere.
2. Cells are passed typically 1:3 to 1:5 upon reaching ~75% subconfluence (*see* **Note 3**).

3.2 Generation of Stable IEC-6 Cell Populations

Retroviral-based method is used to derive IEC-6 cell populations stably expressing TPR-MET or one of its docking-specific variants.

3.2.1 Production of Replication-Deficient Retroviruses

1. Day 1, seed 4×10^5 293 T cells in 10 cm culture petri dishes.
2. Day 2, transfect 293 T cells by Lipofectamine-based method with TPR-MET, the GRB2- or SHC-binding variants, or empty pLXSN retroviral expression vector, along with the pVPack-GP and pVPack-VSV-G packaging plasmids.
3. Day 3, replenish the cells with 7 mL of DMEM supplemented with 10% heat-inactivated FBS (*see* **Note 4**).
4. Day 5, collect the cell conditioned media containing the retroviral particles, and filter it through a 0.45 μm PVDF low protein-binding membrane syringe filter to remove cell debris (*see* **Note 5**).
5. Retroviral particles are used fresh or stored at −80 °C in aliquot.

3.2.2 Infection of IEC-6 Cells

1. Seed the cells at a density of 2,5–5 × 10^4 cells/well in 6-well plates.
2. Wash the cells with serum-free DMEM prior and add 500–1000 μL of viruses stock (*see* **Note 6**) supplemented with 4 μg/mL of polybrene.
3. After an incubation of 4 h, add 3–3.5 mL/well of DMEM supplemented with 10% heat-inactivated FBS.
4. After an incubation of 10–15 h, changed the media for DMEM supplemented with 10% heat-inactivated FBS without polybrene (*see* **Note 7**).
5. Replenish the well with fresh complete DMEM and 400 μg/mL of neomycin as the selection agent 48-h post-infection.
6. Expand IEC-6 cell populations of from a pool of at least 50 -neomycin-resistant colonies, for limiting experimental effects caused by clonal cell line variation.
7. For subsequent experimentation, each modified IEC-6 cell population is paired with that of control (CTRL) IEC-6 cells that have comparable number of passages (±2) and a range between 11 and 25 passages.
8. Evaluate changes in cell morphology by phase contrast microscopy (Fig. 1) (*see* **Note 8**).

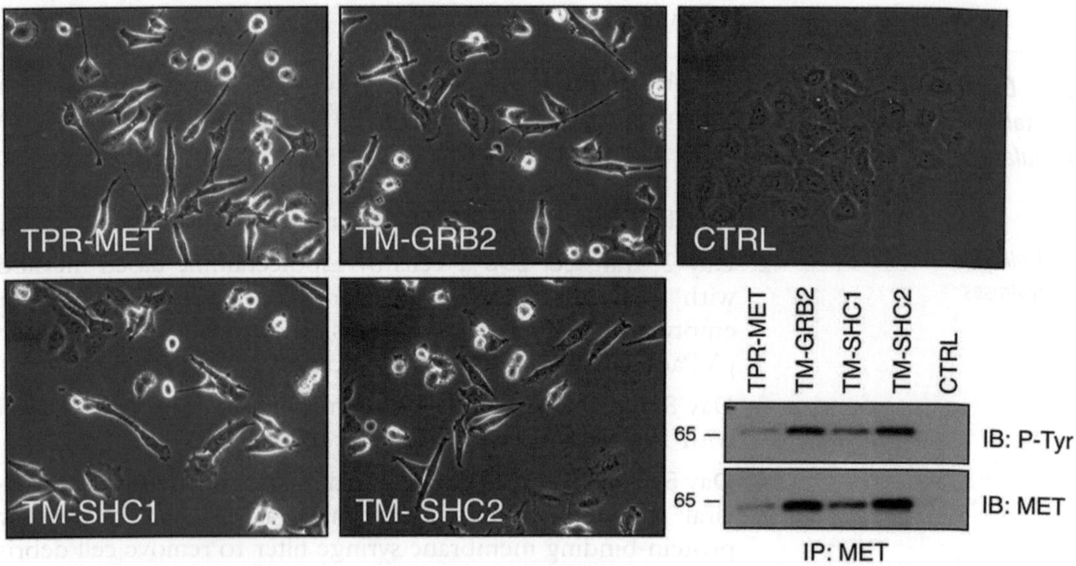

Fig. 1 Photographs show the typical morphology of IEC-6 cells expressing, or not (CTRL), TPR-MET or the GRB2 (TM-GRB2) or SHC (TM-SHC1 or TM-SHC2) docking-specific variants. Expression and phosphorylation levels of these oncoproteins in IEC-6 cell lysates are assessed by immunoblot (IB) analyses following immunoprecipitation (IP) with a MET antibody. Results shown are from a previous published study [19] with permission

9. Expression and phosphorylation levels of the TPR-MET oncoproteins in IEC-6 cells are assessed by standard immunoblot analyses following immunoprecipitation with a MET antibody [18, 19].

3.3 In Cellulo Biological Assays

Biological processes of relevance to tumorigenic and metastatic progression conferred upon the oncogenic engagement of MET signaling, or those downstream of GRB2 and SHC in IEC-6 cells are defined by performing a series of cell-based assays. Each cell-based assay is done usually at least three times in triplicate for obtaining a high degree of confidence in the results.

3.3.1 Cell Growth

For defining whether IEC-6 cell transformation concurs with an increase in cell growth capacity, cell growth assays are performed.

1. Seed the cells in triplicate at a density of 2.5×10^4 in 6-well plates, for each time point tested. Number of cells is then counted daily for up to 6 days.
2. Replace culture medium of the cells by 500 μL of trypsin–EDTA solution/well.
3. Once the cells are fully detached, add 500 μL of serum-free DMEM/well (or more according to the cell density). Count the number of cells in duplicate aliquots of the cell suspension using either a hemacytometer or an automated cell counter (*see* **Note 9**).
4. Cell doubling time is estimated from the growth curves obtained by plotting the number of cells over time using Prism (GraphPad software, Inc).

3.3.2 Focus-Forming Activity

A hallmark of cell transformation is the loss of contact-mediated inhibition of growth. Focus-forming assays allow quantitative assessment of this cell feature.

1. Seed 200 of the tested cells along with 5×10^5 of parental IEC-6 cells to form the monolayer in 6-well plates in triplicate.
2. After ~10–15 days, document the morphology of foci formed by the transformed cells via phase contrast microscopy.
3. For macroscopic revelation of the foci, fix the plates for 20 min at −20 °C in 100% methanol and stain the cells with 0.6% crystal violet.
4. Estimate the average number of foci counted on stained plates using ImageJ software from images acquired at low-magnification, using an imaging system.
5. Express the average number of foci as percentage of those formed by TPR-MET-IEC-6 cells, as CRTL-IEC-6 cells do not form foci.

3.3.3 Anchorage-Independent Growth

Proliferation in the absence of anchorage is associated with oncogenic transformation and is a hallmark of metastatic cancer cells. Cell capacity to grow in an anchorage-independent manner is evaluated by performing soft agar colony formation assays.

1. For each cell population tested, lay out 2 mL of DMEM containing 0.6% agar and 10% FBS in triplicate in 6-well plates (bottom layer). Incubate the plates at 37 °C for ~45 min to allow the soft agar to solidify.
2. To each well, overlay a suspension of 5×10^3 cells in 1 mL of DMEM containing 0.3% agar and 10% FBS on the top of the bottom layer (*see* **Note 10**).
3. Document the morphology of the colonies formed ~10–15 days after seeding the cells by phase contrast microscopy.
4. Stain the cells with 1 mg/mL of MTT for 3 h, for macroscopic visualization of the colonies.
5. Estimate the average the number and size of colonies from images acquired at low-magnification using ImageJ software.
6. Express the results as percentage of those formed by TPR-MET-IEC-6 cells, as CRTL-IEC-6 cells do not form colony in soft agar.

3.3.4 Anoikis Resistance

Growth in soft agar reflects not only the proficiency of cancer cells to proliferate in the absence of extracellular matrix (ECM) attachment, but also to escape anoikis, a prerequisite for tumor cell metastasis [22]. Sensitivity of cells to this form of apoptosis induced by the loss of ECM attachment is measured by performing anoikis assays, which consist of comparing the viability of cells seeded in the absence of serum under adherent and suspension conditions.

1. For growing cells in suspension, coat 24-well plates with 200 μL/well of the polyHEMA solution and let it dry by leaving the plates without the lid under the tissue culture hood for 1.5 h.
2. Repeat **step 1** once.
3. Wash the wells twice with 1 mL of PBS prior to seeding the cells.
4. For each experiment, seed 1.25×10^5 cells in Opti-MEM without serum in triplicate in 24-well plates that are precoated or not with polyHEMA.
5. After 18 h, determine the viability of cells seeded in polyHEMA-coated wells and in noncoated wells by a colorimetric XTT assay.
6. Anoikis sensitivity is reported as the percentage of viable cells in polyHEMA-coated wells (suspension), relative to those seeded in noncoated wells (adherent).

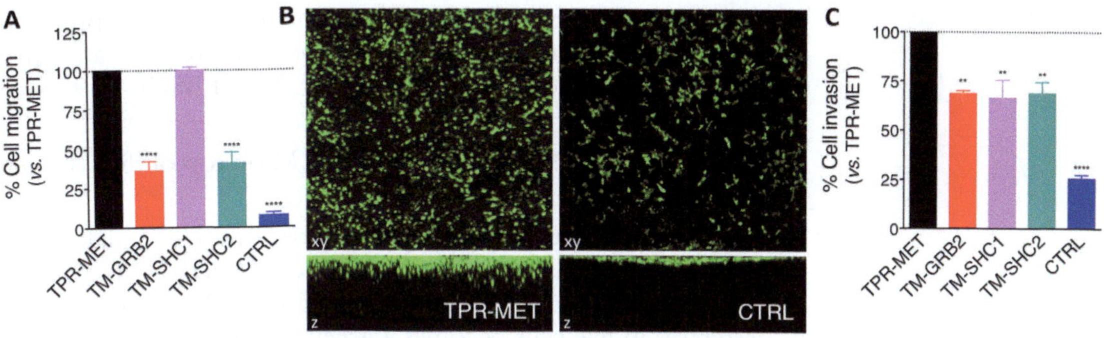

Fig. 2 Quantitative assessment of migration and invasion properties induced by the expression of TPR-MET oncoproteins in IEC-6 cells. (**a**) Migration of cells is evaluated in modified Boyden chambers, as described in the Methods section. Bar graph represents fold induction of migration relative to CTRL IEC-6 cells, expressed in percentage ± S.E.M. of TPR-MET-IEC-6 cells, from four independent experiments done in triplicate. (**b**) A 3D invasion assay in collagen matrix is performed to evaluate the invasive properties of TPR-MET oncoprotein-expressing IEC-6 cells. Representative pictures of TRP-MET and CTRL IEC-6 cells in the z-axis (invasion depth in the collagen matrix) following labeling with CellTrace™ Calcein Green AM. (**c**) Cells that had invaded the collagen layer were imaged and quantified at each 5 μm-layer within the gel. Bar graph shows the fold induction in the mean maximal depth of invasion of cells in the collagen matrix relative to CTRL IEC-6 cells, expressed in percentage ± S.E.M. of TPR-MET-IEC-6 cells. Overall, these results show that signaling pathways engaged by the oncogenic activation of MET in normal IECs, likewise those induced upon the recruitment of GRB2 or SHC, enhances cell growth, loss of growth contact inhibition, anchorage-independent growth, anoikis resistance, migration and invasion

3.3.5 Cell Migration

Dissemination of cancer cells from the primary tumor to distal organs relies on their ability to migrate migration capacity. This capacity can be determined by performing Transwell migration assays.

1. Precoat both sides of the 8.0 μm polycarbonate membrane of chamber inserts of 24-well Transwell® plates with collagen type I (6 $\mu g/cm^2$).
2. In the inner chambers, seed 2×10^5 cells in serum-free DMEM supplemented with 0.1% BSA in triplicate.
3. Add to the lower chamber 600 μL of DMEM supplemented with 10% FBS, as a chemoattractant.
4. After an incubation of 3–6 h, remove nonmigrating cells from the top membrane by scraping with a cotton swab.
5. Fix cells that have migrated through the inserts in 70% ethanol, and stain them with a solution of 0.6% crystal violet.
6. Count the number of migrating cells manually under a phase contrast microscope (Fig. 2a).

3.3.6 Cell Invasion

Cellular invasion through the degradation of ECM is a critical process underlying cancer metastasis. Invasive capacity of cells is evaluated by performing three-dimensional (3D) matrix invasion assays [23].

1. Lay 50 μL/well of fibrillar collagen type-I (2 mg/mL, prepared following manufacturer's instructions), on top of an equal volume an agarose layer containing 20% FBS in a 96-well culture plate.
2. Seed 4×10^4 cells in serum-free DMEM on top of the collagen layer.
3. One hour prior to the end of an incubation of 48 h, label cells invading the collagen matrix with Calcein Green AM. This is a cell permeable agent that once hydrolyzed by intracellular esterases in live cells becomes a green fluorescent molecule.
4. Wash the unincorporated Calcein Green AM with PBS and fix the cells with 3% glutaraldehyde for 30 min.
5. By confocal microscopy, scan the collagen matrix layers along the z-axis, where cells that had invaded the collagen are imaged and quantified at 5-μm intervals, layer by layer within the gel (Fig. 2b).
6. Determine the relative intensity according to the depth of cell penetration into the collagen matrix (Fig. 2c).

3.4 In Vivo Assays

Development of tumors and metastases is dictated by the intrinsic features of cancer cells but also by the intimate crosstalk between cancer and stromal cells. Thus the importance to investigate whether the in cellulo cancer cell features driven by the oncogenic engagement of RTK pathways translate into peculiar tumorigenic and metastatic attributes in vivo. Herein, we described mouse models for assessing the in vivo angiogenic, tumorigenic, and metastatic proficiency of cells [12, 13, 18]. These in vivo cancer assays are performed with 4–5-week-old female CD1 nude mice, under protocols approved by the Université de Sherbrooke Ethics Committee for Animal Care and Use, in accordance with guidelines established by the Canadian Council on Animal Care.

3.4.1 Tumorigenesis

1. Harvest cells by trypsinization and wash them twice in serum-free DMEM.
2. Suspend the cells in serum-free DMEM at a concentration of 10^7 cells/mL.
3. Inject a volume of 100 μL (10^6 cells) subcutaneously into both flanks of mice (*see* **Note 11**).
4. Measure periodically tumor length and width using a digital Vernier caliper.
5. Calculate tumor volume using the modified ellipsoidal formula: $\frac{1}{2}(length \times width^2)$.
6. Euthanize mice prior to the tumor reaching 1 cm^3 or at any signs of ulceration.
7. Tumor growth rate is estimated from curves obtained by plotting the tumors (mm^3) over time (day) (Fig. 3a).

3.4.2 Angiogenesis

Cancer cell capacity to coopt the nearby existing vasculature to form new blood vessels, a process called angiogenesis, is conducive to tumor and metastasis growth, supplying oxygen and nutrients. Furthermore, tumor vascularization fosters metastatic dissemination of cancer cells by providing an escape route by which they can leave the primary tumor site and enter into the blood circulatory system [24]. To assess the ability of cells to induce angiogenesis in vivo, we rely on performing Matrigel plug angiogenesis assays. Matrigel is a liquid at 4 °C, but quickly solidifies once at 37 °C. As such, this confines cells within a Matrigel plug at the injection site, thereby allowing the detection of the newly formed blood vessels in the inoculated gel plugs in mice.

1. Harvest cells by trypsinization and wash them twice in serum-free DMEM.
2. Suspend 4×10^6 cells/mL in ice-cold growth factor-depleted Matrigel (*see* **Note 12**).
3. Inject the 250 μL of Matrigel cell suspension subcutaneously into each flank of at least 3 mice.
4. After ~10 days, photograph the resulting Matrigel plugs containing test cells (Fig. 3b).

3.4.3 Lung Metastatic Activity

A simple method to assess the metastatic capacity of cells is to evaluate their ability to form lung lesions following their intravenous injection into the tail vein of mice. In this assay, the lung is the primary metastatic site because the cells reach the pulmonary capillary bed first post-injection.

1. Harvest cells by trypsinization and wash them twice in serum-free DMEM.
2. Suspend 10^7 cells/mL in serum-free DMEM.
3. Inject 100 μL of the cells suspension (10^6 cells) into the tail vein of mice using a 30 G1/2 inch syringe needle (*see* **Note 13**).
4. Euthanize the animals at any sign of lethargy, respiratory distress or weight loss, or 25–35 days post-cell injection of the cells.
5. Resect and photograph the lungs or any other organs displaying metastases upon macroscopic examination.
6. Fix the lungs in Bouin's staining solution for better macroscopic visualization of pulmonary metastases (Fig. 3c).
7. Proceed on histologic examination of hematoxylin and eosin (H&E)-stained lung sections (5 μm) for the detection of microscopic lung metastatic lesions (Fig. 3c).

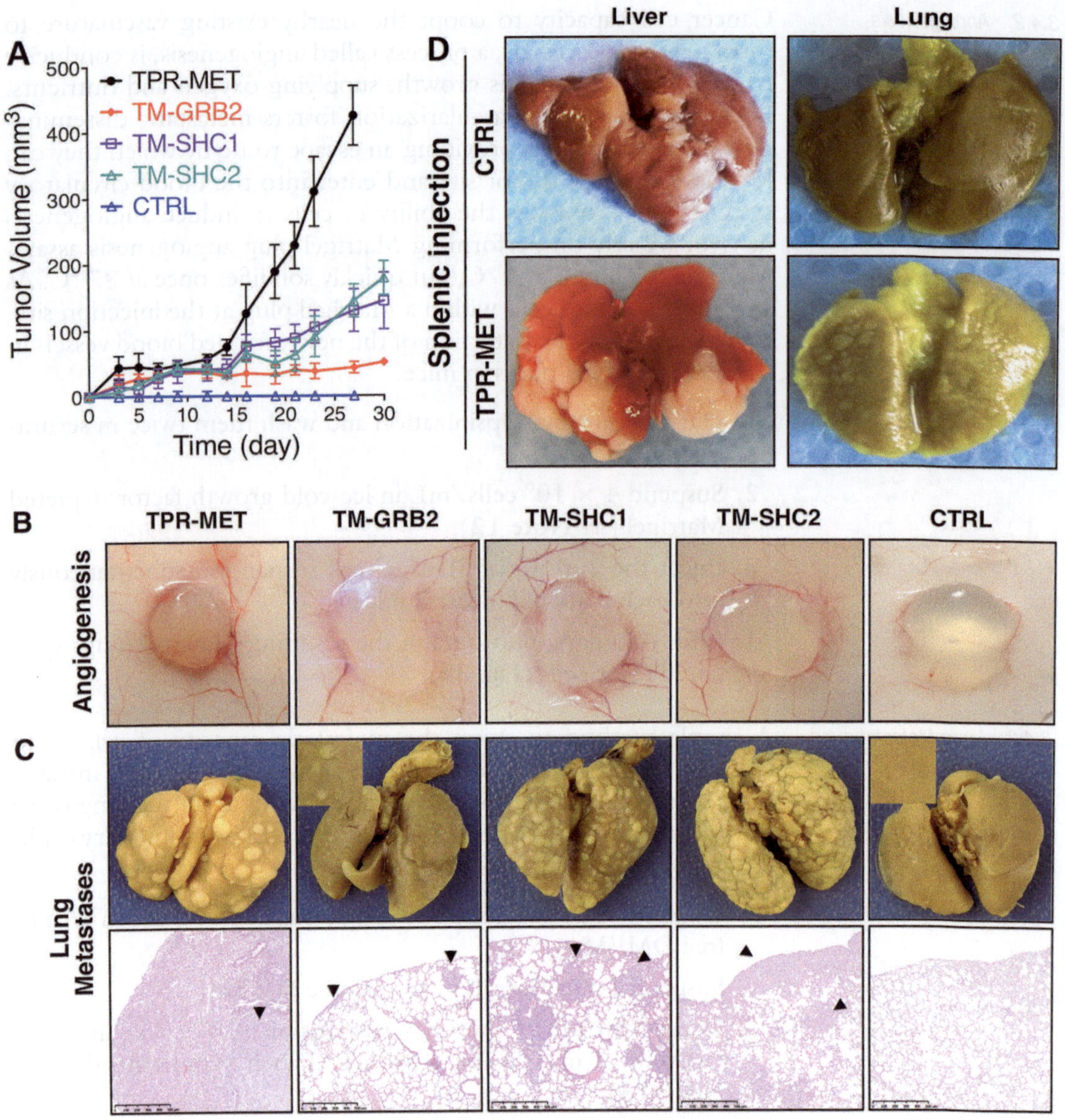

Fig. 3 In vivo evaluation of tumorigenic, angiogenic or metastatic capacity of IEC-6 cells conferred by the expression of TPR-MET oncoproteins. (**a**) Tumor volume (mm^3) over time (day) is measured after the subcutaneous injection of the indicated IEC-6 cell populations (10^6 cells/injection site). Values represent the mean tumor volume of $n = 8$. No tumors were detected after 90 days in mice injected with the CTRL IEC-6 cells. (**b**) Representative photographs of Matrigel plugs formed 10 days post-injection of 10^6 cells mixed with 250 μL of growth factor-depleted Matrigel solution. (**c**) Representative photographs of mice's lungs ~25 days after the tail vein injection of the indicated cells (similar results were obtained in two independent experiments). Small insert corresponds to a magnification of lung tissue, showing microscopic metastases with the TM-GRB2-expressing IEC-6 in comparison to CTRL cells where no metastases are visible. The bottom panel shows representative images of H&E-stained 5 μm lung sections of the mice where metastatic lesions are denoted with a black arrow. (**d**) Representative photographs of liver or lung of mice following the intrasplenic injection of TPR-MET-expressing or CTRL IEC-6 cell populations. In these assays, TPR-MET-IEC-6 cells

3.4.4 Liver Metastatic Activity

The liver is the most common site for CRC metastasis. Thus, we have developed an experimental liver metastasis assay where the cells are delivered into the portal circulation via intrasplenic injection.

1. Prepare cells as described above in Subheading 3.4.3.
2. Anesthetize mice by an intramuscular administration of the anesthesia cocktail at a dose of 0.1 mL/100 g of body weight.
3. Inject the 100 μL of cells (10^6) into the spleen of mice.
4. Allow the cells to disseminate to the liver for 2–3 min prior to splenectomy by suture ligation.
5. Euthanize the animals at any sign of lethargy, respiratory distress or weight loss, or 25–35 days post-cell injection of the cells.
6. Resect and photograph the liver or any other organs displaying metastases upon macroscopic examination (Fig. 3d).

4 Notes

1. The IEC-6 cells exhibit typical features of undifferentiated intestinal crypt cells, including an epithelioid morphology, sparse microvilli, and E-cadherin cell–cell interactions [20]. Notably, they have characteristics of normal untransformed epithelial cells; displaying low plating efficiency when seeded at low density, growing as a monolayer with strong density inhibition of growth, and lacking growth capacity in soft agar and as tumors when injected in nude mice. As such, the IEC-6 cell line represents a widely used model for studying oncogenic pathways of relevance to intestinal epithelial-derived cancer, including CRC [25–30].
2. Generation of the GRB2 and SHC specific docking TPR-MET variants, and their insertion into the pLXSN retroviral expression vector has been previously described [12]. The GRB2-specific TPR-MET variant (TM-GRB2) contains the GRB2

Fig. 3 (continued) develop liver metastases, but also disseminate to the lung and cause severe hemorrhagic ascites [19] (data not shown here). Results presented for CTRL and TPR-MET-expressing IEC-6 cells' capacity to form tumors, and lung and liver metastases in mouse are from an earlier published study [19] with permission. By performing these in vivo cancer assays, we were able to show, for the first time, that the constitutive activation of MET signaling is sufficient alone to confer potent angiogenic, tumorigenic and metastatic proficiency to normal IECs. Notably, although the oncogenic MET-driven downstream engagement of either GRB2 or SHC in IEC-6 cells promoted similar features in cellulo (*see* Figs. 1 and 2), the IEC-6 cells transformed by the SHC-binding MET oncoproteins exhibited much greater in vivo tumorigenic and metastatic activity than those expressing the GRB2-binding MET oncoprotein, which likely a result of their reduced capacity to induce angiogenesis

binding site derived from EGFR. Those selective for the recruitment of SHC encompass either the high affinity SHC binding motif from the TRKA receptor (TM-SHC1) or the lower affinity motif from the EGFR (TM-SHC2). Binding specificity of these TPR-MET variants has been extensively validated in earlier studies [12–17].

3. Since the IEC-6 cells are nontransformed, they display poor seeding efficiency when plated at low density. However, avoid maintaining the cells at high confluence to prevent spontaneous cell transformation.
4. Heat inactivation of serum is done by an incubation of 30 min at 56 °C in a water bath for inactivating heat-labile complement proteins that reduce the viral infection efficiency.
5. Low protein-binding membrane filters are used to prevent virus retention to membranes.
6. For cell infection using frozen virus particles, consider doubling the volume to account for the freeze–thaw reduced transduction efficiency of viruses.
7. Polybrene is a positively charged polymer that increases the transduction efficiency of viruses by enhancing immobilization of negatively charged virus particles to target cellular membranes [31]. However, extended exposure of the IEC-6 cells to polybrene is toxicity.
8. As depicted for IEC-6 cells expressing TPR-MET, or the GRB2- or SHC-docking variants (Fig. 1), the transformation of IEC-6 cells is associated with a breakdown of cell–cell contacts, cell dispersal, the acquisition of a fibroblast-like spindle-shaped morphology, appearance of many cell membrane protrusions typical of lamellipodia and invadopodia-like structures, and a more refractile appearance than the control IEC-6 cells (CTRL), which display typical normal epithelioid morphology [18, 19].
9. Add the impermeable Trypan blue dye at a concentration 0.4% for the specific count of viable cells.
10. Usage of phenol-red-free DMEM enhances the contrast of colonies.
11. For ensuring the injection of the same number of cells, mix the cell suspension well just prior to injection.
12. For handling Matrigel, use tubes, pipet tips, pipettes, and syringes that are precooled at 4 °C to avoid its solidification.
13. For better dilation of the veins, warm up the mice's tail by gentle rubbing, or using an overhead heat lamp, but with extra care to prevent overheating the animals. Start injecting the cells at the distal end of the tail. If the first trial fails, a second attempt can be done at a more proximal region of the tail.

Acknowledgments

This work was supported by an operating grant from the Canadian Institutes of Health Research (CIHR, MOP-106476) awarded to CS.

References

1. Fearon ER, Vogelstein B (1990) A genetic model for colorectal tumorigenesis. Cell 61 (5):759–767
2. Arends JW (2000) Molecular interactions in the Vogelstein model of colorectal carcinoma. J Pathol 190(4):412–416
3. Curley SA (2005) Outcomes after surgical treatment of colorectal cancer liver metastases. Semin Oncol 32(6 Suppl 9):S109–S111
4. Hanahan D, Weinberg RA (2011) Hallmarks of cancer: the next generation. Cell 144 (5):646–674. https://doi.org/10.1016/j.cell.2011.02.013
5. Saucier C, Rivard N (2010) Epithelial cell signalling in metastatic colorectal cancer. In: Huot J, Beauchemin N (eds) Metastasis of colon cancer, Cancer metastasis—biology and treatment, vol 14. Springer, Netherlands, pp 205–241
6. Birchmeier C, Birchmeier W, Gherardi E, Vande Woude GF (2003) Met, metastasis, motility and more. Nat Rev Mol Cell Biol 4 (12):915–925
7. Peschard P, Park M (2007) From Tpr-Met to Met, tumorigenesis and tubes. Oncogene 26 (9):1276–1285
8. Bardelli A, Corso S, Bertotti A, Hobor S, Valtorta E, Siravegna G, Sartore-Bianchi A, Scala E, Cassingena A, Zecchin D, Apicella M, Migliardi G, Galimi F, Lauricella C, Zanon C, Perera T, Veronese S, Corti G, Amatu A, Gambacorta M, Diaz LA Jr, Sausen M, Velculescu VE, Comoglio P, Trusolino L, Di Nicolantonio F, Giordano S, Siena S (2013) Amplification of the MET receptor drives resistance to anti-EGFR therapies in colorectal cancer. Cancer Discov 3(6):658–673. https://doi.org/10.1158/2159-8290.CD-12-0558
9. Van Cutsem E, Eng C, Nowara E, Swieboda-Sadlej A, Tebbutt NC, Mitchell E, Davidenko I, Stephenson J, Elez E, Prenen H, Deng H, Tang R, McCaffery I, Oliner KS, Chen L, Gansert J, Loh E, Smethurst D, Tabernero J (2014) Randomized phase Ib/II trial of rilotumumab or ganitumab with panitumumab versus panitumumab alone in patients with wild-type KRAS metastatic colorectal cancer. Clin Cancer Res 20 (16):4240–4250. https://doi.org/10.1158/1078-0432.CCR-13-2752
10. Eng C, Bessudo A, Hart LL, Severtsev A, Gladkov O, Muller L, Kopp MV, Vladimirov V, Langdon R, Kotiv B, Barni S, Hsu C, Bolotin E, von Roemeling R, Schwartz B, Bendell JC (2016) A randomized, placebo-controlled, phase 1/2 study of tivantinib (ARQ 197) in combination with irinotecan and cetuximab in patients with metastatic colorectal cancer with wild-type KRAS who have received first-line systemic therapy. Int J Cancer 139(1):177–186. https://doi.org/10.1002/ijc.30049
11. Bendell JC, Hochster H, Hart LL, Firdaus I, Mace JR, McFarlane JJ, Kozloff M, Catenacci D, Hsu JJ, Hack SP, Shames DS, Phan SC, Koeppen H, Cohn AL (2017) A phase II randomized trial (GO27827) of first-line FOLFOX plus bevacizumab with or without the MET inhibitor onartuzumab in patients with metastatic colorectal cancer. Oncologist 22(3):264–271. https://doi.org/10.1634/theoncologist.2016-0223
12. Saucier C, Papavasiliou V, Palazzo A, Naujokas MA, Kremer R, Park M (2002) Use of signal specific receptor tyrosine kinase oncoproteins reveals that pathways downstream from Grb2 or Shc are sufficient for cell transformation and metastasis. Oncogene 21(12):1800–1811
13. Saucier C, Khoury H, Lai KM, Peschard P, Dankort D, Naujokas MA, Holash J, Yancopoulos GD, Muller WJ, Pawson T, Park M (2004) The Shc adaptor protein is critical for VEGF induction by Met/HGF and ErbB2 receptors and for early onset of tumor angiogenesis. Proc Natl Acad Sci U S A 101 (8):2345–2350
14. Ishimura A, Lee HS, Bong YS, Saucier C, Mood K, Park EK, Daar IO (2006) Oncogenic Met receptor induces ectopic structures in Xenopus embryos. Oncogene 25 (31):4286–4299
15. Mood K, Saucier C, Ishimura A, Bong YS, Lee HS, Park M, Daar IO (2006) Oncogenic met receptor induces cell-cycle progression in Xenopus oocytes independent of direct Grb2 and Shc binding or mos synthesis, but requires

phosphatidylinositol 3-kinase and raf signaling. J Cell Physiol 207(1):271–285

16. Mood K, Saucier C, Bong YS, Lee HS, Park M, Daar IO (2006) Gab1 is required for cell cycle transition, cell proliferation, and transformation induced by an oncogenic met receptor. Mol Biol Cell 17(9):3717–3728
17. Seiden-Long I, Navab R, Shih W, Li M, Chow J, Zhu CQ, Radulovich N, Saucier C, Tsao MS (2008) Gab1 but not Grb2 mediates tumor progression in Met overexpressing colorectal cancer cells. Carcinogenesis 29 (3):647–655
18. Bernier J, Chababi W, Pomerleau V, Saucier C (2010) Oncogenic engagement of the Met receptor is sufficient to evoke angiogenic, tumorigenic, and metastatic activities in rat intestinal epithelial cells. Am J Physiol 299(3): G677–G686
19. Pomerleau V, Landry M, Bernier J, Vachon PH, Saucier C (2014) Met receptor-induced Grb2 or Shc signals both promote transformation of intestinal epithelial cells, albeit they are required for distinct oncogenic functions. BMC Cancer 14:240. https://doi.org/10.1186/1471-2407-14-240
20. Quaroni A, Wands J, Trelstad RL, Isselbacher KJ (1979) Epithelioid cell cultures from rat small intestine. Characterization by morphologic and immunologic criteria. J Cell Biol 80 (2):248–265
21. Schneider CA, Rasband WS, Eliceiri KW (2012) NIH Image to ImageJ: 25 years of image analysis. Nat Methods 9(7):671–675
22. Vachon PH (2011) Integrin signaling, cell survival, and anoikis: distinctions, differences, and differentiation. J Signal Transduct 2011:738137. https://doi.org/10.1155/2011/738137
23. Arsenault D, Lucien F, Dubois CM (2012) Hypoxia enhances cancer cell invasion through relocalization of the proprotein convertase furin from the trans-Golgi network to the cell surface. J Cell Physiol 227(2):789–800. https://doi.org/10.1002/jcp.22792
24. Folkman J (2002) Role of angiogenesis in tumor growth and metastasis. Semin Oncol 29(6 Suppl 16):15–18. https://doi.org/10.1053/sonc.2002.37263
25. Sheng H, Shao J, Dubois RN (2001) K-Ras-mediated increase in cyclooxygenase 2 mRNA stability involves activation of the protein kinase B1. Cancer Res 61(6):2670–2675
26. Shao J, Evers BM, Sheng H (2004) Roles of phosphatidylinositol 3′-kinase and mammalian target of rapamycin/p70 ribosomal protein S6 kinase in K-Ras-mediated transformation of intestinal epithelial cells. Cancer Res 64 (1):229–235
27. Komatsu K, Buchanan FG, Katkuri S, Morrow JD, Inoue H, Otaka M, Watanabe S, DuBois RN (2005) Oncogenic potential of MEK1 in rat intestinal epithelial cells is mediated via cyclooxygenase-2. Gastroenterology 129 (2):577–590. https://doi.org/10.1016/j.gastro.2005.06.003
28. Nandan MO, McConnell BB, Ghaleb AM, Bialkowska AB, Sheng H, Shao J, Babbin BA, Robine S, Yang VW (2008) Kruppel-like factor 5 mediates cellular transformation during oncogenic KRAS-induced intestinal tumorigenesis. Gastroenterology 134(1):120–130. https://doi.org/10.1053/j.gastro.2007.10.023
29. Voisin L, Julien C, Duhamel S, Gopalbhai K, Claveau I, Saba-El-Leil MK, Rodrigue-Gervais IG, Gaboury L, Lamarre D, Basik M, Meloche S (2008) Activation of MEK1 or MEK2 isoform is sufficient to fully transform intestinal epithelial cells and induce the formation of metastatic tumors. BMC Cancer 8:337
30. Lemieux E, Bergeron S, Durand V, Asselin C, Saucier C, Rivard N (2009) Constitutively active MEK1 is sufficient to induce epithelial-to-mesenchymal transition in intestinal epithelial cells and to promote tumor invasion and metastasis. Int J Cancer 125 (7):1575–1586
31. Davis HE, Morgan JR, Yarmush ML (2002) Polybrene increases retrovirus gene transfer efficiency by enhancing receptor-independent virus adsorption on target cell membranes. Biophys Chem 97(2–3):159–172

Check for updates

Chapter 3

Identification of Response Elements on Promoters Using Site-Directed Mutagenesis and Chromatin Immunoprecipitation

Salah Boudjadi, Julie C. Carrier, and Jean-François Beaulieu

Abstract

Proximal promoters are located upstream of the transcription start sites of genes, and they contain regulatory sequences on which bind different transcription factors for promoting colorectal cancer progression. Here we describe the comprehensive methodology used previously for the identification and functional characterization of MYC-responsive elements in the integrin α1 subunit (ITGA1) gene using a combination of in silico analysis, site-directed mutagenesis, and chromatin immunoprecipitation.

Key words Promoters, ChIP, Response element, Mutagenesis, Transcription factor, MYC, ITGA1

1 Introduction

Identifying the factors involved in the regulation of the expression of a given gene is crucial to understand the mechanism by which a gene is upregulated or downregulated in a specific cellular context. Different valuable tools are available to identify the response elements (REs) for a transcription factor (TF) in the proximal promoters located upstream of the transcription start site. Among these tools, in silico analysis is used to identify the presence of REs which could be the consensus sequence, defined as the most frequent sequence recognized by a transcription factors [1], or incomplete sequences which could be functional and bound by transcription factors [2]. Whether these sequences are functional or not could be demonstrated using promoter reporter assays coupled to selective mutagenesis of the presumed REs [3], despite the fact that these assays remain artificial. To demonstrate that a TF bind to a RE in the context of the in cellulo native chromatin, the chromatin Immunoprecipitation (ChIP) is a valuable and complementary tool confirming the binding of the transcription factor to the promoter area containing the identified REs. In addition to the

Jean-François Beaulieu (ed.), *Colorectal Cancer: Methods and Protocols*, Methods in Molecular Biology, vol. 1765, https://doi.org/10.1007/978-1-4939-7765-9_3,

listing of the needed materials and tools, this protocol details the steps for the analysis of promoter sequence and the identification of REs for transcription factors using the transcription factor MYC and the proximal promoter of the ITGA1 gene as a typical example of an oncogenic pathway potentially involved in colorectal cancer progression [4–6].

2 Materials

2.1 In Silico Analysis

1. MatInspector web-based software (Genomatix, Munich, Germany).

   https://www.genomatix.de/online_help/help_matinspector/matinspector_help.html

2. BLAST© web-based software.
   https://blast.ncbi.nlm.nih.gov/Blast.cgi?PAGE_TYPE=BlastSearch&PROG_DEF=blastn&BLAST_PROG_DEF=blastn&BLAST_SPEC=GlobalAln&LINK_LOC=BlastHomeLink

2.2 Promoter Reporter Assay and Site-Directed Mutagenesis

1. Plasmid vector containing the sequence of the proximal promoter of interest and the reporter gene (i.e., firefly, Renilla).
2. Plasmid construct containing an internal control vector used to assess the transfection efficiency (i.e., pGL4.13 plasmids: luc2/SV40).
3. Plasmid vectors expressing the activators (transcription factors and cofactor, if applicable).
4. 12-well plates.
5. White 96-well assay plate.
6. Effectene transfection reagent.
7. HEK293T cells at low passage.
8. Dual Luciferase Reporter Assay System.
9. GeneArt Site-Directed Mutagenesis Kit.
10. DNase- and RNase-free water.
11. 0.4% trypan blue solution.
12. Fetal bovine serum (FBS).
13. DMEM culture medium for HEK293T cells (10% FBS, 2 mM GlutaMAX, 10 mM Hepes).
14. 1.5 mL tubes.
15. Phosphate buffer saline (PBS).
16. 0.5 M EDTA, pH 8.0.
17. Distilled water.

18. Luminometer (Berthold, Bad Wildbad, Germany).
19. Thermal Cycler for PCR reactions.
20. Water bath.
21. Ice.
22. LB agar plates.
23. Super optimal broth (SOC) medium.
24. Cell culture incubator.

2.3 Chromatin Immunoprecipitation

1. Cell line of interest expressing both the transcription factor and the target gene of interest.
2. 1% paraformaldehyde solution.
3. Protease inhibitor solution.
4. 2.5 M glycine solution: add 1.88 g of glycine to 10 mL of distilled water.
5. Cell lysis Buffer: 50 μL of 1 M HEPES, 850 μL of 1 M KCl, 50 μL of 10% NP40 and complete to 10 mL with distilled water.
6. Nuclear lysis buffer: 0.5 mL of 1 M Tris–HCl pH 8.0, 200 μL of 0.5 M EDTA pH 8.0, 1 mL of 10% SDS and complete to 10 mL with distilled water.
7. ChIP Dilution Buffer: 167 μL of 1 M Tris–HCl pH 8.0, 10 μL of 10% SDS, 110 μL of Triton X-100, 2.4 μL of 0.5 M EDTA pH 8.0, 334 μL of 5 M NaCl and complete to 10 mL with distilled water.
8. Buffer TSE1 solution: 200 μL of 1 M Tris–HCl pH 8.0, 100 μL of 10% SDS, 100 μL of Triton X-100, 40 μL of 0.5 M EDTA pH 8.0, 300 μL of 5 M NaCl and complete to 10 mL with distilled water.
9. Buffer TSE2 solution: 200 μL of 1 M Tris–HCl pH 8.0, 100 μL of 10% of SDS, 100 μL of Triton X-100, 40 μL of 0.5 M EDTA pH 8.0, 1 mL 5 M of NaCl and complete to 10 mL with distilled water.
10. Buffer TSE3 solution: 100 μL of 1 M Tris–HCl pH 8.0, 2.5 mL 1 M of LiCl 1 M, 100 μL of 10% NP 40, 0.10 g of Na-deoxycholate, 20 μL of 0.5 M EDTA pH 8.0 and complete to 10 mL with distilled water.
11. Buffer TE solution: 50 μL 1 M of Tris–HCl pH 8.0, 10 μL of 0.5 M EDTA pH 8.0 and complete to 10 mL with distilled water.
12. Elution solution: Should be prepared fresh, 1 mL of 10% SDS and 0.084 g of $NaHCO_3$ and complete to 10 mL with distilled water.
13. 5 mg/mL RNase A solution.

14. 10 mg/mL proteinase K solution.
15. DNA purification kit (QIAquick PCR purification Kit, or similar).

3 Methods

3.1 Promoter Analysis

This step provides preliminary data and indications about the possibility that a transcription factor could bind to the promoter of interest. Finding REs in the promoter sequence could be done either with basic analysis or using software.

1. Basic analysis consists of the comparison between the consensus REs and the sequence of the positive and negative strands of the promoter.
2. Using software, such as Matinspector, the proximal promoter sequence could be directly uploaded or found using the search function of the website. Once the analysis is finished, select the transcription factor of interest and check the corresponding response element sequences (*see* **Note 1**).

3.2 Site-Directed Mutagenesis

Once the REs selected, the next step is to evaluate their functionality using selective mutations rendering them unrecognized by the TF of interest.

1. Selective mutations could be introduced using the GeneArt Site-Directed Mutagenesis Kit.
2. For the primer design, change the nucleotides shared by the RE and the consensus RE in order to alter completely the sequence of the RE (*see* **Note 2**).
3. If there is two REs (or more) for the transcription factor of interest, mutations should be done separately to evaluate their functionality (*see* **Note 3**).
4. Perform the PCR reaction using the PCR mix (Table 1) and incubate in a thermocycler:
   (a) Step 1: incubate for 20 min at 37 °C for plasmid methylation and then 2 min at 94 °C.
   (b) Step 2 (20 cycles): incubate for 20 s at 94 °C, then at 57 °C for 30 s followed by incubation for 30 s/kb at 68 °C.
   (c) Step 3: terminate the reaction with incubation at 68 °C (elongation) for 5 min and then hold at 4 °C. The PCR product can be stored at −20 °C.
5. For the recombination reaction (*see* **Note 4**):

Table 1
PCR MIX for mutagenesis reaction

10× AccuPrime™ Pfx reaction mix	5 μL	1×
10× enhancer	5 μL	1×
Primer mix (10 μM each)	1.5 μL	0.3 μM each
Plasmid DNA (20 ng/μL)	1 μL	20 ng
DNA methylase (4 U/μL)	1 μL	4 units
25× SAM	2 μL	1×
AccuPrime™ Pfx (2.5 U/μL)	0.4 μL	1 unit
PCR water	To 50 μL	

(a) Add 4 μL of 5× reaction buffer to 4 μL of the PCR product (**step 3** above) and 2 μL of 10× Enzymer mix, and incubate for 10 min at RT.

(b) Stop the reaction by adding 1 μL of 0.5 M EDTA.

6. For the transformation reaction (*see* **Note 5**):

   (a) Transfer 2 μL of the recombination reaction directly into the vial of DH5α competent cells (Reaction 1), mix by gentle tapping and then incubate for 12 min.

   (b) Immediately incubate the vials at 42 °C for exactly 30 s and then reincubate on ice for 2 min.

   (c) Add 250 μL of SOC medium to the Reaction 1 creating the Reaction 2 and then incubate at 37 °C for exactly 1 h with 225 rpm shaking.

   (d) Add 10 μL from Reaction 2 to 90 μL of SOC medium, then spread 100 μL onto LB plates and incubate overnight (*see* **Note 6**).

   (e) Select 5–10 colonies and isolate DNA from the bacteria using a plasmid purification kit.

   (f) Sequence the DNA product to ensure that the plasmid contains the mutations introduced in the promoter and compare to the original promoter using Align software (*see* **Note 7**).

   (g) DNA can be stored at −20 °C.

3.3 Transient Transfection and Promoter Reporter Assays

1. Keep HEK293T cells (*see* **Note 8**) in DMEM media supplemented with 10% FBS (without antibiotics).
2. Plate 50,000 cells per well in 12-well plates and add a total of 1 mL of DMEM 10% FBS media to each well and the transfection will be started the following day.

Table 2
Plasmid preparation for showing the responsiveness of the promoter to the TF of interest

	Condition	
Plasmids	**Control**	**TF**
Wild-type plasmid	100 ng	100 ng
Plasmid expressing the activator (TF)	×	100 ng
Empty vector (EV)	200 ng	100 ng
pGL4.13 (firefly)	2 ng	2 ng

Table 3
Plasmid mix for the comparison between wild-type and mutated promoters

	Wild-type promoter		Mutated promoter	
Plasmids	**EV**	**TF**	**EV**	**TF**
Wild-type promoter	100 ng	100 ng	×	×
Mutated promoter	×	×	100 ng	100 ng
Plasmid expressing the activator (TF)	×	100 ng	×	100 ng
Empty vector	100 ng	×	100 ng	×
pGL4.13 (firefly)	2 ng	2 ng	2 ng	2 ng

3. Transient transfection is performed using (as example) the Effectene Kit©:
   (a) For each well, add equal amounts of the plasmid mix for exactly 5 min. The amounts of plasmids are indicated in Table 2 for testing the wild-type promoter responsiveness to the TF, and in Table 3 for comparing wild-type and mutated promoters.
   (b) Add Effectine reagent (2 μL/ well), mix gently and incubate for 10 min.
   (c) Change the media in the 12-well plates, add the plasmid mix to each well and incubate for 48 h.
4. For cell lysis, rinse the wells with cold PBS and then add 250 μL of Passive Lysis Buffer 1× to each well of the 12-well plates and incubate for 15 min with gentle shaking.
5. For the promoter reporter assay, transfer 10 μL from each PLB lysate in wells of a 96-well plate and run dual reported

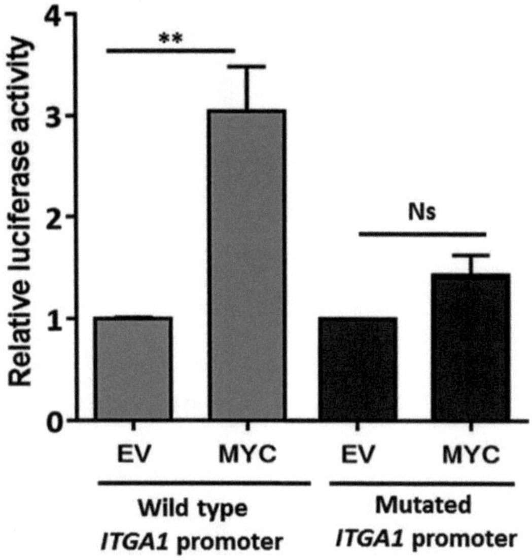

Fig. 1 c-MYC controls the ITGA promoter activity. Promoter gene reporter assay showing the relative luciferase activity presented as fold change. The wild-type *ITGA1* promoter vector, or the mutated promoter (dark gray columns) were separately transfected into HEK293T cells, together with the empty vector, or MYC expressing vector (MYC). Experiments were repeated three times and performed in triplicate. T test. $^{**}P < 0.01$, $^{***}P < 0.001$. Original data are from [6]

detection with a luminometer. Using the Orion Microplate (Berthold Detection Systems, Huntsville, Alabama, USA), we set injectors one and two to dispense 50 μL of LARII and Stop & Glo solutions, respectively, and use 10 s for reading time and 2 s as a delay (*see* **Note 9**).

6. Results are expressed as relative luciferase activity (luciferase–renilla ratio) (Fig. 1)

3.4 Chromatin Immunoprecipitation

3.4.1 Day 1

1. If needed, perform any specific treatment to the cells prior to the ChIP assay, or use the cells directly grown in their adapted medium.
2. Cross-linking:
   (a) Remove the medium from the dishes and add fresh medium (without serum) containing 1% paraformaldehyde (final concentration) and incubate for 15 min at room temperature (RT) (*see* **Note 10**).
   (b) Stop the cross-linking by adding one part of the 2.5 M glycine solution to nine part of medium and incubating for 5 min at RT.

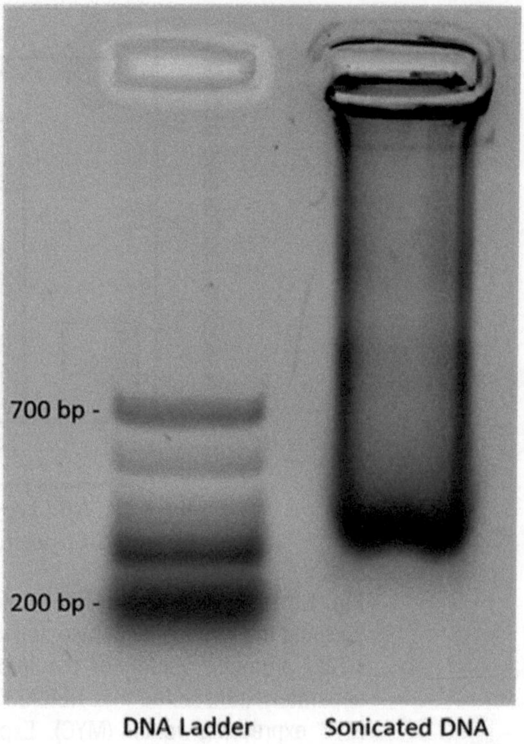

Fig. 2 DNA sonication pattern extracted from HT29 cell line. After nuclear lysis step, DNA was sonicated three times during 10 s separated by a 30 s pause on ice. 10 μL of the sonicated DNA (right) were migrated on agarose gel (1%) and show that most of the DNA migrates at the level of 300 bp, compared to the DNA ladder (left)

3. Cell lysis:
   (a) Remove the medium and rinse twice with cold PBS containing protease inhibitors (PIs) (*see* **Note 11**).
   (b) Scrape the cells and transfer to a 1.5 mL tube using PBS with PIs, microfuge at 1000 rpm for 5 min, remove the PBS, resuspend the pellet in the cell lysis buffer (with PIs) and incubate for 20 min at 4 °C with gentle agitation.
   (c) Microfuge and resuspend the pellet in 500 μL of PBS containing PIs, incubated with gentle rocking for 5 min, wash again twice in PBS with PIs.
4. Nuclear lysis and DNA sonication
   (a) Resuspend the pellet in 400 μL of nuclear lysis buffer (with PIs) and incubated with gentle rocking at 4 °C for 20 min.
   (b) DNA is fragmented into ~300–500 bp segments by sonication using a cycle of 10 s pulses followed by a pause of 30 s (*see* **Note 12**).

   (c) Check DNA size (Fig. 2, *see* **Note 13**).
   (d) DNA can be stored at −80 °C.
5. DNA preclearing:
   (a) To prepare the samples for ChIP, microfuge the sonicated DNA at full speed for 10 min at 4 °C and prepare 100 μL aliquot into new 1.5 mL tubes and add 900 μL of the ChIP dilution buffer (with PIs) in each tube.
   (b) Add 40 μL of 50% slurry protein A agarose beads (*see* **Note 14**) to each tube containing the diluted DNA and incubate with gentle rocking for 1 h at 4 °C. Subsequently, microfuge (2000 rpm, 5 min) the tubes and transfer the supernatants into new tubes, and discard the beads (*see* **Note 15**).
   (c) Keep aside 20 μL of the precleared DNA and store it at −80 °C. This represents the input DNA (2%) and will be used for the calculation of the chromatin enrichment after incubation with the antibodies (*see* below).
6. For DNA–antibody complexing, incubate precleared DNA samples with antibodies used at a 1/100 dilution of the 1 μg/mL antibody preparation incubated overnight with gentle rocking at 4 °C:
   (a) Antibodies targeting the TF of interest.
   (b) Antibodies targeting the RNA POL-II.
   (c) Control anti-IgG antibodies (*see* **Note 16**).

3.4.2 Day 2

1. DNA–protein–antibody complex precipitation:
   (a) Add 40 μL of 50% slurry protein A agarose beads protein to each tube and incubate for 1 h at 4 °C with gentle rocking in order to allow beads to bind the DNA–protein–antibody complex.
   (b) Microfuge the beads at 6000 rpm for 3 min at 4 °C and discard the supernatant.
2. Washing steps: The beads are washed using the buffer TSE1, TS2, TSE3, and TE in order to remove unbound DNA and weak nonspecific bindings.
   (a) Add 1 mL of buffer TSE1 to the beads, mix gently and incubate at 4 °C with rocking for 5 min and microfuge at 2000 rpm for 3 min and discard the supernatant.
   (b) Repeat the wash a second time (*see* **Note 17**).
   (c) Perform the (a) and (b) steps for each of the TSE2, TSE3, and TE buffers.

3. Elution and reverse cross-linking step:
   (a) Add 200 μL of fresh elution buffer and incubate for 20 min at 60 °C. Mix gently every 2 min to dissociate the beads from the DNA–protein–antibody complex.
   (b) Microfuge full speed for 1 min to pellet the beads and transfer the supernatant in a new tube. Add 10 μL of 5 M NaCl to each tube and mix well.
   (c) Taw the input sample prepared earlier (**step 5c**) and add 180 μL of elution buffer and 10 μL of 5 M NaCl, mix well.
   (d) Incubate all the tubes at 65 °C overnight.

3.4.3 Day 3

1. DNA purification:
   (a) Mix the samples and add 2 μL of RNase A (5 mg/mL) and incubate at 37 °C for 30 min (*see* **Note 18**).
   (b) Add 2 μL of proteinase K (10 mg/mL) and incubate for 2 h at 42 °C (*see* **Note 19**).
   (c) Use a DNA purification kit and follow the manufacturer's instructions (*see* **Note 20**).
   (d) Samples with purified DNA are now ready for the PCR reaction.
2. PCR reaction:

   Use real-time PCR to quantify and compare genomic DNA enrichment among all the conditions: Input DNA, anti-TF antibody, RNA-POL-II antibody, and the control IgG. Design primer in order to target the DNA sequence containing the response element on the studied promoter (*see* **Note 21**). Design another set of primers to target a DNA negative control region. This region should be at least 5 kb distant from the targeted promoter, and will not contain any binding sites for the TF studied (*see* **Note 22**).
3. DNA enrichment calculation reaction:

   In the condition using the anti-TF antibody, two amplification values are obtained: (a) the amplification value obtained by targeting the region of interest on the promoter; (b) the value obtained from the amplification of the DNA negative control region. These two values are subtracted from the value of the amplification of the Input DNA. The log 2 of the difference between the two resulting values will correspond to the enrichment product of the promoter region (of the gene of interest) immunoprecipitated using the anti-TF antibody compared to the loading DNA and to the negative control region (*see* Fig. 3 as an example). The same calculation is performed for the conditions using anti-RNA POLII antibody and using anti-IgG antibody as negative control.

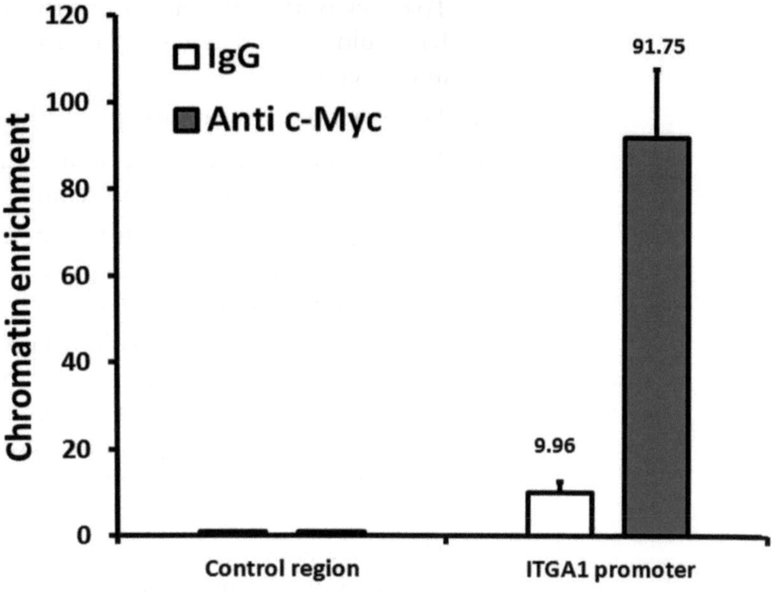

Fig. 3 c-MYC occupies the ITGA1 promoter in HT29 colon cancer cells. ChIP assay was performed in HT 29 cells, using human c-MYC-specific antibody (black columns) and using rabbit anti-IgG (white columns) as negative control. Data were calculated with PCR quantification of DNA fragments containing c-MYC response element relative to a negative control DNA fragment

4 Notes

1. Response elements identified should be selected according to their nucleotide sequence. Keep only sequences that match the consensus response element as well as sequences close to the consensus sequence. The latter can be functional despite the fact that they are considered as imperfect sequences.
2. Make sure that the sequence of the RE is centrally located in the sequence of both foreword and reverse primers, to ensure proper annealing. For the two MYC response elements E-box sites found on the ITGA1 promoter (named EBOX-S1 and EBOX-S2, [6]), we have used the following primers for EBOX-S1: forward 5′-CGACTTCACGGTGAATTTGGACAATCCG CAGGGGATGGAAGG-3′ and reverse 5′-CCTTCCATCCCC TGCGGATTGTCCAAATTCACCGTGAAGTCG-3′ and EB OX-S2: forward 5′-CACCCTCTCAATGAAAGGGGGACCT CCCTTTAAGGTTTGCTT-3′ and reverse 5′-AAGCAAACC TTAAAGGGAGGTCCCCCTTTCATTGAGAGGGTG-3′. Mutations of these promoter regions were confirmed by DNA sequencing.

3. To check both at the same time, the plasmid with one disrupted RE could be used as a template to create the second mutations in the second RE.
4. This reaction converts the plasmid to a circular form.
5. This allows the production of high quantities of the plasmid of interest using competent bacteria.
6. Avoid mix the bacterial vials by pipetting up and down. During incubation at 37 °C, the LB plate should be inverted to avoid condensation and contamination.
7. Align the sequence of the original promoter to the sequence of the new promoter containing the introduced mutations, and make sure that this is the only difference between the promoter sequences. Other changes in the sequence (polymerase errors) could modify the functionality of the promoter or create unneeded responsive sequences.
8. This assay is performed using HEK293T cells, for their high transfection efficiency [7].
9. The enzymatic activity of luciferase (which reflects the promoter activity) is quantified using a luminometer measuring the light produced by the luciferase activity. The two values obtained indicate the activity of the promoter of interest and the activity of the control promoter which reflects the transfection efficiency. For each well, the final value is the ratio between the first and the second values.
10. This step allows the protein–DNA cross-linking (including TFs).
11. Protease inhibitors are added at the time of using the solution. Add: 1 mM PMSF, 1 μg/mL aprotinin, 1 μg/mL leupeptin, and 1 μg/mL pepstatin.
12. The tube should be kept in contact with ice during the sonication.
13. For each cell line, sonication cycles should be adjusted to obtain the optimum DNA size needed for the ChIP assay. DNA size should be verified by loading 20 μL (add appropriate amount of loading buffer) of the sonicated DNA on agarose gel and can be compared to the nonsonicated DNA and the DNA ladder as illustrated in Fig. 2.
14. When pipetting the beads, it is useful to cut the top of the tip of the pipette (about 5 mm) to be able to easily pipet the beads.
15. This is an important step which prevents nonspecific DNA binding to the beads during the incubation with the antibodies.
16. Control antibodies should be isotype- and species-matched with specific antibodies.

17. To validate the IP reaction, resuspend the TSE1 washed beads in equal volume of 2× Laemmli sample buffer and add β-2-mercaptoethanol to a final 5% concnetration. Add also 20 μL of 2× Laemmli sample buffer to 20 μL to the input. Incubate both samples at 95 °C for 7 min and then centrifuge at 6000 rpm. Transfer the supernatant in a new tube and blot in SDS-PAGE gel in order to detect the proteins of interest and the IgG control.
18. Removing RNA can prevent the competition with the DNA for the binding to the column.
19. Proteinase K will help to disrupt the cross-links between proteins and DNA, and will improve the DNA purification.
20. Using the QIAquick spin kit, add five volumes of buffer PB to each simple and then transfer to a column and microfuge full speed for 1 min. Repeat this step two times using 600 μL each time and discard the flow-through. Add 750 μL of the buffer PE and full speed microfuge for 1 min and discard the flow-through. Transfer the filters in the collecting tubes, add 30 μL of elution buffer (EB) or water and incubate for 1 min at RT. Repeat this last step using 20 μL of water or buffer EB.
21. For instance, in our study, the ITGA1 promoter region including the two sites identified for MYC was targeted for amplification using the forward 5′-CAGTGAGATTTCAGAGACC AAG-3′ and reverse 5′-CTGGCTGGGCCACTTATC-3′ primers [6].
22. For instance, in our study [6], the negative control segment without a MYC response element, we used a sequence located 5-kb upstream from the ITGA1 initiation start site; the primers were: forward 5′-GGAGGGAGAAACACCTATTTTA-3′ and reverse 5′-GGAACTTAAACTTCACCATGAG-3′.

Acknowledgments

The original work was supported by the Canadian Institute of Health Research Grants MOP-97836 and MOP-123415. J-FB was the recipient of the Canadian Research Chair in Intestinal Physiopathology. JCC is a scholar of the Fonds de la Recherche du Québec-Santé (FRQS). SB is a recipient of the FRQS postdoctoral fellowship.

References

1. Zambelli F, Pesole G, Pavesi G (2013) Motif discovery and transcription factor binding sites before and after the next-generation sequencing era. Brief Bioinform 14(2):225–237. https://doi.org/10.1093/bib/bbs016
2. Osada M, Park HL, Nagakawa Y, Yamashita K, Fomenkov A, Kim MS, Wu G, Nomoto S, Trink B, Sidransky D (2005) Differential recognition of response elements determines target gene specificity for p53 and p63. Mol Cell Biol 25(14):6077–6089. https://doi.org/10.1128/MCB.25.14.6077-6089.2005
3. Boudjadi S, Bernatchez G, Beaulieu JF, Carrier JC (2013) Control of the human osteopontin promoter by ERRalpha in colorectal cancer. Am J Pathol 183(1):266–276. https://doi.org/10.1016/j.ajpath.2013.03.021
4. Boudjadi S, Beaulieu JF (2016) MYC and integrins interplay in colorectal cancer. Oncoscience 3 (2):50–51. https://doi.org/10.18632/oncoscience.293
5. Boudjadi S, Carrier JC, Beaulieu JF (2013) Integrin alpha 1 subunit is up-regulated in colorectal cancer. Biomarker Res 1(16):1–7
6. Boudjadi S, Carrier JC, Groulx JF, Beaulieu JF (2016) Integrin alpha1beta1 expression is controlled by c-MYC in colorectal cancer cells. Oncogene 35(13):1671–1678. https://doi.org/10.1038/onc.2015.231
7. Thomas P, Smart TG (2005) HEK293 cell line: a vehicle for the expression of recombinant proteins. J Pharmacol Toxicol Methods 51 (3):187–200. https://doi.org/10.1016/j.vascn.2004.08.014

Chapter 4

Identification and Functional Analysis of Gene Regulatory Sequences Interacting with Colorectal Tumor Suppressors

Katja Dahlgaard and Jesper Thorvald Troelsen

Abstract

Several tumor suppressors possess gene regulatory activity. Here, we describe how promoter and promoter/enhancer reporter assays can be used to characterize a colorectal tumor suppressor proteins' gene regulatory activity of possible target genes. In the first part, a bioinformatic approach to identify relevant gene regulatory regions of potential target genes is presented. In the second part, it is demonstrated how to prepare and carry out the functional assay.

We explain how to clone the bioinformatically identified gene regulatory regions into luciferase reporter plasmids by the use of the quick and efficient In-Fusion cloning method, and how to carry out transient transfections of Caco-2 colon cancer cells with the produced luciferase reporter plasmids using polyethyleneimine (PEI). A plan describing how to set up and carry out the luciferase expression assay is presented. The luciferase/β-galactosidase (Dual Light) assay presented is a highly sensitive assay that can monitor small changes in the promoter/enhancer activity and includes an internal control monitoring transfection efficiency.

Key words CDX2, *GPA33*, Enhancer, Promoter, Transcription factor, Promoter reporter assay, Transfection, Luciferase

1 Introduction

Several tumor suppressor proteins act as regulators of transcription. Well-known examples are p53 and Rb. Conversely, in the colon, some of the key intestinal specific transcriptional activators and drivers of normal cellular differentiation have been demonstrated to act as tumor suppressors [1, 2]. A prominent example is the caudal homeodomain protein, CDX2. It has been demonstrated using mouse *Cdx2* gene knock out models that Cdx2 is essential for normal development of an intestinal epithelium and that *Cdx2*-null colon epithelial cells exhibit a transformed phenotype [3]. In humans, metastasizing colon cancer cells at the invasive front of the cancer downregulate their CDX2 expression [4]. Furthermore, stage 2 colon cancer patients having a low CDX2 expression are at

Jean-François Beaulieu (ed.), *Colorectal Cancer: Methods and Protocols*, Methods in Molecular Biology, vol. 1765, https://doi.org/10.1007/978-1-4939-7765-9_4,

an increased risk for relapse and will benefit from adjuvant chemotherapy [5].

CDX2 is a transcriptional activator that regulates hundreds of intestinal expressed genes. Target genes of CDX2 have been extensively characterized in colon cancer cell lines. We and other groups have shown that CDX2 regulates the expression of genes encoding proteins involved in the WNT pathway (e.g., *APC*, *AXIN2*, *HBP1* and *Mucdhl*) [6–8]. In order to understand the molecular mechanisms behind the tumor suppressor activity executed by some transcription factors (TFs), it is important to identify target genes and functionally characterize their transcriptional regulation of relevant oncogenic target genes. Candidate target genes of transcriptional regulators are often identified using genome-wide techniques, e.g., RNA expression profiling with microarray or RNA-Seq. In this chapter, we will demonstrate how to identify active promoters and gene regulatory enhancer regions of potential tumor suppressor target genes using a bioinformatic strategy with publicly available genomic information and optimally combining it with own genomic experimental data.

We will further demonstrate, how to functionally characterize the transcriptional regulation of potential target genes by tumor suppressors with the use of a promoter/enhancer reporter gene assay. As an example of a candidate target gene, we are using a well-known colon cancer surface antigen, Glycoprotein A33 (*GPA33*) [9]. By using bioinformatic information about the *GPA33* gene, we demonstrate how to identify its promoter and a potential enhancer binding CDX2. The identified *GPA33* promoter and enhancer are subsequently functionally characterized in the colon cancer cell line Caco-2, demonstrating that *GPA33* promoter activity is increased by CDX2 overexpression.

2 Materials

2.1 Bioinformatical Identification of Regulatory Genomic Regions

1. The FANTOM5 Human promoterome in the Zenbu browser (http://fantom.gsc.riken.jp/zenbu/).
2. UCSC Genome Browser (https://genome.ucsc.edu).

2.2 Functional Analysis of Gene Regulatory Regions

2.2.1 Promoter Reporter Gene Construction

1. pGL4.10 plasmid (Promega).
2. PCR reagents:
   (a) Template for PCR amplification of gene regulatory region (Human genomic DNA).
   (b) Phusion Hot Start II polymerase (Thermo Fisher Scientific).
   (c) dNTPs.
   (d) In-Fusion-cloning primers designed for specific amplification of gene regulatory regions.

3. Thermo cycler.
4. Gel electrophoresis apparatus to run agarose gels.
5. Agarose (Molecular Biology Grade).
6. 1 × TAE (Tris–acetate–EDTA) buffer.
7. DNA molecular weight marker.
8. Ethidium bromide.
9. Restriction enzymes and buffers.
10. Gel extraction kit, e.g., E.Z.N.A. Gel Extraction Kit (Omega Bio-tek Inc.).
11. In-Fusion HD Cloning Kit (Clontech Laboratories) including 5× In-Fusion HD enzyme Premix.
12. Competent cells, e.g., DH5α competent cells with a transformation efficiency >1.0×10^{-8} cfu/μg.
13. Antibiotics for bacterial selection according to vector. pGL4.10 requires Ampicillin 100 mg/mL stock.
14. Luria–Bertani liquid (LB) medium.
15. LB plates containing antibiotics for selection.
16. Mini-preparation of plasmids DNA, e.g., PureLink Quick Plasmid Miniprep Kit (Thermo Fisher Scientific).
17. Maxi-preparation for high quality plasmid DNA, e.g., NucleoBond Xtra Midi/Maxi (MACHEREY-NAGEL GmbH & Co. KG).

2.2.2 Cell Work

1. Mammalian colon cancer cell line such as Caco-2 (ATCC: HTB-37).
2. Supplemented DMEM: Dulbecco's modified Eagle medium with 4.5 g/L glucose and with UltraGlutamine (Lonza), 10% fetal bovine serum (FBS), and 100 U/mL Penicillin–Streptomycin (P/S).
3. Cell incubator with a humidified atmosphere containing 5% CO_2 at 37 °C.
4. 0.085 M Sodium citrate, sterile filtered.
5. 1× trypsin–EDTA Solution: 0.05% trypsin, and 0.02% EDTA.
6. Hematocyte counting chamber.
7. Tissue culture vessels such as Nunc Cell Culture Treated EasY Flasks (Thermo Fisher Scientific).

2.2.3 Overexpression of TF

1. Mammalian expression vector as pcDNA3.1 (Invitrogen) or pHIV-dTomato (unpublished by Bryan Welm, Addgene plasmid #21374) with insert for overexpression of TF of interest.

2.2.4 Promoter Reporter Assay

1. 24-well plates Nunclon Delta treated (Thermo Fisher Scientific).
2. Standard plasmids for promoter reporter assays:
   (a) pCMV-*lacZ* (Clontech).
   (b) Plasmid without eukaryotic gene regulatory sequence, e.g., pBluescript SK+ (pBSK+) or pUC18.
3. 150 mM NaCl, sterile filtered.
4. Polyethyleneimine (PEI) (Alfa Aesar). Kept as 1 mM stock solution at −20 °C.
5. Centrifuge with plate adapters to spin 24-well plates.
6. Phosphate buffered saline (PBS).
7. Tropix Dual-Light Luciferase and β-Galactosidase Reporter Gene Assay System (Thermo Fisher Scientific). Including:
   (a) Lysis Solution.
   (b) Buffer A.
   (c) Buffer B.
   (d) Galacton-Plus Substrate.
   (e) Accelerator II.
8. Dithiothreitol (DTT) 1 M stock solution.
9. GloMax-96 Microplate Luminometer with dual injectors (Promega).
10. White 96-well plates with flat bottom.
11. Seventy percentage ethanol.

3 Methods

3.1 Bioinformatic Identification of Gene Regulatory Genomic Regions

For analysis of potential target genes for a TF it is crucial to identify the active promoter in the cell type of investigation while binding sites for specific TFs can be identified by ChIP-Seq analysis.

3.1.1 Identifying the Sequences of the Active Promoter of Interest

1. For analysis of potential target genes for a TF it is crucial to identify the active promoter in the cell type of investigation. A large fraction of genes has multiple promoters that are differentially active in different tissues and under different physiological conditions. Consequently, the transcriptional start site (TSS) active in the selected cell type has to be identified in order to perform functional studies for promoter/enhancer activity. The UCSC Genome Browser shows when a gene has multiple annotated TSSs, while genomic data on the TSSs from the cell type of interest might be available from genomics repositories or own experiments. The FANTOM5 Human

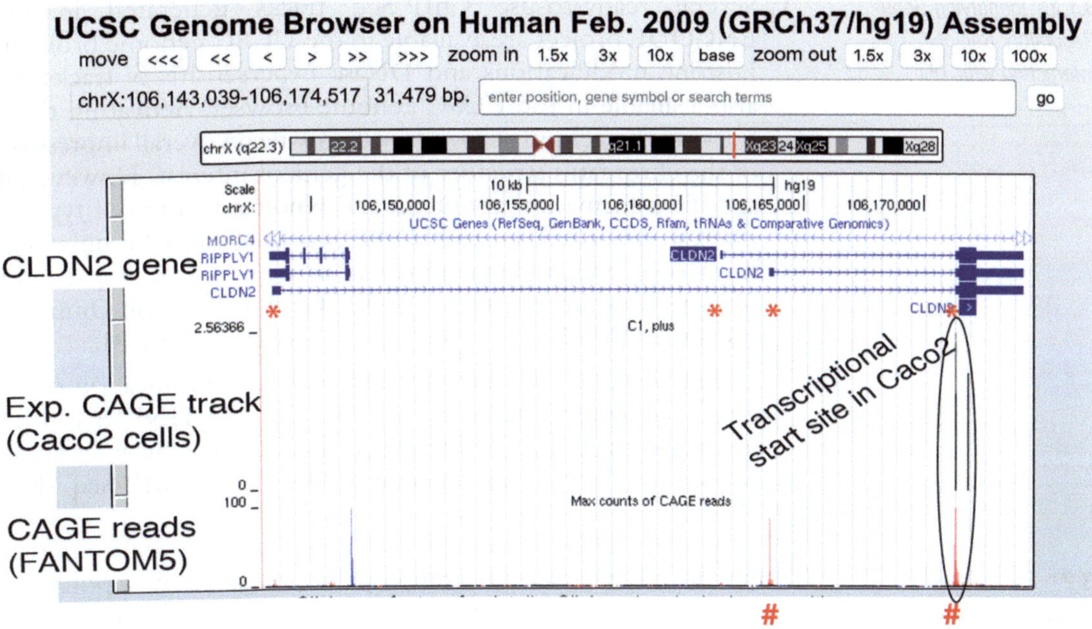

Fig. 1 Bioinformatic identification of the active promoter in the *CLDN2* gene in the colon cancer cell line Caco-2 using the UCSC Genome Browser (http:/genome.ucsc.edu/). The identification is based on public available cap analysis of gene expression (CAGE) data from the FANTOM5 hub on the USCS Genome Browser (https:/genome.ucsc.edu/cgi-bin/hgHubConnect?hubUrl=http%3A%2F%2Ffantom.gsc.riken.jp%2F5%2Fdatahub%2Fhub.txt&hgHubConnect.remakeTrackHub=on) combined with experimental CAGE data from Caco-2 cells (Exp. CAGE track (Caco-2) available at Gene Expression Omnibus (GEO) at NCBI (accession GSE54074). The *CLDN2* gene in the human reference genome is annotated with four different TSSs (shown with red "*"). The FANTOM5 CAGE track demonstrates that only two of these TSSs (marked with red "#") are frequently used and the Caco-2 CAGE track identifies that only one TSS (marked with the circle) is used in this colon cancer cell line. The promoter sequence for the colonic active promoter can easily be obtained by zooming in on the promoter region (e.g., 500 bp upstream) and use the Genome Browser function "DNA"

promoterome in the Zenbu browser has an extensive list of hundreds of human cell and tissue samples that have been analyzed for transcriptional start sites (TSSs) using the cap analysis of gene expression (CAGE) technique. These data can be imported as custom tracks into the UCSC Genome Browser (Fig. 1). Once the TSS of interest has been identified, the active promoter in most genes is located within an approx. 300 bp region upstream of the TSS [10].

2. Claudin 2 (*CLDN2*) is an example of a gene with multiple TSSs annotated in the human reference genome. This gives rise to a complex picture when visualized with the UCSC Genome Browser (Fig. 1). However, FANTOM5 CAGE data can be used to determine the generally preferred promoter usage over several cell types. As it can be seen in Fig. 1, only two of the four annotated TSSs are frequently used, while the Caco-2 CAGE data limits the number of used TSSs, and thus active promoter, to only one in this colon cancer cell line (Fig. 1).

3.1.2 Identifying Gene Regulatory Regions Interacting with TFs

1. Several ready-to-use ChIP-Seq tracks generated in the ENCODE project are available in the UCSC genome browser. Histone modifications and DNase hypersensitivity tracks are also available in the UCSC genome browser. Activating these tracks in the genome browser will provide an overall impression of the chromatin structure of the gene of interest. However, if specific information about the TF binding in the cell type of interest is needed, custom ChIP-Seq tracks can be uploaded from own experimental research or from ChIP-Seq dataset from a genomics repository like the Gene Expression Omnibus (GEO) at NCBI or the Array Express database at EBI.
2. In Fig. 2 it is shown how promoter usage and location of an enhancer region interacting with CDX2 and HNF4A can be identified using standard tracks in the Genome Browser combined with own experimental CAGE and ChIP-Seq data [8, 11].

3.2 Functional Analysis of Gene Regulatory Regions

To functionally characterize transcriptional regulation of potential target genes by a TF and assess the cis-regulatory effects of promoter and enhancer regions, the promoter/enhancer reporter gene assays is ideal. The activity of gene regulatory regions can be studied by linking them to an easily detectable reporter gene, such as *luciferase*, and transfecting the plasmid constructs into mammalian cells. A chemiluminescent assay is used to measures amount of synthesized luciferase and thus monitor the activity of the gene regulatory regions in the given setting. Further manipulation of the level of TF in the promoter/enhancer reporter assays can be used characterize the functionality of the TF (Fig. 3).

3.2.1 Promoter Reporter Construction by In-Fusion cloning

Based on the bioinformatic analysis, decide which TSS and thus potential target promoter region to use for construction of the basic promoter reporter constructs based on pGL4.10. The basic promoter construct should contain the potential target gene promoter (PTG-Pro) in front of the *luciferase* reporter gene (pGL4.10-PTG-Pro). If a predicted TF binding site is in a potential enhancer region, design a basic promoter/enhancer reporter construct including the potential target gene promoter and enhancer (PTG-Pro/Enh) based on the pGL4.10 vector (pGL4.10-PTG-Pro/Enh) (*see* **Notes 1** and **2**).

1. Primer design: For the generation of promoter and promoter/enhancer reporter constructs, we recommend to use the quick, efficient, and ligation-free In-Fusion technique where a PCR-generated DNA fragment with 15 bps vector sequences at the ends fuses to linearized vector. Design and order In-Fusion primers for the potential target gene regulatory sequences of interest to be cloned into pGL4.10. Primers should in their 5′ end contain a 15–16 nt sequence with

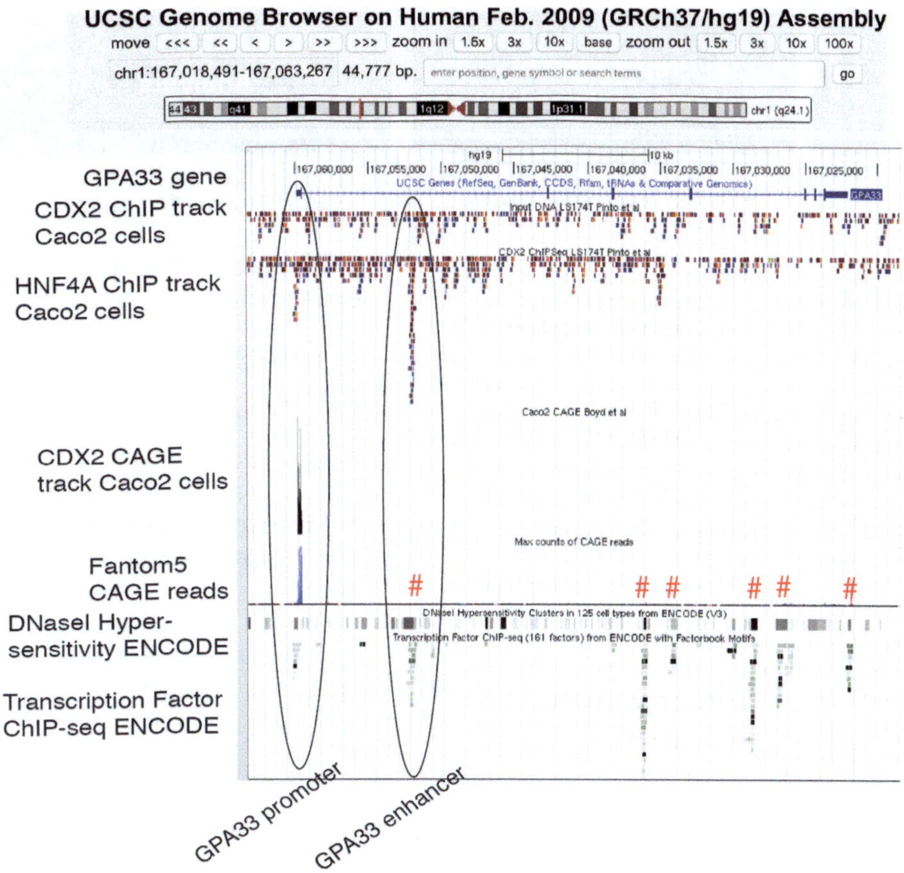

Fig. 2 Bioinformatic analysis using the UCSC Genome Browser to identify the promoter usage (**a**) and an CDX2 binding enhancer region (**b**) in the *GPA33* gene. **a**) As shown in Fig. 1, promoter usage can be identified by using TSS data from CAGE analysis. In the case of the *GPA33* gene, it is simple to identify the colonic active promoter as only one TSS has been identified in the FANTOM5 project and in the experimental Caco-2 CAGE analysis [11]. This is in accordance with the human reference genome annotation. **b**) A possible active enhancer in intron 1 of the *GPA33* gene (marked with a circle) interacting with CDX2 and HNF4A has been identified using a combination of standard ENCODE data tracks from the UCSC genome browser and own experimental ChIP-Seq data [8]. The DNaseI Hypesensitivity (ENCODE) track shows which regions in the *GPA33* gene that have an open and accessible chromatin structure, which is a potential sign of gene regulatory activity. The Transcription Factor ChIP-Seq (ENCODE) shows regions in the *GPA33* gene where multiple TFs bind in different cell lines (191 TFs have been ChIP analyzed in 91 cell lines). From these two ENCODE tracks, five potential enhancer regions can be identified in the *GPA33* gene (marked with red #). In order to identify enhancers regulated by CDX2, experimental CDX2 ChIP-Seq data (Caco-2 cells) is added. As CDX2 often binds in combination with HNF4A [12], experimental HNF4A ChIP-Seq data (Caco-2 cells) is also added. When combining this information, it is possible to identify one CDX2 binding site in an enhancer region in intron 1 in the *GPA33* gene (marked with a circle), which is possibly active in Caco-2 cells

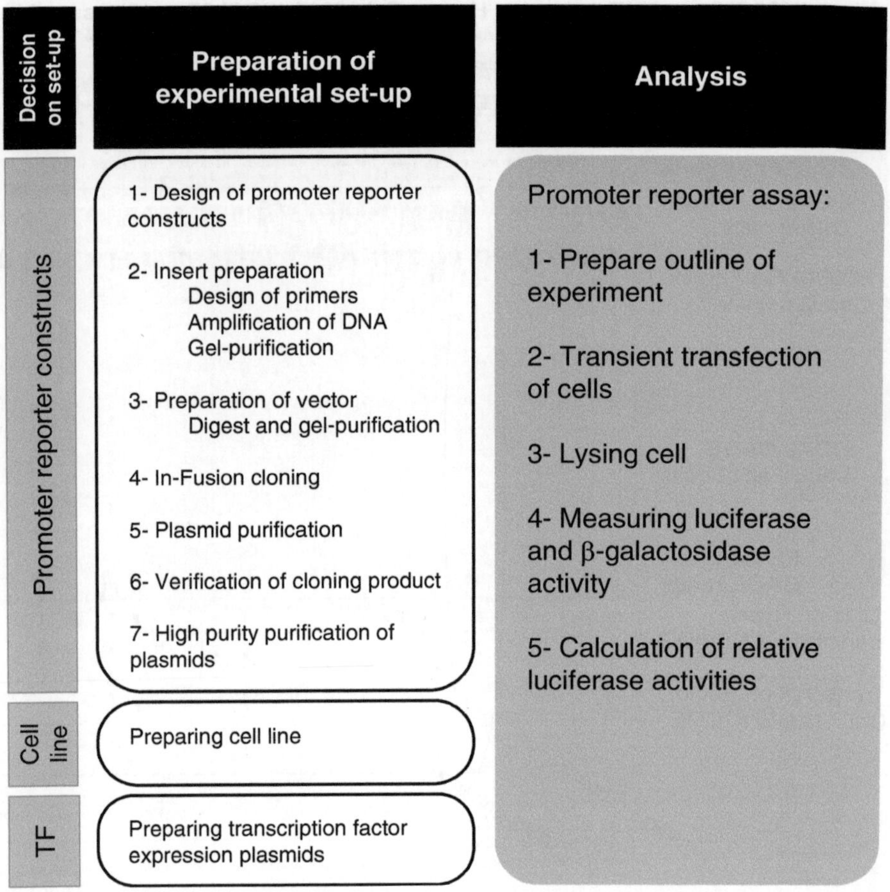

Fig. 3 Outline of the main steps for the experimental characterization of TFs regulatory effect on expression of potential target genes using Dual-light Luciferase promoter reporter assay. Make decisions on the experimental setup based on these questions: Which reporter promoter constructs to use for the analysis of the TF's ability to regulate expression of the potential target gene? Which cell type to use? And, how to change the level of active TF? With these decisions, prepare for the analysis by: (1) Cloning of promoter and promoter-enhancer constructs (Subheading 3.2.1). (2) Grow up cells for transfection (Subheading 3.2.2). (3) Prepare plasmids for expression of TF (Subheading 3.2.3). (4) Carry out the promoter reporter analysis (Subheading 3.2.4)

homology to the vector insertion point and in the 3′ end contain a 18–25 nt target-specific sequence for amplification of your gene regulatory region of interest (Figs. 4 and 5).

(a) When deciding on the vector insertion point keep in mind that it is not important to choose a restriction site not present in the target sequence to be cloned, as the insert sequence will not be exposed to restriction enzymes before cloning.

(b) Linearization of vector with one restriction enzyme is sufficient. The directionality of the insertion is defined by the primers and the cloning is ligation-free.

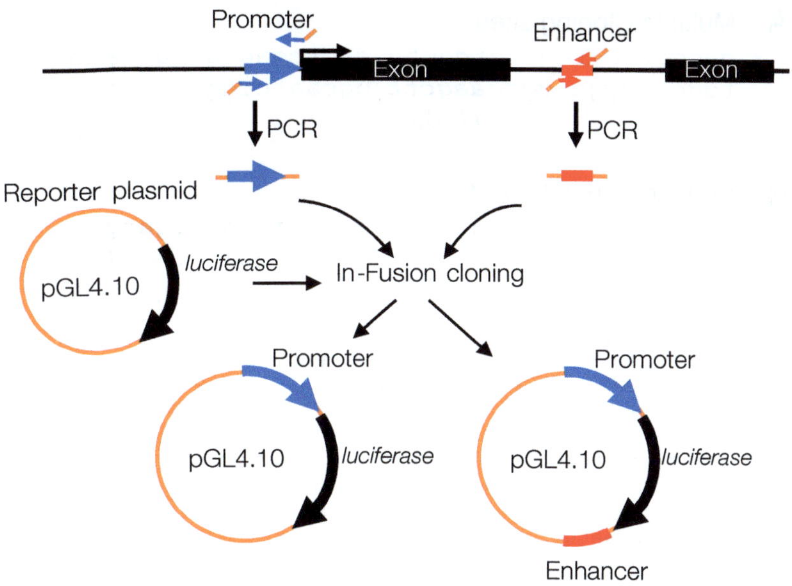

Fig. 4 Insertion of gene regulatory regions into the pGL4.10 reporter plasmid. Identified gene regulatory regions, active promoter and TF binding enhancer of potential target genes, can be amplified from genomic DNA for In-Fusion cloning by PCR, and cloned into pGL4.10, a promoterless reporter plasmid encoding firefly luciferase for measuring of activities from promoter and enhancer sequences

(c) The promoter sequence to be amplified can be added into any of the restriction sites in the multiple cloning sites upstream of *luciferase* in pGL4.10 (Figs. 4 and 5). If it is desired to clone into the *Hin*dIII site, the forward primer should be 5′ *ctcggcggccaagctt target-specific sequence*, and the reverse primer should be 5′ *ccggattgccaagctt target-specific sequence*.

(d) The potential enhancer region to be amplified can be cloned into the *Bam*HI or *Sal*I restriction sites downstream of *luciferase* in pGL4.10 (Fig. 5).

(e) To identify robust target-specific primers for the potential gene regulatory region of interest use NCBI primer Blast tool (https://www.ncbi.nlm.nih.gov/tools/primer-blast/). Aim for primers 18–20 nt long with a Tm of 60 °C. Use the identified primer sequences as the 3′ target-specific sequence of the In-Fusion primers.

2. DNA amplification by PCR: PCR amplify the gene regulatory regions with a thermostable DNA polymerase with high proof-reading activity. We recommend Phusion Hot Start II High-Fidelity DNA polymerase.

(a) Prepare reaction mix according to manufacturers' protocol. For Phusion Hot Start II High-Fidelity DNA polymerase with CG buffer mix: 9.4 μL H_2O, 4.0 μL 5×

A Multiple Cloning sites

gccggtacct gagctcgcta gcctcgagga tatcaagatc
tggcctcggc ggcc***aagctt*** ggcaatccgg tactgttggt
*Hin*dIII

B Enhancer Insertion sites

atgtggtaaa atcgataagg atccg***tcgac*** ***cgatgc***cctt
gagagccttc aacccagtca *Sal*I *Bam*HI

C GPA33 enhancer sequence

TCTTTAGCCCCTTTGGGATTgaagaaggagaaatggaggtgggtttgtag
gttatagggaaggtgctgccagcaaggaagagtctgaaagtgcagcagac
accagatggagcaagaccttagcctgggaggggacccgagaggaggggaa
gggccagggcacagttggaaagccagctttgctcacggcaagtgtcacct
gttccccaaatgcagatggagatacattggtggacacgtgcagggcgtga
gctctagccaacagatatacgttttatgctcctctcccagtgaactttgt
gacggccctaatgggaagcgtctgtctgtcgccatgttctgcccatgcct
ggtgtttatggcatccctgactcaccagggcagaaaatgaggaagcagtc
caaaggtcactgggtaggagaggagagggaaacacctcaggaaggaggcg
ggttccaagcttgacggttggtgccccaggcagaaaggggacagggtgat
ctgggaacagagacaagccccacagagcaggcagagagaagacgatggag
ggcaaaacctgagtgctgccaacccggggtggcttgaggggcaactgaac
ttcccccaagtccactATGTCCTCCACCAGCTCTTG

D In-Fusion primers

Forward: ataaggatccg***tcgac***TCTTTAGCCCCTTTGGGATT
Reverse: aagggcatcgg***tcgac***CAAGAGCTGGTGGAGGACAT

PCR product size: 637 bp
Restiction sites: *Sal*I
Target specific primers anneal at 63ºC

Fig. 5 Design of primers for In-Fusion cloning. (**a**) Multiple Cloning region of pGL4.10 for insertion of promoter regions upstream of *luciferase* coding region. The *Hin*dIII site highlighted in bold is often used as insertion site. (**b**) Sequence of pGL4.10 at the enhancer insertion site downstream of *luciferase*. Both the *Sal*I and the *Bam*HI sites are marked with bold. (**c**) Sequence of the 637 bp *GPA33* enhancer region binding CDX2 in Fig. 2. The target-specific sequences of the primers/annealing to the primer are in upper case. (**b**) In-Fusion primers for amplification of the 637 bp *GPA33* enhancer region. The 5′ sequences of 16 nts with homology to the vector ends are in lower case. The *Sal*I sites are in bold and italics, and the 3′ target-specific sequences for the enhancer are in upper case

Phusion GC buffer, 0.4 μL 10 mM dNTP, 1.0 μL F primer (10 μM), 1.0 μL R primer (10 μM), 2.0 μL Template Human Genomic DNA (20 ng/μL), 1.0 μL Phusion Hot start II DNA polymerase.

(b) Establish cycling conditions for the PCR reaction. Use manufacturers' protocol and determine the optimal annealing temperatures using the online tool (http://tmcalculator.neb.com/#!/). In the initial cycles, it is only the 3′ target-specific part of the In-Fusion primers that anneals to template, and thus the estimated annealing temperature should be based on only this part of the primers.

(c) Program your Thermo Cycler with your PCR reaction conditions, e.g., initial denaturation at 98 °C for 2 min, seven cycles with step-down (98 °C for 15 s, 70 °C–1 °C/cycle for 15 s, 72 °C for 60 s/kb), 22 regular cycles (98 °C for 15 s, 63 °C for 15 s, 72 °C for 60 s/kb), final elongation at 72 °C for 5 min.

(d) Run the PCR reaction.

(e) Analyze the PCR amplification product by agarose gel electrophoresis.

(f) Excise the PCR-generated gene regulatory regions having 15 bp vector sequence at both ends from the gel and purify the DNA.

(g) Measure the concentration of the gel-purified PCR product, which is now ready for insertion in In-Fusion cloning (*see* Subheading 3.2.1.4).

3. Vector preparation

(a) Digest the pGL4.10 based vector with restriction enzyme according to the cloning strategy. For cloning of potential target enhancer region into the *SalI* restriction site downstream of *luciferase* in pGL4.10-PTG-Pro set up the following reaction:1 μg pGL4.10-PTG-Pro, 1 μL *SalI* (10 U/μL), 2 μL 10× Restriction enzyme buffer, MilliQ H_2O up to 20 μL

(b) Mix the restriction digest reaction and incubate for 4 h at 37 °C to increase the efficiency of the digestion.

(c) Analyze the restriction digest by agarose gel electrophoresis and excise the linearized vector fragment.

(d) Gel-purify the vector fragment to reduce background from unlinearized plasmid.

(e) Measure the concentration of your vector fragment. The vector is now ready for In-Fusion cloning. No further treatment is required as the reaction is ligase free.

4. In-Fusion cloning

(a) The ideal molar ratio of insert to vector in In-Fusion cloning is two with a minimum of 50 ng insert. For cloning with a 4200 bp vector and a 700 bp use 150 ng of vector to 50 ng of insert. For more information refer to Clontech Online tools or User Manual for In-Fusion Cloning.

(b) Mix vector and PCR product and add MilliQ H_2O up to 8 μL.

(c) Add 2 μL 5× In-Fusion HD enzyme Premix and incubate the reaction at 50 °C for 15 min and place on ice. The In-Fusion reaction is now ready for transformation.

(d) Add 2 μL of your In-Fusion reaction to 50 μL of competent cells kept on ice for transformation and incubate for 10 min.

(e) Heat-shock at 42 °C for 30 s, and place back on ice for 3 min.

(f) Spread on LB agar plates with antibiotics for selection (100 μg/mL Ampicillin for pGL4.10 based plasmids).

(g) Incubate the plates overnight at 37 °C.

(h) Pick colonies for purification of plasmids and make mini-preparations.

(i) Determine presence of insert in purified plasmids by restriction digest.

(j) Sequence selected positive clones in order to verify correct construction of the plasmids (*see* **Note 3**).

(k) Make maxi-preparation of your verified plasmid to yield high purity plasmids required for the promoter/enhancer reporter assay.

3.2.2 Cell Work

1. Choice of cell line: Regulation of transcription depends not only on one TF but on an orchestra of TFs being present in the cells at the right levels. Consequently, it is important to carry out the promoter reporter assays in a suitable cell line, and to remember that results depend on the cell line used. Use a cell line:
   (a) Which is easily transfected.
   (b) That relates to the tissue and gene regulation of interest.
   (c) In which the target gene is expressed to some extent or in which it is expected that all other components except for the targeting TF required for expression is present.
   (d) In which manipulation of the amount of active TF potentially makes a difference to the activity of the target promoter.
2. In this chapter, the Caco-2 cell line is chosen for the promoter reporter assay (*see* **Note 4**).
3. Grow up Caco-2 cells in advance of the promoter reporter assay in cell culture treated flasks with supplemented DMEM in a cell incubator with a humidified atmosphere containing 5% CO_2 at 37 °C to ensure enough well-growing cells for the experiment.
4. Split cells before they reach 70% confluency (*see* **Note 5**).
5. To split the cells, remove the media and wash three times in 85 mM sodium citrate (*see* **Note 6**).

6. Remove the sodium citrate and add 1 mL 1 × Trypsin-EDTA Solution. Let the trypsination proceed in the incubator (*see* **Note 7**).
7. As soon as a tap on the side of the culture flask loosens the cells, the trypsination has proceeded long enough. Add 9 mL supplemented DMEM to the flask and pipet up and down with the tip of the serological pipette tilted on the plastic to get cell clumps disrupted into single cells.
8. Count the cell concentration in the Hematocyte counting chamber. For sub-culturing twice a week, seed at 4–5 × 10^{-5} cells per T75 flask.

3.2.3 Overexpression of TF

To analyze the gene regulatory effect of a TF on gene expression it may be desired to change the amount of active TF. A common way to change the amount of active TF is to use cotransfection of the promoter reporter construct along with mammalian expression plasmids expressing the TF of interest (*see* **Note 8**).

1. TF expression plasmids might be obtained from Addgene (https://www.addgene.org/). Alternatively, cDNA can be cloned into the mammalian expression plasmids as pHIV-dTomato or pcDNA3.1
2. Use the in Subheading 3.2.1 described In-Fusion cloning technique to design and construct TF expression plasmids.

3.2.4 Promoter Reporter Assay

1. Outline of the promoter reporter assay: The number of conditions in the experiment depends on the number of pGl4.10 based promoter reporter constructs to analyze, and the number of ways TF activity is manipulated, but also include a control of untransfected cells (*see* a setup of conditions in Table 1). Setup conditions for promoter activity measurement from:
   (a) pGL4.10 empty vector, if this vector's activity is desired for normalization of results.
   (b) pGL4.10-PTG-Pro at endogenous TF level.
   (c) pGL4.10-PTG-Pro/Enh to analyze if presence of the potential enhancer influences the promoter activity at endogenous TF level.
   (d) Each of the pGL4.10 based vectors cotransfected with TF expression plasmid manipulating the TF activity level.
   (e) Remember controls: For cotransfections, transfect with empty expression plasmid to analyze if the expression plasmid in its self has unintended effects in the assay and include untransfected cells to measure background activity of the assay.

Table 1
Experimental design for functional characterization of CDX2's regulation of *GPA33*

Conditions:	pGL4.10 based plasmid (μg)	pHiv(EV)	pCMV-*lacZ* (μg)	pBSK+ (μg)	Total (μg)	Per well (μg)
1. pGL4.10	0.20		0.100	0.90	1.20	0.30
2. pGL4.10 *GPA33Pro*	0.20		0.100	0.90	1.20	0.30
3. pGL4.10 *GPA33ProEnh*	0.20		0.100	0.90	1.20	0.30
4. pGL4.10 + pHIV (EV)	0.20	0.100 μg	0.100	0.80	1.20	0.30
Conditions:	**pGL4.10 based plasmid (μg)**	**pHiv-CDX2 (μg)**	**pCMV-*lacZ* (μg)**	**pBSK+ (μg)**	**Total (μg)**	**Per well (μg)**
5. pGL4.10 *GPA33Pro* + pHIV-CDX2	0.20	0.100	0.100	0.80	1.20	0.30
6. pGL4.10 *GPA33ProEnh* + pHIV-CDX2	0.20	0.100	0.100	0.80	1.20	0.30
7. Untransfected						

An example of the conditions to use in a promoter/enhancer reporter assay monitoring effects of cotransfection with TF expression plasmid. Condition 1 is used to analyse the activity of pGL4.10 and is used for reference. Condition 2 is used to monitor the activity of the *GPA33* promoter at cell endogenous CDX2 levels. Condition 3 is used to monitor if the addition of identified CDX2 binding region acts as an enhancer for the *GPA33* promoter. Condition 4 is used to analyze if presence of expression plasmid by itself influences the baseline activity. Condition 5 and 6 are used to characterize if overexpression of CDX2 influences the activity of the *GPA33* gene regulatory regions. Each condition is tested with four replicates. For each condition a DNA mix of 1.2 μg DNA in 100 μL 150 mM NaCl is required (0.3 μg DNA per replicate). These 1.2 μg includes: 0.2 μg pGL4.10 based vector (pGL4.10 in condition 1, pGL4.10 *GPA33Pro* in condition 2...), 0–0.1 μg expression plasmid (pHIV-CDX2 in condition 4 and 5, and pHIV empty vector in condition 3), 0.1 μg pCMV-*lacZ* for internal transfection control, and for each condition pBSK + to fill up to 1.2 μg

2. Transient transfections of cells: Transfection of plasmid DNA into mammalian cells can, depending on cell line, be carried out in a number of ways. Many transfection reagents are commercially available. For most experiment, we use the linear polyethyleneimine (PEI) with the molecular weight of 25 kDa. It functions well in our preferred cell lines and is cheaper than other reagents sold as transfection reagent.
   (a) One day prior to transfection trypsinize 70% confluent Caco-2 cells. Count the cells and seed at 4×10^{-4} cells/well in 24-well plates. Set up four wells for each condition.
   (b) At the day of transfection: Prepare 2 μM PEI in 150 mM NaCl from a 1 mM PEI stock. Vortex the mixture intensely for minimum 5 min to get PEI into solution (*see* **Note 9**).

(c) For each transfection condition (four wells) a total of 1.2 μg DNA is needed in 100 μL 150 mM NaCl. Predilute plasmid DNA down to 20–50 ng/μL in 150 mM NaCl and remeasure concentrations. For each transfection condition (four wells) mix, with the diluted plasmids: 200 ng of pGL4.10 based promoter reporter plasmid (pGL4.10 (EV), pGL4.10-PTG-Pro or pGL4.10-PTG-Pro/Enh), 200 ng of endogenous transfection control plasmid pCMV-*lacZ* plasmid, 100 ng of expression plasmid (this could be pHIV (EV) or pHIV-TF), pBSK+ plasmid to normalize the DNA mix to a total amount of 1.2 μg DNA (*see* **Note 10**), fill up with 150 mM NaCl to 100 μL. (*see* setup in Table 1).

(d) One hour prior transfection, mix the 100 μL 1.2 μg DNA solution with 100 μL 2 μM PEI. Vortex briefly and let the reaction stand to form precipitate at room temperature.

(e) Remove media of cells seeded before transfection and add 1 mL fresh supplemented DMEM media to each well (*see* **Note 11**).

(f) Add in small droplets, 49 μL of the 200 μL DNA–PEI mixture to each of four wells in the plate (*see* **Note 12**).

(g) Spin the plate at 200 × *g* for 5 min to force the DNA–PEI precipitate down onto the cells.

(h) Place the plates in the cell incubator and leave them with the transfection media for minimum 4 h before changing the medium of the cells to fresh supplemented DMEM media.

3. Preparing cell lysate

(a) Lyse the cells 48 h post transfection.

(b) Before lysing the cells, prepare 130 μL of Lysis buffer per well by adding DTT to 0.5 mM final concentration in Lysis Solution (0.5 μL 1 M DTT/ 1 mL Lysis Solution), and equilibrate Lysis buffer and 1 × PBS to room temperature.

(c) Wash each well with 200–300 μL 1 × PBS. Remove all PBS from wells.

(d) Add 130 μL Lysis buffer to each well and incubate for approximately 5 min on shaker or by tapping the plate once in a while by hand.

(e) The cell lysate is now ready for analysis of luciferase and β-galactosidase activities.

(f) Place the plates with cell lysate on ice until further analysis. For later analysis, which will slightly decrease the luciferase activity, wrap plates with paraffin and store at −20 °C for a week or −80 °C for longer storage.

4. Measuring luciferase and β-galactosidase activity

The measurement of promoter activities is done with the Tropix Dual-light assay, which is a highly sensitive assay as it enables accurately monitoring of small changes both in the experimental and in the control reporter gene assays in the same cell lysate sample. The experimental reporter gene is *luciferase,* while the CMV-promoter-driven *lacZ* gene, encoding β-galactosidase, is used as a control reporter gene to measure variation in transfection efficiency. First, the activity of luciferase is measured. This is a flash-type luciferase assay in which most of the luminescence signal is emitted within 10 s after addition of substrate. The luciferase signal decays after a few minutes, and does thus not affect measurement of β-galactosidase activity to be conducted 30–45 min after the first luciferase measurement. During the 30–45 min incubation period, β-galactosidase catalyzes formation of product, but the luminescence signal is suppressed by low pH. The luminescence signal from the β-galactosidase catalyzed reaction is initiated by adding Accelerator II reagent, which provides a luminescence enhancer and raises the pH. The light emission from the β-galactosidase reaction exhibit a glow kinetics with a half-life of 180 min. The assay can be run using any machine capable of quickly measuring light emission. We use the GloMax Luminometer, with two injectors.

(a) For each sample transfer 10 μL of cell lysate to a well in a white flat bottom 96-well plates that is appropriate for the luminometer.

(b) Prepare buffers in reagent bottles and equilibrate to room temperature: Buffer A (25 μL is required per sample plus 1.5 mL extra for tubing), Buffer B (dilute Galacton-Plus Substrate 1:100 in Buffer B, 100 μL is required per sample plus 1.5 mL extra for tubing), Accelerator-II (100 μL is required per sample plus 1.5 mL extra for tubing).

(c) Turn on the GloMax Luminometer, and open the GloMax software on the computer.

(d) For measurement of luciferase activity prepare a protocol which first injects 25 μL of Buffer A, without delay (0 s) injects 100 μL Buffer B with Galacton-Plus Substrate, and finally with a delay of 2 s measures luminescence for 5 s.

(e) Place Buffer A and Buffer B with Galacton-Plus Substrate at appropriate injectors and prime the tubing.

(f) Insert the 96 well plate with cell lysate in the luminometer.

(g) Define in the protocol which wells contain lysate to be measured and start the protocol.

(h) When all the samples have been measured, save the data.

(i) Reverse purge both injectors and save leftover Buffer A for other experiments. Throw away Buffer B.

(j) Clean the tubing with MilliQ H_2O and 70% ethanol by "flushing" both injectors.

(k) Incubate samples at room temperature for 30–45 min from the measurement of the first sample.

(l) Prepare a protocol for measurement of β-galactosidase activity. A protocol that injects 100 μL Accelerator II and with a delay of 2 s measures luminescence for 5 s (*see* **Note 13**).

(m) Place Accelerator II at appropriate injector and prime the tubing.

(n) Place the 96-well plate back in the luminometer—again choose which wells are to be measured and start the protocol.

(o) When all samples have been measured, save the data.

(p) Clean the tubing with MilliQ H_2O and 70% ethanol by "flushing" the used injector.

5. Analysis of data

(a) Inspect the raw data. Make sure the data makes sense. Check that there is a marked difference in the luminescence measurements obtained from the background (untransfected cells) and the transfected cells, both from the experimental reporter luciferase and the control reporter β-galactosidase.

(b) It is preferable that the β-galactosidase activity counts are fairly stable across all measurements (*see* **Note 14**).

(c) To calculate the relative activity in each sample: Calculate the "ratio of luminescence" from each sample by dividing the luminescence signal from luciferase with the luminescence signal from β-galactosidase.

(d) The "average ratio of luminescence for the experimental reference condition" is calculated from the "ratio of luminescence" of the four samples from the experimental reference condition. The experimental reference condition can be the condition in which cells were transfected with pGL4.10 empty vector.

(e) The "relative ratio of luminescence" in each sample is calculated by dividing "ratio of luminescence" from each sample with the "average ratio of luminescence for the experimental reference condition" (often pGL4.10 empty vector).

(f) For each condition (four samples) in the reporter assay the average and the standard deviation of the "relative ratio of luminescence" can be calculated from the "relative ratio of luminescence" in the four samples and presented in a bar diagram (Fig. 6).

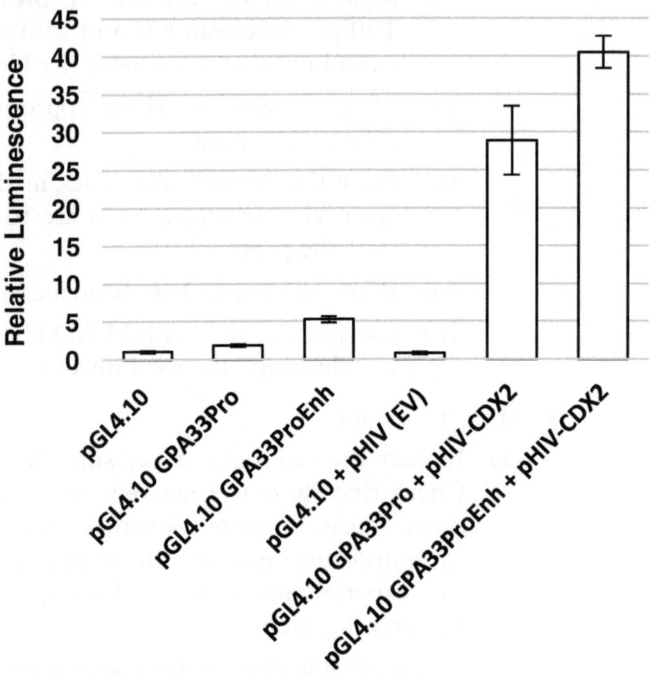

Fig. 6 Functional characterization of CDX2's regulation of *GPA33* in Caco-2 cells. Bar diagram representing results from a promoter/enhancer reporter assay experiment with conditions as described in Table 1. The relative luminescence activity was calculated with pGL.4.10 (condition 1, Table 1) for normalization. Error bars indicate standard deviations. The *GPA33* promoter (pGL4.10 *GPA33Pro*) provides less than twice the activity of pGL4.10. Addition of the identified enhancer (pGL4.10 *GPA33ProEnh*) provides an activity 5 times the activity of pGL4.10, and does thus verify that it contains enhancer activity. Addition of empty expression plasmid pHIV (pGL4.10 + pHIV (EV)) has a minor inhibiting effect in the assay; however, cotransfection with pHIV-CDX2 increases relative luminescence activities both for pGL4.10 *GPA33Pro* and pGL4.10 *GPA33ProEnh* (pGL4.10 *GPA33Pro* + pHIV-CDX2 and pGL4.10 *GPA33ProEnh* + pHIV-CDX2 respectively). This shows that CDX2 functions as a transcriptional activator of *GPA33*

4 Notes

1. If it is desired to analyze the importance of a specific target sequence predicted to directly bind the TF, consider mutagenizing or deleting the potential TF binding sites in the basic construct, pGL4.10-PTG-Promut or pGL4.10-PTG-Pro/Enhmut. If known, compare the characterized consensus TF binding sequence with the TF binding site in the potential target gene regulatory region. Identify the important bases in the binding site. To reduce the possibility of interaction between the potential binding site and the TF, change important Adenine and Thymine bases with Cytosine and Guanine to change groups available for protein interactions at both major and minor groove. To be able to easily recognize the mutated plasmid insert a restriction site that by introduction into the gene regulatory sequence will provide the intended A/T-C/G changes. As an example, the CDX2 binding sites, the seven-base-pair sequence a/cATAAAa/t can be disrupted by replacing it with GGAATTC containing an *Eco* RI cleavage site.
2. For cloning, the pGL4.10-PTG-Promut or pGL4.10-PTG-Pro mut we also recommend to use the ligation free In-Fusion technique. Introduce changes in the potential TF binding sites by In-Fusion primers. Amplify the gene regulatory region in two PCR fragments, one fragment with the gene regulatory region upstream and the other with the gene regulatory region downstream of the potential TF binding sites. In addition, the two fragments should contain 15–16 nt with homology to the vector insertion point in one end and 15–16 nucleotides with mutated TF binding site and homology to the other PCR product in the other end. This enables the two PCR products to be fused together and inserted back into the pGL4.10 based construct. Reuse the two primers designed for In-Fusion cloning of the gene regulatory region and design two new primers for the mutagenesis. The two mutagenesis primers should contain 15 nt with homology to each other in their 5′ end and the target-specific region in their 3′ end counting from the changed nt.
3. For sequencing of pGL4.10 inserts, the two standard primers: Reporter Vector primers RVPRIMER3 and RVPRIMER4 can respectively be used for sequencing of promoter inserts in the multiple cloning site upstream of luciferase and for sequencing of potential enhancers inserted downstream of luciferase.
4. Colon cancer cell lines we recommended to use are Caco-2, LS174T, and SW480. Alternatively, we recommend using the epithelial cell line HEK293. These are all examples of the cell lines that are relatively easy to transfect.

5. If Caco-2 cells become more than 80% confluent they start a differentiation process and will be less efficiently transfected. This effect cannot be reverted so Caco-2 cells from flasks 80% or more confluent should not be carried forward.
6. Caco-2 adhere stronger together than most other cell lines. Sodium citrate is used to bind Ca^{2+} and weaken the Ca^{2+} dependent cell adhesion molecules, making it possible to obtain single cells with gentler treatment.
7. Let the trypsination proceeds for around 5 min, but no more than 10 min to ensure viability of cells.
8. The amount of active TF can be manipulated in many ways (e.g., by use of expression plasmids activating or inhibiting upstream signal transduction pathway components or expressing shRNA silencing endogenous TF expression or by genetic manipulation).
9. The rigorous vortexing of 2 μM PEI in 150 mM NaCl is important for the ability of the PEI to form optimal transfection precipitate with DNA. If available, it can be mixed on a ThermoMixer for 30 min. Larger batches can be prepared and kept at 4 °C.
10. Any plasmid DNA without eukaryotic gene regulatory elements can be used to fill up.
11. Even though, many protocols carry out transfections in serum free media, we do not find it necessary for transfections with PEI.
12. To get even amounts of DNA–PEI in the four wells remember to mix it by pipetting up and down before taking first aliquot out.
13. It is important that Accelerator II is not running in same tubing as Buffer B. If the two solutions are run in same tubing precipitate is likely to appear even though the tubing has been cleaned in between.
14. We have observed systematic downregulation of β-galactosidase activity under conditions with high amount of certain expression plasmids, and we speculate that the CMV promoter of expression plasmids might compete with the CMV promoter of pCMV-*lacZ*. Under such conditions test if same reduction in β-galactosidase is observed using an empty expression plasmid, and use a condition with same amount of total expression without insert (empty vector (EV)) as reference condition to calculate the relative ratio of luminescence. A systematic increase in β-galactosidase activity can also be observed. We observed this when overexpressing p65 (NFkB). In such cases β-galactosidase activity cannot be used as control of transfection efficiency between conditions with or

without TF and the analysis should be made based on the luciferase counts only. If your DNA preparations are not of high quality they can potentially also effect transfection efficiency (make new plasmid preparations or carry out an extra ethanol precipitation step).

Acknowledgment

This work was supported by The Danish Council for Independent Research (4004-00140B). We would like to thank Johanne Davidsen and Sylvester Larsen for reagents and fruitful discussions on the method and Louise Torp Dalgaard for constructive comments.

References

1. Olsen J, Espersen ML, Jess P, Kirkeby LT, Troelsen JT (2014) The clinical perspectives of CDX2 expression in colorectal cancer: a qualitative systematic review. Surg Oncol 23 (3):167–176
2. Yao HS, Wang J, Zhang XP, Wang LZ, Wang Y, Li XX, Jin KZ, Hu ZQ, Wang WJ (2016) Hepatocyte nuclear factor 4alpha suppresses the aggravation of colon carcinoma. Mol Carcinog 55(5):458–472
3. Chawengsaksophak K, James R, Hammond VE, Kontgen F, Beck F (1997) Homeosis and intestinal tumours in Cdx2 mutant mice. Nature 386:84–87
4. Brabletz T, Spaderna S, Kolb J, Hlubek F, Faller G, Bruns CJ, Jung A, Nentwich J, Duluc I, Domon-Dell C, Kirchner T, Freund JN (2004) Down-regulation of the homeodomain factor Cdx2 in colorectal cancer by collagen type I: an active role for the tumor environment in malignant tumor progression. Cancer Res 64(19):6973–6977
5. Dalerba P, Sahoo D, Paik S, Guo X, Yothers G, Song N, Wilcox-Fogel N, Forgo E, Rajendran PS, Miranda SP, Hisamori S, Hutchison J, Kalisky T, Qian D, Wolmark N, Fisher GA, van de Rijn M, Clarke MF (2016) CDX2 as a prognostic biomarker in stage II and stage III colon cancer. N Engl J Med 374(3):211–222
6. Hinkel I, Duluc I, Martin E, Guenot D, Freund JN, Gross I (2012) Cdx2 controls expression of the protocadherin Mucdhl, an inhibitor of growth and beta-catenin activity in colon cancer cells. Gastroenterology 142 (4):875–885 e873
7. Olsen AK, Coskun M, Bzorek M, Kristensen MH, Danielsen ET, Jorgensen S, Olsen J, Engel U, Holck S, Troelsen JT (2013) Regulation of APC and AXIN2 expression by intestinal tumor suppressor CDX2 in colon cancer cells. Carcinogenesis 34(6):1361–1369
8. Boyd M, Hansen M, Jensen TG, Perearnau A, Olsen AK, Bram LL, Bak M, Tommerup N, Olsen J, Troelsen JT (2010) Genome-wide analysis of CDX2 binding in intestinal epithelial cells (Caco-2). J Biol Chem 285 (33):25115–25125
9. Garin-Chesa P, Sakamoto J, Welt S, Real F, Rettig W, Old L (1996) Organ-specific expression of the colon cancer antigen A33, a cell surface target for antibody-based therapy. Int J Oncol 9(3):465–471
10. Cooper SJ, Trinklein ND, Anton ED, Nguyen L, Myers RM (2006) Comprehensive analysis of transcriptional promoter structure and function in 1% of the human genome. Genome Res 16(1):1–10
11. Boyd M, Coskun M, Lilje B, Andersson R, Hoof I, Bornholdt J, Dahlgaard K, Olsen J, Vitezic M, Bjerrum JT, Seidelin JB, Nielsen OH, Troelsen JT, Sandelin A (2014) Identification of TNF-alpha-responsive promoters and enhancers in the intestinal epithelial cell model Caco-2. DNA Res 21(6):569–583
12. Verzi MP, Shin H, San Roman AK, Liu XS, Shivdasani RA (2013) Intestinal master transcription factor CDX2 controls chromatin access for partner transcription factor binding. Mol Cell Biol 33(2):281–292

Check for updates

Chapter 5

Methods for In Vivo Functional Studies of Chromatin-Modifying Enzymes in Early Steps of Colon Carcinogenesis

Martine Chevillard-Briet and Fabrice Escaffit

Abstract

Since chromatin-modifying enzymes are involved in most processes needing to access the DNA fiber such as transcription, replication or DNA repair, their involvement in the regulation of gene expression in numerous physiopathological contexts is widely studied. Most of these enzymes are essential for cell growth and survival due to their pleiotropic roles and studying their impact in vivo on organ development or tissue physiopathology is challenging. In this chapter, we describe a chemically-mediated method to induce colorectal carcinogenesis that we have used to identify in vivo the role of two chromatin modifying enzymes belonging to the same multimolecular complex, the histone acetyltransferase Tip60 and the histone variant-incorporating ATPase p400.

Key words Chromatin, Aberrant crypt foci, Adenomas, Colon cancer, Mouse models, Chemically induced carcinogenesis, Azoxymethane (AOM), Dextran sodium sulfate (DSS), Wnt pathway

1 Introduction

Multiple epigenetic alterations are involved in colorectal cancer progression [1] by deregulating the expression of oncogenes, tumor suppressors or factors involved in key signaling pathways. Most enzymes controlling the deposition of chromatin marks are essential for the survival and growth of cells, due to their pleiotropic involvement in many physiological processes. Thus, studying their impact in vivo is difficult and needs the use of heterozygous or inducible transgenic animal models. Here, we describe a method in which we can study the impact of such heterozygosities for components of the Tip60 complex on the formation of early preneoplastic lesions [2]. We take advantage of a largely used chemical-based strategy [3–6] to rapidly induce aberrant crypt foci (ACF) [7] (Fig. 1) or adenomas (Fig. 2) on the colon mucosae. This strategy allowed us to highlight significant effects of the reduction of the chromatin-modifying enzymes Tip60 and p400 on early steps of colon tumorigenesis, in less than one (for ACF) or three

Jean-François Beaulieu (ed.), *Colorectal Cancer: Methods and Protocols*, Methods in Molecular Biology, vol. 1765,
https://doi.org/10.1007/978-1-4939-7765-9_5,

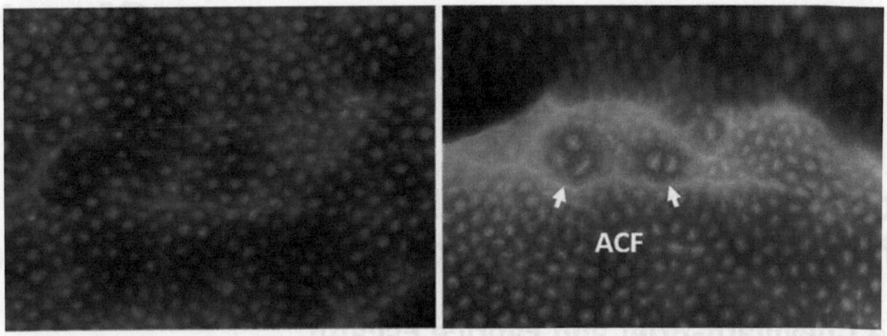

Fig. 1 Observation of ACF on colon mucosae after AOM injections. The methylene blue staining of the normal (left) or ACF-containing (right) epithelium is a critical step for the correct visualization of ACF. The number of ACF per colon is an important parameter, as well as the multiplicity of crypts in each ACF, to evaluate the incidence of such preneoplastic lesions

(adenomas) months [2]. The efficiency of azoxymethane (AOM) and the short time needed for the appearance of preneoplastic lesions allows us to avoid adaptative phenomena. Moreover, it is also possible to administer in vivo inhibitors for key signaling pathways, concomitantly with AOM, to decipher the involvement of such pathways in preneoplastic lesion formation (Fig. 3).

2 Materials

Prepare all injectable solutions in medicine-grade physiological saline (NaCl 9 g/L). Store all reagents at room temperature during the experiment and freeze (−20 °C) until next use, for a maximum of 2 months.

2.1 AOM Manipulations

1. Preparation: Ampoule of pure AOM (25 mg), a colon genotoxic carcinogen, ampoules of medicine-grade physiological serum, 50 mL conic tubes, 5 mL syringe, and 21G × 2 needle.
2. Injection: 1 mL syringes, 26G × ½ needles.
3. Neutralization: 12% sodium hypochlorite.

2.2 DSS and C59 Inhibitor Treatments

1. Dextran sodium sulfate (DSS), a nongenotoxic colon carcinogen.
2. Wnt-C59 to be diluted in DMSO (2.5 mg C59 in 250 μL DMSO). C59 decreases the activity of the Wnt pathway by inhibiting the PORCN enzyme.
3. Drinking water.

2.3 Tissue Preparation

1. Mouse dissection: ethanol 70%, scissors, clamps, and scalpel.
2. Tissue fixation: prepare formalin solution as 500 mL of 4% formaldehyde in phosphate buffered saline (PBS), 140 mm petri dishes, 110 mm diameter Whatman discs and pencil, clamps.

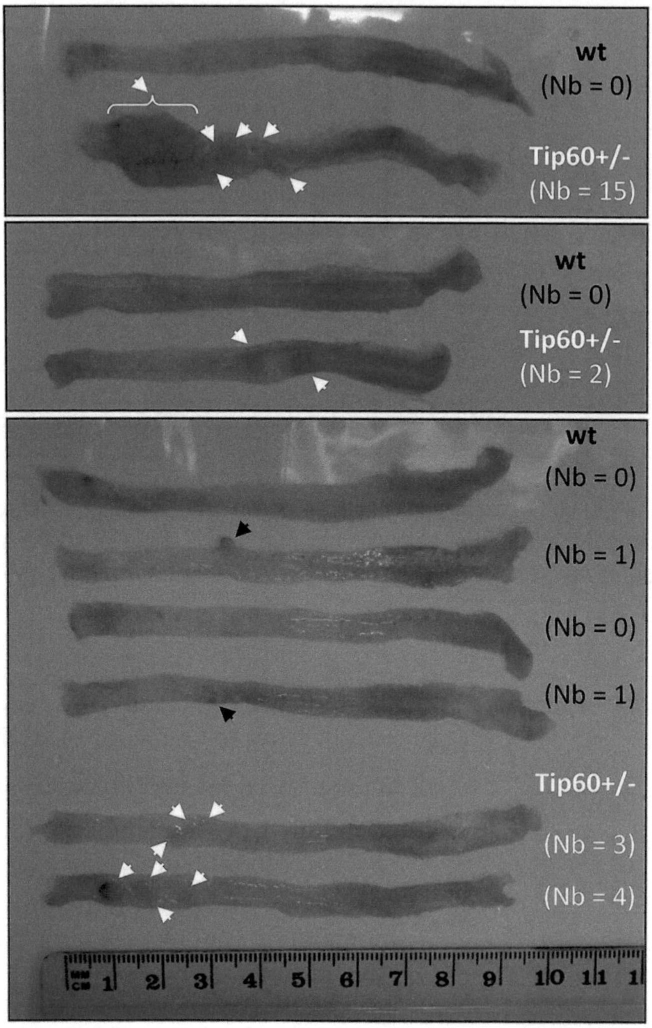

Fig. 2 Observation of adenomas on colon mucosae after AOM injections upon DSS administration via the drinking water. DSS strongly reduces the latency and greatly increases the speed of appearance of adenomas under favorable conditions. Thus, this protocol highlights the differences and reveals the favorable effects of a specific context (here, an obvious increase is observed in Tip60 heterozygous mice versus wild-type). Note that such a protocol induces a very low number of adenomas (at least with this timing) in wild-type control mice. (*Reproduced from ref.* [2] *with permission from Oxford University Press*)

3. Tissue coloration for ACF counting: methylene blue solution: dissolve 0.05 g of methylene blue in 100 mL water.

3 Methods

It is absolutely necessary to prevent any dissemination (aerosol) of AOM or contamination of reusable materials (caution, *see* **Note 1**).

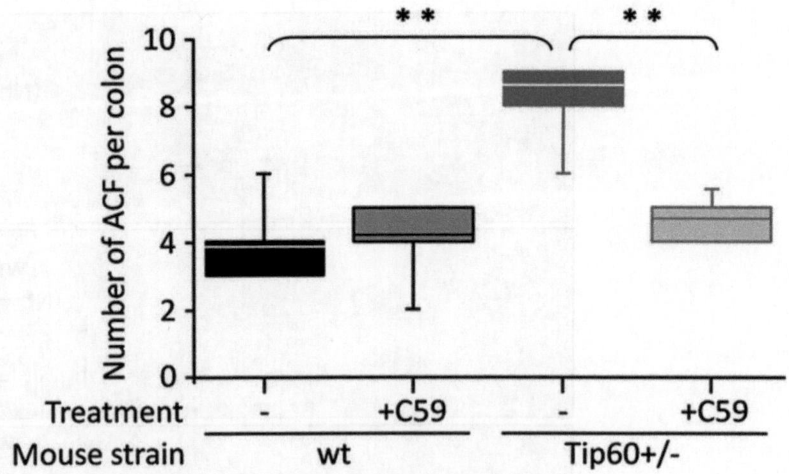

Fig. 3 Analysis of the role of signaling pathways in genotype-dependent early steps of carcinogenesis. The use of inhibitors (here, C59 Wnt pathway inhibitor) allows deciphering the involvement of such pathways in the formation of ACF, after AOM injections. (*Reproduced from ref.* [2] *with permission from Oxford University Press*)

3.1 AOM Preparation

For homogeneity of results, it is fundamental to do all experiments of a study using the same lot of AOM (*see* **Note 2**).

1. Dispense 15 mL physiological saline into a 50 mL conic tube.
2. Carefully open the ampoule of pure AOM and dilute it with 1.7 mL physiological saline.
3. Pipet the contents of the ampoule and add it to the tube containing the physiological saline. After homogenization, the final concentration of AOM is 1.5 mg/mL. Such a dilution will allow the injection of a reasonable volume into the mice (around 0.2 mL for a 20 g mouse).
4. Eliminate all containers and materials which have been in contact with AOM (*see* **Note 3**).
5. Prepare a tube containing only physiological saline for control injections.

3.2 Carcinogen Injections

1. Genotype and select a cohort of six- to eight-week-old animals, with appropriate genotypes, that will receive two intraperitoneal injections of AOM or vehicle (physiological saline) alone, 1 week apart.
2. Prepare the syringe with the appropriate volume of AOM preparation to inject a dose of 15 mg AOM per kg live weight. A preliminary experiment needs to be performed to determine the optimal dose to efficiently induce lesions with an acceptable survival rate for the mice (*see* **Note 2**).

3. Carefully constrain the mouse and relax the animal by caressing its belly. This will avoid any excessive reaction upon needle penetration and risk for the worker.
4. Inject i.p. the appropriate volume of AOM solution (*see* **Note 4**) or physiological saline alone for controls.
5. Repeat the injection 1 week later.
6. Regularly check the weight of the animals to be sure to not reach the endpoint of the experiment, according to animal practices and protocols.
7. Three weeks after the second injection, the mice are euthanized and colons are dissected and analyzed for ACF detection (Fig. 1).

3.3 Advanced Lesion Appearance: Acceleration by DSS Treatment

To accelerate the formation of advanced lesions, mice can be cotreated with 1% DSS, a proinflammatory reagent which dramatically shortens the latency period for the induction of colorectal cancer. This improves the efficiency of AOM and accelerates the ACF–adenoma–carcinoma sequence.

1. Proceed with AOM or physiological saline injections (as described in Subheading 3.2).
2. Immediately after the second injection, dilute 1% DSS in the drinkable water of the mice.
3. The colon can be dissected 10 weeks later, fixed, and observed under a binocular microscope (2× magnification) for adenoma detection (Fig. 2).

3.4 Mechanistic Investigations

The in vivo administration of specific inhibitors of key signaling pathways can help to decipher the mechanisms surrounding the observed effects. For example, we used [2] the Wnt pathway inhibitor C59 to modulate the "activation" of this pathway and thus, to demonstrate that this pathway is involved in the Tip60/p400 effect on preneoplastic lesion formation.

1. Proceed with AOM or physiological serum injections (as described in Subheading 3.2).
2. Immediately after the second injection, dilute the resuspended Wnt inhibitor C59 in drinking water to treat mice with 5 mg C59 per kg per day. Note that the control treatment is done using DMSO-containing drinking water without inhibitor.
3. Three weeks later, the animals are euthanized and the colons are dissected and analyzed for ACF detection (Fig. 3).

3.5 Tissue Fixation

1. Dissected colons are cleaned by flushing the lumen contents using a syringe containing PBS.
2. The cleaned colon is then opened longitudinally using appropriate scissors.

3. Tissues are fixed in formalin, carefully unfolded and spread out on Whatman paper using clamps and then stored in formalin before analysis. Note that such fixed tissues are suitable for ACF detection after coloration and direct adenoma observation (as described here), and also for tissue immunohistochemistry after paraffin inclusion and sectioning.

3.6 Tissue Coloration and ACF Observation

1. Dissected and fixed colons are colored using 0.05% methylene blue for 10 min.
2. After coloration, tissues are rinsed with water (*see* **Note 5**) and observed under a binocular device or microscope (40× magnification) (Fig. 1).
3. The number and characteristics of ACF (localization in the organ and multiplicity of crypts within each ACF) are collected for each colon (*see* **Note 6**).

4 Notes

1. Wear a mask, gloves, and jacket when preparing AOM dilutions. For the safety of workers, AOM must be prepared under a hood. Carefully avoid dispersal of AOM and inactivate any trace of the carcinogen as described in *see* **Note 3**.
2. Each lot of AOM has its own activity level. Two samples of different lots can have very different effects, at the same dose, on ACF formation and mouse survival. Thus, it is required to (1) use the same AOM lot all along the study and (2) set-up the protocol by first testing the activity of the AOM lot with a dose-dependent analysis of ACF induction and mouse survival.
3. All AOM-containing solutions, as well as AOM-contaminated materials, must be treated with sodium hypochlorite before being eliminated, in order to inactivate all traces of AOM.
4. Be very careful when injecting i.p. the AOM solution! AOM is a powerful carcinogen in humans and it is essential not to take any risk during injections. Thus, be sure that the mouse is correctly constrained, that the mouse and the worker are calm and relaxed, and that movements are controlled. Once injected, replace the mouse in its cage and carefully eliminate the syringe and needle.
5. The coloration step has to be strictly controlled, as well as the rinsing time to ensure the reproducibility of the staining between tissue samples.
6. The number of ACF is higher in the distal than in the proximal colon, and is nearly nil in AOM-untreated animals.

Acknowledgments

We thank Pr Denis Corpet for teaching us the AOM injections and ACF analysis.

The original work described in this chapter [2] was supported by the *Ligue Nationale Contre le Cancer* as an "*Équipe labellisée*," by the *Fondation of the Association pour la Recherche contre le Cancer* and by the *Fondation de France.*

References

1. Fullgrabe J, Kavanagh E, Joseph B (2011) Histone onco-modifications. Oncogene 30:3391–3403
2. Chevillard-Briet M, Quaranta M, Grezy A, Mattera L, Courilleau C, Philippe M et al (2014) Interplay between chromatin-modifying enzymes controls colon cancer progression through Wnt signaling. Hum Mol Genet 23:2120–2131
3. Parnaud G, Tache S, Peiffer G, Corpet DE (1999) Polyethylene-glycol suppresses colon cancer and causes dose-dependent regression of azoxymethane-induced aberrant crypt foci in rats. Cancer Res 59:5143–5147
4. Tanaka T, Kohno H, Suzuki R, Yamada Y, Sugie S, Mori H (2003) A novel inflammation-related mouse colon carcinogenesis model induced by azoxymethane and dextran sodium sulfate. Cancer Sci 94:965–973
5. Pierre FH, Santarelli RL, Allam O, Tache S, Naud N, Gueraud F et al (2010) Freeze-dried ham promotes azoxymethane-induced mucin-depleted foci and aberrant crypt foci in rat colon. Nutr Cancer 62:567–573
6. De Robertis M, Massi E, Poeta ML, Carotti S, Morini S, Cecchetelli L et al (2011) The AOM/DSS murine model for the study of colon carcinogenesis: from pathways to diagnosis and therapy studies. J Carcinog 10:9
7. Lopez-Ceron M, Pellise M (2012) Biology and diagnosis of aberrant crypt foci. Color Dis 14: e157–e164

Check for updates

Chapter 6

The Colorectal Cancer Microenvironment: Strategies for Studying the Role of Cancer-Associated Fibroblasts

Rahul Bhome, Massimiliano Mellone, Katherine Emo, Gareth J. Thomas, A. Emre Sayan, and Alex H. Mirnezami

Abstract

Colorectal cancer (CRC) is a key public health concern and the second highest cause of cancer related death in Western society. A dynamic interaction exists between CRC cells and the surrounding tumor microenvironment, which can stimulate not only the development of CRC, but its progression and metastasis, as well as the development of resistance to therapy. In this chapter, we focus on the role of fibroblasts within the CRC tumor microenvironment and describe some of the key methods for their study, as well as the evaluation of dynamic interactions within this biological ecosystem.

Key words Colorectal cancer, Tumor microenvironment, Cancer-associated fibroblasts, Extracellular vesicles

1 Introduction

Colorectal cancer (CRC) is of significant public health concern, and represents 9% of all cancer incidence, and the third highest cause of cancer-related death in Western civilizations [1, 2]. CRC is a multipart cellular entity composed of malignant cancer cells, surrounded by a variety of non-transformed cell types, bound together by an extracellular matrix. These components assemble together to form the tumor microenvironment (TME), and interact with one another by a variety of means to create a functional and dynamic ecosystem, able to promote and enhance tumor initiation, growth, invasion, metastasis, and resistance to therapy [3, 4].

The seminal observations of Paget more than a century ago in his seed (cancer cells) and soil (the microenvironment) hypothesis demonstrate that the importance of the TME has long been appreciated [5]. Nevertheless, the underlying mechanisms for the importance of the TME and its constituents in promoting the hallmarks of cancer remained opaque for many years, as the enabling methods

Jean-François Beaulieu (ed.), *Colorectal Cancer: Methods and Protocols*, Methods in Molecular Biology, vol. 1765, https://doi.org/10.1007/978-1-4939-7765-9_6,

and techniques for dissecting the different inter-cellular and cell-matrix signalling systems were not available. Over the last few decades however, several innovative methods for the study of the different components of the TME, and more importantly their dynamic interactions with one another have been identified, and have dramatically enhanced our understanding of these complex interactions.

These techniques are helping decipher the processes taking place within the TME, and provide significant promise also for highlighting opportunities to manipulate the TME for therapeutic gain in the future. Many current treatment strategies directly targeting CRC cells remain disadvantaged by the high genetic and chromosomal instability in CRC and the resistance to therapy that develops from the outgrowth of impervious clones under selective pressure [6, 7]. In stark contrast, the genetically stable stromal cells are therefore a more attractive alternative for therapeutic targeting and modulation of the TME [8].

In the present manuscript, we describe some of the key methods for the study of colorectal cancer-associated fibroblasts, and their interactions with cancer cells. Our focus is on methods for their isolation and in vitro culture; direct isolation and molecular profiling from human tumor tissue; examination of their signaling output via extracellular vesicles (EVs); their utility in 3-dimensional in vitro coculture assays; and finally evaluation of their role in in vivo models of CRC.

Deciphering the complex cross talk and interplay that exists between components of the TME with these methods will advance our understanding of tumor behavior, and help pinpoint novel opportunities for therapeutic manipulation, facilitating continued progression toward more personalized treatment approaches.

2 Materials

2.1 Isolation and Culture of Fibroblasts

1. 10 cm diameter dish.
2. Forceps and scalpel.
3. 12-well plate.
4. Phosphate buffered saline (PBS) supplemented with 2% (double-strength) penicillin–streptomycin (penicillin, 200 units/mL—streptomycin, 200 μg/mL) and 0.1% amphotericin B (Fungizone) (*see* **Note 1**).
5. Dulbecco's Modified Eagle's Medium (DMEM) supplemented with 20% fetal calf serum (FCS), 2% penicillin–streptomycin, and 0.1% amphotericin B.
6. Ciprofloxacin (BIOMYC-3 100×).
7. Trypsin–EDTA solution (0.25%).

2.2 Molecular Profiling by Laser Capture Microdissection

1. Cryostat.
2. Mounted slides.
3. Microtome.
4. Xylene.
5. Ethanol (75%, 100%).
6. Cresyl Violet.
7. Laser microdissection (LMD) platform (e.g., Leica AS, Leica Microsystems).
8. Lysis buffer.
9. RNAqueous®-Micro Kit.
10. RecoverAll™ kit.
11. NanoDrop™ 1000 spectrophotometer.
12. Agilent 2100 Bioanalyzer with RNA 6000 PicoChip.

2.3 CRC Fibroblast EVs

2.3.1 Isolation of EVs from CRC Fibroblasts

1. EV-depleted FCS (FCS ultracentrifuged at 100,000 × *g* for 16 h).
2. 50 mL falcon tubes.
3. Polycarbonate ultracentrifuge tubes.
4. Ultracentrifuge/rotor (e.g., Sorvall Discovery 100 s/TYP TFT 50.38 rotor).
5. Appropriate solvent for downstream analysis: PBS/protein lysis buffer/RNA lysis buffer/sterile water.

2.3.2 Labelling and Transfer of EVs

1. Protein Lysis Buffer
2. Vybrant Cell-Labeling Solution (Molecular Probes).
3. BCA Protein Assay Kit.

2.3.3 Extraction of RNA from EVs

1. RNase-free water.
2. 100% ethanol.
3. RNase-free 1.5–2 mL tubes.
4. miRNeasy Micro Kit (Qiagen).

2.4 Organotypic Coculture Systems with CRC Fibroblasts

1. Culture medium components: Collagen type I (rat-tail), Matrigel, FCS, 10× DMEM, 1× DMEM.
2. Other components: Fibroblasts/stromal cells of choice, 25% glutaraldehyde, 24- and 6-well plates, steel grids, nylon mesh, full keratinocyte growth medium (KGM) of choice (without cholera toxin).

2.5 Cancer-Associated Fibroblasts In Vivo

1. 6–8-week-old immuno-incompetent mice, e.g., SCID or nude mice.
2. Sterile hood with laminar flow and oxygen, and inhalational anesthetic agent, e.g., Isoflurane.
3. Operating surgical loupes with 2.5–3.5× magnification.
4. Sterile small animal surgery equipment: sterile drapes and skin prep, e.g., 10% Povidine–iodine, small animal clipper, warming pad.
5. 1 mL Micro-Fine 29–30 Gauge syringe (or Hamilton syringe), sterile saline, sterile 4/0 absorbable suture material (e.g., polyglactin 910 suture).

3 Methods

3.1 Isolation and Culture of Colorectal Fibroblasts

1. Collect fresh tumor and normal colorectal mucosa (ensure institutional ethical approval and patient consent) in PBS supplemented with antimicrobials (*see* **Note 2**).
2. Wash three times with PBS and do not aspirate after final wash.
3. Divide sample into 2 mm sections using sterile scalpel and forceps.
4. Score the bottom of a 12-well plate with a cross ("X").
5. Place tissue sections on to the center of each cross.
6. Add 750 μL medium (DMEM supplemented with 20% FCS and antimicrobials) to each plate, while ensuring the specimen fragment is not dislodged.
7. Incubate at 37 °C/5% CO_2.
8. Change medium at 24 h and every 72 h thereafter, checking for outgrowth of fibroblasts and microbial infection at each interval (Fig. 1a, b).
9. When 70% confluent, expand into a T25 flask (usually 4–6 weeks). Add BIOMYC-3 (1/100) to the growth medium for the first expansion.

3.2 Laser Microdissection of CRC Stroma

1. Fresh frozen specimens: use cryostat to divide specimen into 8–10 μm thickness sections on to membrane mounted slides.
2. FFPE specimens: use microtome to section specimen and deparaffinize in xylene for 1 min.
3. Fix tissue sections in 75% ethanol for 30 s.
4. Stain with Cresyl Violet for 1 min.
5. Dehydrate in 100% ethanol for 1 min.
6. Leave sections to air dry.

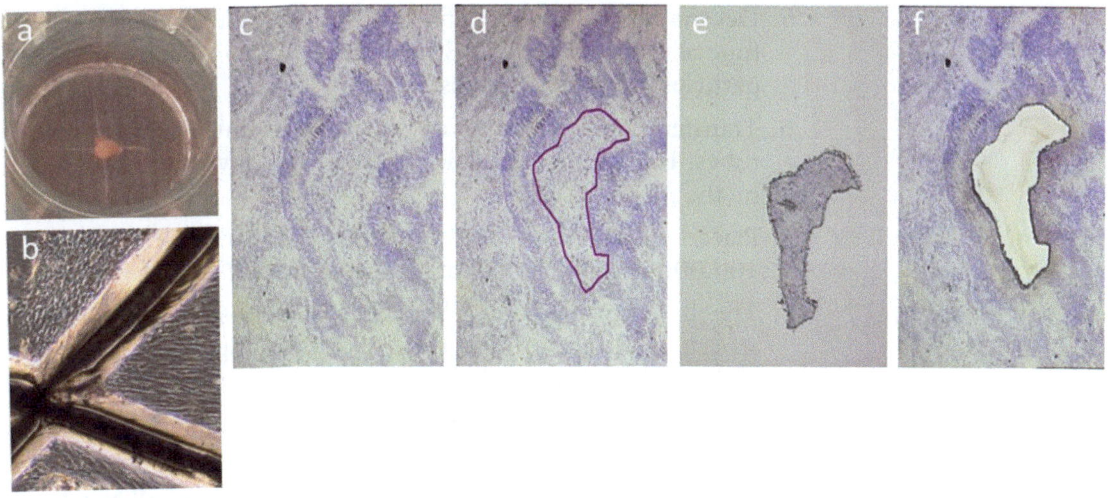

Fig. 1 Normal and cancer associated ex vivo fibroblasts and laser microdissection. (**a**) Low power magnification showing dissected human CRC tumor tissue in a 12-well plate on the "X" made in the bottom of the plate; (**b**) 10x magnification of ex vivo cancer associated fibroblasts in culture next to the "X" (**c**–**e**) Laser capture microdissection of the stromal component of fresh frozen human colorectal cancer tumor tissue. The tumor is stained with Cresyl Violet to highlight epithelial tumor and stromal compartments and visualized (**c**), marked for microdissection (**d**), and captured (**e**). Tumor after microdissection (**f**)

7. Use LMD platform according to manufacturer's instructions to separate epithelial from stromal layers, producing a 1 × 106 μm^2 cut from each layer.
8. Collect microdissected specimen in 50 μL lysis buffer (Fig. 1c–e).
9. Proceed immediately to total RNA extraction using RNAqueous®-Micro Kit for fresh-frozen tissue or Recover-All™ kit for FFPE in accordance with the manufacturer's instructions.
10. Assess yield and purity of RNA using spectrophotometer and/or bioanalyzer.

3.3 Isolation of EVs from Primary Ex Vivo CRC Fibroblasts

1. Primary fibroblasts should be cultured in FCS-depleted medium for 48–72 h prior to isolation of exosomes (*see* **Notes 3–5**).
2. Harvest the conditioned media from cells being studied, and transfer to a 50 mL falcon tube.
3. Centrifuge at 500 × *g* for 5 min at room temperature to pellet out floating cells. It is not necessary to decant supernatant at this step (*see* **Note 6**).
4. Centrifuge again at 2000 × *g* for 10 min at room temperature to pellet out debris.

5. Decant supernatant into fresh 50 mL falcon tubes and centrifuge at 10,000 × *g* for 30 min at 4 °C to pellet out microparticles/apoptotic bodies.
6. Transfer equal volumes of supernatant into ultracentrifuge tubes. Ensure tubes balance each other to within limits stated by the manufacturer.
7. Place tubes into ultracentrifuge rotor. Centrifuge at 100,000 × *g* for 70 min at 4 °C (*see* **Note 7**).
8. The 1–2 mm diameter EV pellet will be visible on the radial aspect of ultracentrifuge tube. Carefully aspirate supernatant without disturbing pellet.
9. Resuspend the EV pellet in 200 μL PBS and pool samples together in one ultracentrifuge tube.
10. In the event that you cannot see a pellet, aspirate all but 1 mL of supernatant, mix well, and add this to the pool.
11. Fill tube to capacity with PBS.
12. Ultracentrifuge again at 100,000 × *g* for 70 min at 4 °C and aspirate supernatant as above.
13. Resuspend washed EV pellet in 200 μL PBS (for cell transfer), 200 μL protein lysis buffer (western blotting), 700 μL QIAzol Lysis Reagent (RNA extraction), or 50 μL sterile water (for imaging by transmission electron microscopy) (*see* **Note 8**).
14. Store samples at 4 °C for short term (<1 week) or −80 °C for longer term. Samples for electron microscopy should not be frozen (*see* **Note 9**).
15. EV samples should be validated as follows: transmission electron microscopy with negative staining (e.g., 5% ammonium molybdate/1% trehalose) for size and morphology (Fig. 2a); western blotting for presence of transmembrane (e.g., CD63 and CD81) and endosomal (e.g., ALIX and TSG101) markers, and absence of other organelle markers (e.g., GM130 and cytochrome C); as well as nanoparticle tracking analysis (Nanosight™; Fig 2b).

3.4 Organotypic Coculture with CRC Fibroblasts

3.4.1 Day 1—Gels

1. Prepare a cell suspension of fibroblasts at 250,000 cells/gel in 1× DMEM.
2. Make up gels in the following ratio:

(a) Collagen: matrigel (1:1)	7 volumes
(b) 10× DMEM	1 volume
(c) FCS	1 volume
(d) CRC fibroblasts	1 volume

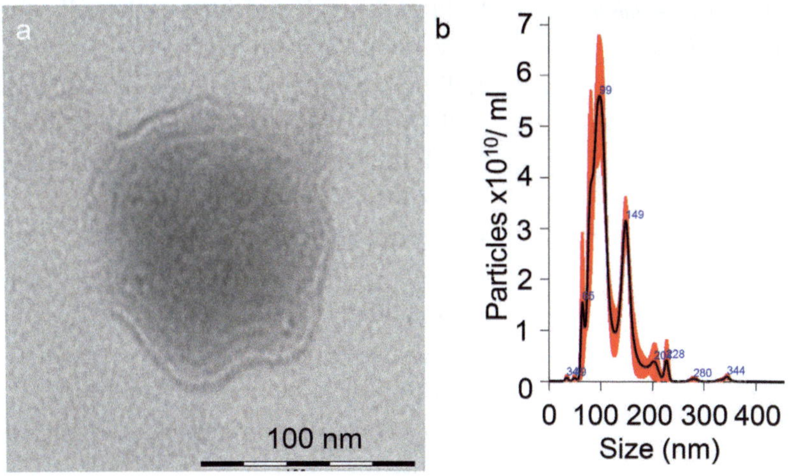

Fig. 2 Characterisation of EVs. Transmission electron micrograph (120,000 ×) of a single EV demonstrating bilayered morphology and size in the order of 100 nm (**a**); Size distribution of EVs by Nanoparticle Tracking Analysis: modal size 99 nm (**b**)

3. Add 1 mL of the above mix into each well of a 24-well plate.
4. Incubate at 37 °C for 1 h.
5. Add 1 mL of 1× DMEM on top and incubate overnight at 37 °C.

3.4.2 Day 2—Plating out CRC Cells

1. Aspirate medium from the top of the gels.
2. Plate out desired number of tumor cells (usually 500,000 per gel in 1× DMEM).
3. Incubate overnight at 37 °C.
4. Place required number of sterile nylon sheets in a 10 cm dish.
5. Make up gel coat for nylon sheets (250 μL of mix per sheet):

(a) Collagen	7 volumes
(b) 10× DMEM	1 volume
(c) FCS	1 volume
(d) 1× DMEM	1 volume
NB If the solution is yellow, neutralize with 0.1 M NaOH until it turns pink	

6. Add 250 μL gel coat to each nylon sheet and incubate at 37 °C for 15–30 min.
7. Make up 1% glutaraldehyde (in PBS) and add 10 mL to each dish. Incubate at 4 °C for 1 h.
8. Wash three times with PBS and once with 1× DMEM and leave in 1× DMEM overnight at 4 °C.

3.4.3 Day 3—Raising Gels on to Grids

1. Place a steel grid into each well of a 6-well plate and place a gel-coated nylon sheet on it (with sterile forceps).
2. Remove gel from 24-well plate using a sterile spatula and place it on the nylon sheet (*see* **Note 10**).
3. Fill the well with KGM such that it reaches the undersurface of the grid (4.8 mL KGM).
4. Replace medium every two days.
5. Harvest after 14 days of culture (or less if RNAi or treatments are added).
6. Remove whole organotypic from well and cut in half with disposable scalpel on cling film.
7. Fix both halves in a universal container filled with 10% formol saline for 24 h.
8. Replace formol saline with 70% ethanol after 24 h and leave overnight.
9. Section and mount as required (Fig. 3).

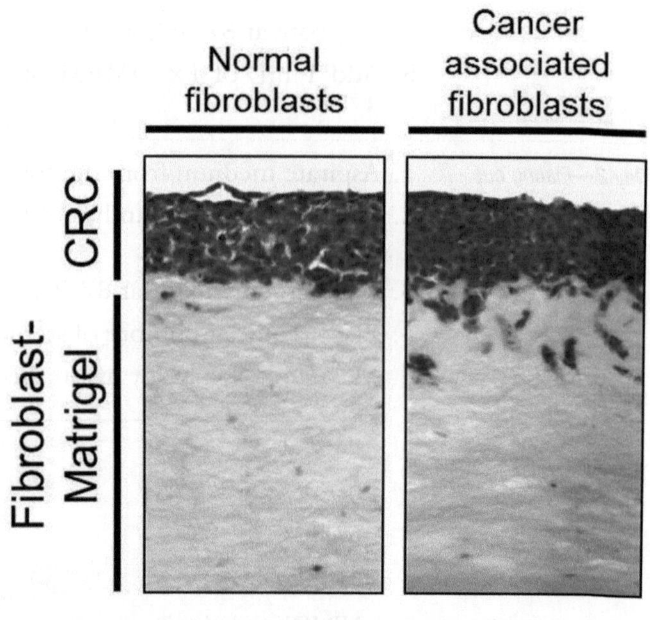

Fig. 3 Haematoxylin and Eosin staining of typical three-dimensional organotypic cocultures of CRC cells and ex vivo CRC fibroblasts (normal and cancer-associated fibroblasts) in a 1:1 Rat-Tail Collagen:Matrigel matrix (Fibroblast-Matrigel). Cancer-associated fibroblasts can enhance invasion of CRC into the simulated stromal model

3.5 Coinjection of Colorectal Fibroblasts in Subcutaneous Location

1. Mix CRC cells and fibroblasts at desired ratio for experimental protocol.
2. Add Matrigel to the cell mixture (1:1 volume)
3. Transfer to container of choice and keep on ice until ready for injection.
4. Clip the hair on the intended surgical site on 6–8-week-old SCID mice (*see* **Note 11**).
5. Anesthetize under sterile conditions in a laminar flow hood.
6. Position on a warming pad, perform skin preparation over the operative field with 10% povidine–iodine, and drape the skin to expose the surgical site.
7. Inject 0.5 mL of sterile saline subcutaneously at desired site to raise a skin bleb.
8. Inject cell-Matrigel suspension into bleb.
9. Compress for 1 min and recover animal in recovery chamber.
10. Observe until fully recovered from anesthesia.
11. Monitor for tumor growth or metastasis by physical (size of tumor, weight loss, general health, etc.) or radiological parameters (e.g., small animal imaging units).

3.6 Coinjection of Colorectal Fibroblasts in Orthotopic Location

1. Mix CRC cells and fibroblasts at desired ratio for experimental protocol.
2. Add Matrigel to the cell mixture (1:1 volume).
3. Transfer to container of choice and keep on ice until ready for injection.
4. Clip the hair on the intended surgical site on 6–8-week-old SCID mice (*see* **Note 11**).
5. Anesthetize under sterile conditions in a laminar flow hood.
6. Position on a warming pad, perform wide abdominal skin preparation with 10% povidine–iodine, and drape the skin to expose the surgical site.
7. Lift the skin in the midline with a pair of toothed forceps and perform a careful incision longitudinally with a sharp pair of dissecting scissors.
8. Lift the incised area and extend the incision cephalad and caudally to desired length for adequate exposure (Fig. 4a).
9. With a pair of small atraumatic bowel grasping forceps (e.g., DeBakey or Tuttles forceps) gently grasp the cecum which is located typically in the left iliac fossa in mice and deliver into the wound area where it can be visualized (*see* **Note 12**).
10. Gently grasp the cecum to steady it and inject the cell suspension prepared earlier just under the surface of the colon to raise a bleb in the submucosal plane (*see* **Note 13**; Fig. 4b).

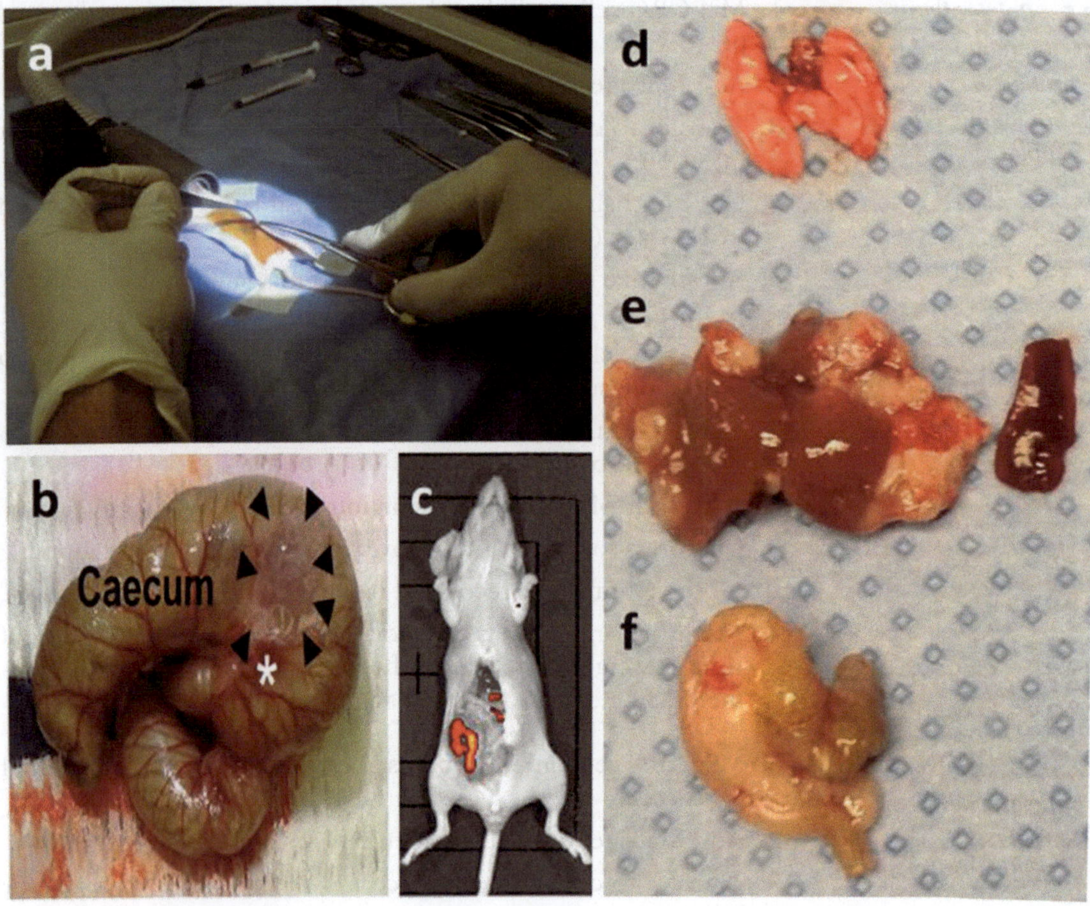

Fig. 4 Orthotopic in vivo model to study the role of colonic fibroblasts in tumor formation and metastasis. Mice are anesthetized by inhalational anesthesia and skin preparation and draping conducted. In a sterile laminar flow cabinet with full aseptic measures, a midline laparotomy is performed under magnified vision with operating loupes and a headlight (**a**). The cecum and terminal ileum are identified and exteriorized, and the cell suspension injected under direct vision to raise a clearly demarcated bleb on the surface of the cecum (**b**). After a variable length of time, mice are humanely culled and evaluated for distant metastases by imaging (**c**) and/or gross (**d–f**) or microscopic pathological analysis. Typical organs harvested include the lungs (**d**); the liver and spleen (**e**) (containing CRC metastases in the former but not latter); and the primary site of tumor injection in the cecum (**f**)

11. Press with a sterile cotton bud on the injection site for 1 min.
12. Return the bowel to the abdominal cavity and close the midline incision in layers with a continuous 4/0 suture.
13. Recover animal in recovery chamber and observe until fully recovered from anesthesia.
14. Monitor for tumor growth or metastasis by physical (weight loss, general health, etc.) or radiological parameters (e.g., small animal imaging units; Fig. 4c), or by evaluate metastatic pattern by organ collection and histological analysis at the end of the experiment (Fig. 4d).

4 Notes

1. Penicillin–streptomycin usually comes as penicillin (10,000 units/mL) and streptomycin (10 mg/mL). Fungizone comes as amphotericin B 250 μg/mL. Working concentrations are given in the "Materials" section.
2. Ensure rapid transfer from theater to laboratory to diminish cold ischemia time.
3. Each "T175" flask should contain 16–18 mL medium to concentrate exosomes without depriving cells.
4. 12× "T175" flasks of confluent fibroblasts (3–4 × 10^6 cells/flask) will produce EVs from which approximately 300–400 ng RNA can be extracted. This is adequate for most downstream analyses.
5. Cancer cells produce approximately 3–4 times more EVs than fibroblasts.
6. Serial centrifugation is carried out to avoid lysing cells and releasing organelles into the supernatant.
7. We use a fixed angle rotor because the EV pellet is seen clearly on the radial aspect of the tube. A swinging bucket rotor can also be used.
8. The final EV pellet is resuspended in whichever solvent is most appropriate for downstream analysis.
9. Samples for electron microscopy should not be frozen as this leads to artifact from ice crystals.
10. This is a critical step—be gentle with the gel and make sure it is orientated the right way up.
11. To avoid cells staying on ice too long, shaving of the operative site and other set up aspects should be done prior to splitting/mixing of the cells.
12. The bowel wall in mice is thin and can be damaged if grasped too firmly leading to a postoperative perforation. Where possible push and manipulate without actual grasping of the bowel and never use toothed forceps.
13. It is important to avoid intra-luminal injection of the cell suspension as this will not lead to tumor development. Using operating loupes for magnification, and ideally a head light and careful injection to raise a bleb are critical.

Acknowledgments

This work was supported by grant funding from Cancer Research UK.

References

1. Haggar FA, Boushey RP (2009) Colorectal cancer epidemiology: incidence, mortality, survival, and risk factors. Clin Colon Rectal Surg 22:191–197
2. Siegel R, Desantis C, Jemal A (2014) Colorectal cancer statistics. CA Cancer J Clin 64:104–117
3. Bhome R, Bullock MD, Al Saihati HA, Goh RW, Primrose JN, Sayan AE, Mirnezami AH (2015) A top-down view of the tumor microenvironment: structure, cells and signalling. Front Cell Dev Biol 3:33. https://doi.org/10.3389/fcell.2015.00033
4. Bullock MD, Pickard KM, Nielsen BS, Sayan AE, Jenei V, Mellone M, Mitter R, Primrose JN, Thomas GJ, Packham GK, Mirnezami AH (2013) Pleiotropic actions of miR-21 highlight the critical role of deregulated stromal microRNAs during colorectal cancer progression. Cell Death Dis 4:e684. https://doi.org/10.1038/cddis.2013.213
5. Paget S (1889) The distribution of secondary growths in cancer of the breast. Lancet 1:571–573
6. Zhai Z, Yu X, Yang B, Zhang Y, Zhang L, Li X, Sun H (2017) Colorectal cancer heterogeneity and targeted therapy: clinical implications, challenges and solutions for treatment resistance. Semin Cell Dev Biol 64:107–115. https://doi.org/10.1016/j.semcdb.2016.08.033
7. De Roock W, De Vriendt V, Normanno N, Ciardiello F, Tejpar S (2011) KRAS, BRAF, PIK3CA, and PTEN mutations: implications for targeted therapies in metastatic colorectal cancer. Lancet Oncol 12:594–603
8. Bhome R, Al Saihati HA, Goh RW, Bullock MD, Primrose JN, Thomas GJ, Sayan AE, Mirnezami AH (2016) Translational aspects in targeting the stromal tumour microenvironment: from bench to bedside. New Horiz Transl Med 3:9–21
9. Bhome et al. (2017) Methods Mol Biol. 1509:115–122

Check for updates

Chapter 7

Methods for Assessing Apoptosis and Anoikis in Normal Intestine/Colon and Colorectal Cancer

Pierre H. Vachon

Abstract

Caspase-dependent apoptosis, including its distinct cell death subroutine known as anoikis, perform essential roles during organogenesis, as well as in the maintenance and repair of tissues. To this effect, the continuous renewal of the human intestinal/colon epithelium is characterized by the exfoliation by anoikis of differentiated cells, whereas immature/undifferentiated cells may occasionally undergo apoptosis in order to evacuate daughter cells that are damaged or defective. Dysregulated epithelial apoptosis is a significant component of inflammatory bowel diseases. Conversely, the acquisition of a resistance to apoptosis represents one of the hallmarks of cancer initiation and progression, including for colorectal cancer (CRC). Furthermore, the emergence of anoikis resistance constitutes a critical step in cancer progression (including CRC), as well as a limiting one that enables invasion and metastasis.

Considering the implications of apoptosis/anoikis dysregulation in gut physiopathology, it therefore becomes incumbent to understand the functional determinants that underlie such dysregulation—all the while having to monitor, assess, or evidence apoptosis and/or anoikis. In this chapter, methodologies that are typically used to assess caspase-dependent apoptosis and anoikis in intestinal/colonic normal and CRC cells, whether in vivo, ex vivo, or in cellulo, are provided.

Key words Anoikis, Apoptosis, Caspase, Cell line, Cell survival, Colon, Colorectal cancer, DNA laddering, Small intestine, Regulated cell death

1 Introduction

Regulated cell death (RCD) is one of the manifold regulatory systems that are required for the ontogenesis, and subsequent upkeep, of the various organs and tissues that enable multicellular organisms to function, survive, adapt, and reproduce [1–6]. Largely defined as "*a sequence of events based on cellular metabolism that lead to cell destruction*" [1], RCD is composed of a number of distinct subtypes of cell death processes (e.g., apoptosis, autophagic cell death, necroptosis) that may be caspase-dependent or -independent, in addition to being contingent upon the deathly stimulus, the initiating transduction events that activate the executioner mechanisms, and the molecular make-up of the executing

Jean-François Beaulieu (ed.), *Colorectal Cancer: Methods and Protocols*, Methods in Molecular Biology, vol. 1765,
https://doi.org/10.1007/978-1-4939-7765-9_7, © Springer Science+Business Media, LLC, part of Springer Nature 2018

machinery [1, 3, 4, 7–10]. The present chapter will focus upon a single subtype of RCD, namely caspase-dependent apoptosis [3, 4, 9, 11, 12], along with its distinct subroutine known as *anoikis* ("detachment-induced apoptosis" or "integrin-mediated death"), the latter being defined primarily as caspase-dependent apoptosis that is induced by inappropriate, or loss of, cell–extracellular matrix (ECM) interactions [4, 9, 13–19].

Apoptosis performs crucial roles in embryogenic, ontogenic, and physiological processes, such as tissue development, sculpting, and homeostasis, as well as in the removal of defective, infected, damaged, and/or obsolete cells [1–3, 5, 8, 9, 11–13, 20]. Regardless of their state of being, normal cells are intrinsically wired by default to enter apoptosis—therefore, apoptosis must be kept in a suppressed mode when not needed and, consequently, survival signals are required in order for cells to stay alive [1, 3–5, 8, 9, 11, 12]. Aside from the loss of survival signals, apoptosis can be induced by a variety of stimuli that impede, or damage, the integrity and proper functionality of a given cell, such as endoplasmic reticulum (ER) stress, plasma membrane injury by free radicals, or radiation-induced DNA damage [1–5, 8, 9, 11, 12]. Concordantly, a dysregulation of apoptosis is implicated in numerous disorders and diseases [2, 4, 5, 8, 11–13, 20].

Like apoptosis, anoikis performs essential roles during organogenesis, as well as in the maintenance and renewal of tissues [5, 13, 14, 16–19, 21–23]. To this effect, not only do normal cells require anchorage to their ECM to survive, but also any such cell that strays from its assigned position within its given tissue, either by interacting with a "wrong" ECM or by losing anchorage altogether, is targeted for death-by-anoikis [13–19, 21–23]. In other words, anoikis constitutes a critical defense mechanism that serves to prevent detached cells from readhesion to an ECM that is different than that of their assigned one, or to avert straying cells from wandering toward incorrect locations, and thus ensuring a healthy continuity of tissue integrity [13–19, 21–23]. Consequently, the dysregulation of anoikis is likewise implicated in various physiopathologies [13, 14, 16–19, 21, 23].

In the case of an average adult human being, some sixty billion cells are produced each day, while a comparable number of cells are eliminated by apoptosis or anoikis, principally—therefore underlying the importance of these two cell death processes for the functional upholding of tissues [13, 20, 21, 23]. This, of course, applies to the epithelium of the gastrointestinal tract [13, 19, 24–33]. For instance, the continuous renewal of the human small intestinal epithelium occurs along a well defined and compartmentalized histological unit, the crypt–villus axis; this axis is essentially comprised of two cell populations: (1) the proliferative, immature/undifferentiated cells of the crypt; and (2) the differentiated (non-proliferative) cells of the villus [13, 25, 26, 28, 30]. The latter are ultimately exfoliated by anoikis [13, 19, 26, 28, 31, 32], whereas the former may occasionally undergo apoptosis in order to evacuate daughter cells that are damaged or defective [25–30, 33]. Illicit, dysregulated epithelial apoptosis is a significant component of inflammatory bowel diseases, such as ulcerative colitis [24–30]. Conversely, the acquisition of means to evade apoptosis represents one of several hallmarks of colorectal cancer (CRC) initiation and progression [25–30, 34]—as in the case of all known types of cancer [1, 8, 11, 12]. Furthermore, the emergence of a resistance to anoikis constitutes not only a critical step in cancer progression overall, but furthermore a limiting one that roughly coincides with cancer cells undergoing epithelial–mesenchymal transition, subsequently enabling invasion and metastasis [14, 16–19, 23, 35–38]. Once again, this likewise applies to CRC [13, 19, 28, 31, 34, 39].

Hence, considering the cancer-therapeutic caveats of chemo-, radiation- and/or drug-resistance encountered from aggressive cancer cells (due in large part to their acquired resistance to apoptosis), as well as the additional problem of circulating/metastasing ones and the metastases that they have already established (thanks principally to their acquired resistance to anoikis), it therefore becomes incumbent to identify functionally and diagnostically the microenvironmental, as well as molecular, determinants that underlie the resistance to apoptosis and/or anoikis exhibited by cancer cells. Herein, detailed descriptions of the methodologies typically used in our laboratory to assess caspase-dependent apoptosis and anoikis in intestinal/colonic normal and CRC cells, whether in vivo, ex vivo, or in cellulo, are provided to further stimulate their (preferably combined) use in clinical and experimental investigations that focus on the dysregulation of apoptosis, and/or anoikis, in gut physiopathologies.

2 Materials

2.1 Cell Lines

The normal human intestinal epithelial crypt-like cell strain HIEC-6 was established by Perreault and Beaulieu [40–42]. The Caco-2/15 cell line, a clone of the parental CRC Caco-2 cells, was established by Beaulieu and Quaroni [43, 44]. The HT-29, SW480 and SW620 CRC cell lines were from the American Type Culture Collection (ATCC; Manassas, VA).

2.1.1 Cell Culture

1. Complete Dulbecco's Modified Eagle's medium (DMEM): DMEM culture medium supplemented with 10 mM 4-(2-hydroxyehtyl)-1-1piperazineethanesulfonic acid HEPES, 2 mM GlutaMAX, and 10% (v/v) fetal bovine serum (FBS) (*see* **Note 1**).
2. Complete OPTI-minimum essential medium (OPTI-MEM) culture medium supplemented with 10 mM HEPES, 2 mM

GlutaMAX, 5 ng/mL epidermal growth factor (EGF), and 5% (v/v) FBS (*see* **Note 2**).

3. Corning Falcon™ standard tissue culture dishes, 12 mm circular coverslips, 12-well Corning Falcon™ tissue culture plates.
4. Phosphate-buffered saline (PBS), pH 7.4: 137 mM NaCl, 2.7 mM KCl, 8.1 mM Na_2HPO_4, and 1.5 mM KH_2PO_4, in autoclaved, bidistilled H_2O (*see* **Note 3**).
5. 0.25% trypsin–ethylenediaminetetraacetic acid (EDTA) solution.
6. Sterile 15 mL Falcon™ conical centrifuge tubes.
7. 0.1 mg/mL poly-L-lysine solution in sterile PBS (pH 7.4) (*see* **Note 4**).

2.2 Tissues

Jejunum and/or colon tissues, varying in age from 18 to 20 weeks of gestation (postfertilization), were obtained from normal elective pregnancy terminations. No tissue was collected from cases associated with known fetal abnormality or fetal death. Studies were approved by the Institutional Human Subject Review Board.

2.2.1 Cryo-Embedding for Cryostat Sectioning (See Note 5)

1. Washing and dissecting solution: PBS (pH 7.4).
2. Embedding agent: Tissue-Tek® optimum-cutting temperature (OCT) compound, in 10 mm cylindrical aluminum holders.
3. Liquid nitrogen (*see* **Note 7**).

2.2.2 Ex Vivo Explant Culture (See Note 6)

1. Washing solution: PBS (pH 7.4) (*see* **Note 3**).
2. Substratum for dissection into explants: solidified Leibovitz's L-15 medium with 1% (w/v) agar, in plastic culture dishes Petri style.
3. Dissection and explant culture medium: Leibovitz's L-15 medium supplemented with 40 μg/mL gentamicin sulfate and 200 U/mL Gibco™ Nystatin.
4. Falcon™ organ culture dishes.
5. Preembedding washing solution: PBS (pH 7.4).
6. Embedding agent: Tissue-Tek® OCT compound in 10 mm cylindrical aluminum holders.
7. Liquid nitrogen (*see* **Note 7**).

2.3 Apoptosis Induction

1. Dimethylsulfoxide (DMSO).
2. 300 mM genistein solution in DMSO (*see* **Notes 8** and **9**).

2.4 Anoikis Induction

1. Poly-2-hydroxyethylmethacrylate (PolyHEMA; Sigma-Aldrich).
2. Absolute (100%) ethanol.
3. PBS (pH 7.4) (*see* **Note 3**).

2.5 Apoptosis/Anoikis Assays

2.5.1 ISEL (In Situ TUNEL [Terminal Deoxynucleotidyl Transferase (TdT) dUTP-Mediated Nick-End Labeling])

1. ApopTag® fluorescein (FITC) in situ apoptosis detection kit (Millipore).
2. PBS (pH 7.4) (*see* **Note 3**).
3. Fixation: 2% formaldehyde solution in phosphate buffer (PB; *see* next item).
4. PB: 0.2 M Na_2HPO_4 solution in autoclaved bidistilled H_2O (pH 7.4) (*see* **Note 10**).
5. Quenching: 100 mM glycine solution in PBS (pH 7.2) (*see* **Note 10**).
6. Cell permeabilization: 0.1% (w/v) Triton™ X-100 solution in PBS (pH 7.4) (*see* **Note 11**).
7. 5% sodium azide (NaN_3) solution in bidistilled H_2O (*see* **Note 12**).
8. Blocking: 10% (w/v) nonfat dry milk (Blotto) solution in PBS, with 0.01% (v/v) of 5% sodium azide solution (*see* **Note 13**).
9. Nuclei staining: 10 mg/mL 4′,6-diamidino-2-phenyl-indole (DAPI) solution in bidistilled water (*see* **Note 14**).
10. Cell/tissue staining: 1% Evans Blue staining solution in PBS (*see* **Note 15**).
11. Mounting medium: 0.1% *p*-phenylenediamine solution in a 9:1 glycerol–PBS mix (*see* **Note 16**).

2.5.2 Annexin V Staining

1. Annexin V-FITC apoptosis detection kit (Sigma-Aldrich).
2. Evens Blue and DAPI staining as above.

2.5.3 DNA Laddering Assays

1. DNA isolation
   - (a) PBS (pH 7.4) (*see* **Note 3**).
   - (b) Sterile 15 mL Falcon™ conical centrifuge tubes.
   - (c) Cell lysis—TE–Triton buffer: 0.2% (v/v) Triton™ X-100 in TE buffer (*see* **Note 17**).
   - (d) 10 mg/mL RNase A-, DNase-, and protein-free solution.
   - (e) 10% (w/v) sodium dodecyl sulfate (SDS) in autoclaved bidistilled water.
   - (f) 20 mg/mL proteinase K, PCR grade solution.
   - (g) 5 M NaCl in autoclaved bidistilled H_2O (*see* **Note 18**).
   - (h) Isopropanol, molecular biology grade.
   - (i) TE buffer (pH 8.0).
2. DNA agarose gel electrophoresis
   - (a) Loading buffer: 0.25% (w/v) bromophenol blue to 50% glycerol in TE buffer (pH 8.0)

(b) TBE buffer (pH 8.3): 89 mM Tris, 89 mM boric acid, and 2 mM EDTA in bidistilled H_2O (*see* **Note 19**).

(c) 10 mg/mL ethidium bromide (EtBr) solution.

(d) 2% separating gel: 2% (w/v) UltraPure™ agarose (Thermo Fisher Scientific) in TBE buffer (pH 8.3), with 0.0001% (v/v) of 10 mg/mL EtBr solution.

(e) Running buffer—Tris–acetate buffer (TAE; pH 8.3): 40 mM Tris, 20 mM glacial acetic acid and 1 mM EDTA in distilled H_2O (*see* **Note 20**).

(f) 1 Kb Plus DNA ladder.

2.5.4 SDS-PAGE and Western Blotting

1. Mini-Protean® handcast, electrophoresis, and trans-blot, systems (Bio-Rad, Mississauga, ON).
2. Laemmli solubilization buffer: 56.25 mM Tris–HCl (pH 6.8), 2.3% (w/v) SDS, 10% (v/v) glycerol, 0.005% bromophenol blue. 5% (v/v) β-mercaptoethanol is added at the time of lysis.
3. 12% separating gel: mix 2.7 mL 30% acrylamide solution (29:1, Acrylamide/Bis-Acrylamide), 1.7 mL 1.5 M Tris–HCl (pH 8.8), 66 μL 10% (w/v) SDS, 2.3 mL bidistilled H_2O, 66 μL 10% (w/v) ammonium persulfate (APS), and 6.6 μL of N,N,N′,N-tetramethylethylenediamine (TEMED).
4. Overlay: isopropanol (*see* **Note 21**).
5. 5% Stacking gel: mix 335 μL 30% acrylamide solution (29: 1, Acrylamide/Bis-Acrylamide), 630 μL 0.5 M Tris–HCl (pH 6.8), 25 μL 10% (w/v) SDS, 1.5 mL bidistilled H_2O, 25 μL 10% (w/v) APS, and 5 μL TEMED.
6. Running buffer: 25 mM Tris, 0.1% (w/v) SDS, and 192 mM glycine in distilled H_2O.
7. Precision Plus Protein™ Dual Color Standards.
8. Transfer buffer: 25 mM Tris, 192 mM glycine, and 20% methanol in distilled H_2O (*see* **Note 22**).
9. Nitrocellulose membrane.
10. Ponceau S solution: 0.2% (w/v) Ponceau S and 20% trichloroacetic acid (TCA) in distilled H_2O.
11. PBS (pH 7.4).
12. Blocking solution: 10% (w/v) nonfat dry milk (Blotto) in PBS (pH 7.4), with 0.1% (v/v) Tween 20 and 0.01% (v/v) of 5% sodium azide solution.
13. Washing buffer: 0.05% Tween 20 in PBS (pH 7.4).
14. Primary anti-human antibodies: rabbit polyclonal, anti-activated Caspase-3 (CASP-3), which recognizes the long 17/19 kDa subunit of activated CASP-3 (dilution: 1/1000; Ab9661; New England BioLabs, Ipswich, MA); rabbit

polyclonal anti-polyADP-ribose polymerase (PARP), which recognizes both native PARP (116 kDa) and its CASP-3-cleaved (89 kDa) fragment (dilution: 1/1000; Ab9542; Cell Signaling, Danvers, MA); rabbit polyclonal anti-β-actin (dilution 1/20000; Ab8229; Abcam, Cambridge, MA) (*see* **Note 23**).

15. Secondary antibody: anti-rabbit IgG conjugated to horseradish peroxydase (*see* **Note 24**).
16. ECL Immobilon™ reagents.
17. LI-Cor Odyssey Fc imaging system with LI-Cor Image Studio (v2.1) software (Mandel Scientific, Guelph, ON).

2.5.5 Fluorogenic Caspase Activity Assays

1. PBS (pH 7.4).
2. 1 M DTT stock solution.
3. Lysis buffer (pH 7.0–7.2): 50 mM Tris–HCl (pH 7.2), 150 mM NaCl, 1 mM dithiothreitol (DTT), 0.5 mM EDTA, 1% (v/v) Nonidet P-40, 0.5% (v/v) sodium deoxycholate, 0.1% (v/v) SDS, 100 μM orthovanadate, 1 mM phenylmethylsulfonyl fluoride (PMSF), 0.5 μg/mL leupeptin, 0.5 μg/mL aprotinin, 0.7 μg/mL pepstatin, and 40 mM β-glycerophosphate in bidistilled H_2O (*see* **Notes 11** and **25**).
4. Reaction buffer: 0.2% (w/v) 3-[(3-cholamidopropyl)dimethylammonio]-1-propanesulfonate (CHAPS), 100 mM HEPES (pH 7.4), 200 mM NaCl, 2 mM EDTA, and 20% (v/v) glycerol in bidistilled H_2O (*see* **Note 26**).
5. Fluorogenic standard: 10 mM 7-amino-4-trifluoromethyl coumarin (AFC) solution in DMSO (*see* **Note 27**).
6. Caspase 10 mM fluorogenic substrate storage-stock solutions in DMSO: CASP-3, Ac-DEVD-AFC (N-acetyl-Asp-Glu-Val-Asp-AFC); CASP-8, Ac-LETD-AFC (N-acetyl-Leu-Glu-Thr-Asp-7-amido-4-AFC); CASP-9, Ac-LEHD-AFC (N-acetyl-Leu-Glu-His-Asp-7-amino-4-AFC) (*see* **Note 28**).
7. BrandTech® Puregrade™ 96-well black F-bottom microplates (Ultident Scientific, Saint-Laurent, QC).
8. VICTOR X multilabel plate reader spectrophotometer with PerkinElmer 2030 Workstation software (PerkinElmer, Waltham, MA).

3 Methods

The methods described below outline: (1) the detection of apoptosis by ISEL in vivo, ex vivo, and in cellulo, (2) the detection of apoptosis by the Annexin V approach, (3) the visualization of CASP-3-dependent internucleosomal DNA degradation, (4) the assessment of CASP-3 activation and/or activity, and (5) the fluorogenic measurement of CASP-8, CASP-9 and/or CASP-3 activities. Furthermore, these approaches are provided with examples of application under normal physiological conditions, as well as following the experimental induction of caspase-dependent apoptosis or anoikis.

3.1 ISEL Detection of Apoptosis

Initially developed by Gavrieli et al. [45], this approach relies on a specialized DNA polymerase, TdT, which adds nucleotides to DNA fragments. Although quite useful and rather easy to perform, great care must be taken in the interpretation of ISEL-positive staining: indeed, DNA degradation occurs in both caspase-dependent and -independent apoptosis, and may likewise occur in other subtypes of RCD [1, 3, 4, 9, 10]. Hence, it is recommended [3, 4, 9] that at least one or more additional means of detecting/evidencing/measuring caspase-dependent apoptosis be undertaken alongside ISEL. What follows is the indirect immunofluorescence method of ISEL application, where dUTP is coupled to dioxigenin (DIG) and its incorporation into DNA fragments by the TdT is revealed with an FITC-coupled, anti-DIG antibody. We have found this approach to provide for minimal background and nearly nonexistent false-positive staining (see for example [46]).

3.1.1 Twenty-Week-Old Human Fetal Small Intestine (See Note 29)

1. For the purpose herein, use one microscope slide, already holding at least two, 4–6 μM-thick transverse cryosections grouped together at both its left and right sides (thus, at least four cryosections in total). Sections on the left side are to be used as negative reaction controls (i.e., no TdT; *see* Fig. 1a) and those on the right side as experimental (i.e., with TdT; *see* Fig. 1b).
2. Fix the cryosections with 2% formaldehyde for 45 min at 4 °C.
3. Wash 3 × 10 min in PBS, at room temperature (RT).
4. Quench with glycine–PBS solution for 45 min at 4 °C.
5. Wash 3 × 10 min in PBS, at RT.
6. Block potential reactive sites by incubation with 10% Blotto for 15 min at RT (*see* **Note 30**).
7. Prepare the TdT+ reaction mix (75 μL/section is required, thus, herein, 150 μL for the right side of the slide will be needed as follows: 62.5 μL TdT added to 87.5 μL of reaction buffer; vortexed gently). These reagents are supplied by the ApopTag® kit. In parallel, set aside 150 μL of the reaction buffer alone (TdT− reaction mix, for the left side). Preincubate both TdT+ and TdT− reaction mixes for 15 min at 37 °C.
8. Add the ApopTag® equilibration buffer (50 μL/section required, thus 100 μL for the left side and 100 μL for the right side). Incubate for 15 min at RT (*see* **Note 30**).

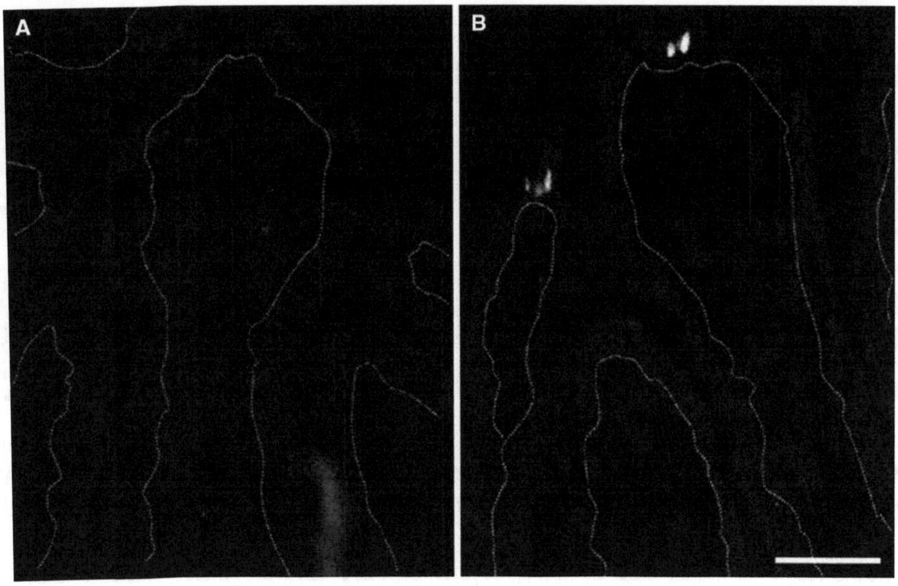

Fig. 1 In situ detection of villus-apex enterocyte exfoliation by apoptosis/anoikis in 20-week-old (postfertilization) human fetal jejunum. Representative micrographs of indirect immunofluorescence ISEL (**a**) without TdT, or (**b**) with TdT. The epithelial–mesenchymal interface is emphasized by a fine dotted line ($n = 3$). Bar = 40 μM. Adapted in part from [32]

9. Remove the equilibration buffer, then add the preincubated TdT+ reaction mix on the right side and the preincubated TdT− reaction mix on the left side. Incubate for 2 h at 37 °C (*see* **Note 30**).
10. Remove the TdT+ and TdT− reaction mixes and wash once, for 10 min at RT, with the ApopTag® stop-wash buffer (stock solution diluted 1/34 in autoclaved, bidistilled water as working solution).
11. Block potential reactive sites again by incubation with 10% Blotto for 30 min at RT (*see* **Notes 30** and **31**).
12. Prepare the anti-DIG antibody reaction mix (again, 75 μL/section is required, thus, herein, 300 μL total for both sides of the slide will be needed as follows: 159.24 μL of the anti-DIG antibody added to 140.76 μL of the 10% Blotto solution; vortex gently). Incubate for 1 h at RT (*see* **Note 30**).
13. Wash 3 × 10 min in PBS, at RT.
14. Stain sections with working Evans Blue–PBS solution for 30 s at RT (*see* **Notes 32** and **33**).
15. Wash 2 × 5 min in PBS, at RT.
16. Place a drop of mounting medium onto the sections and then cover with square coverslips.
17. View sections under a microscope equipped for epifluorescence (*see* Fig. 1).

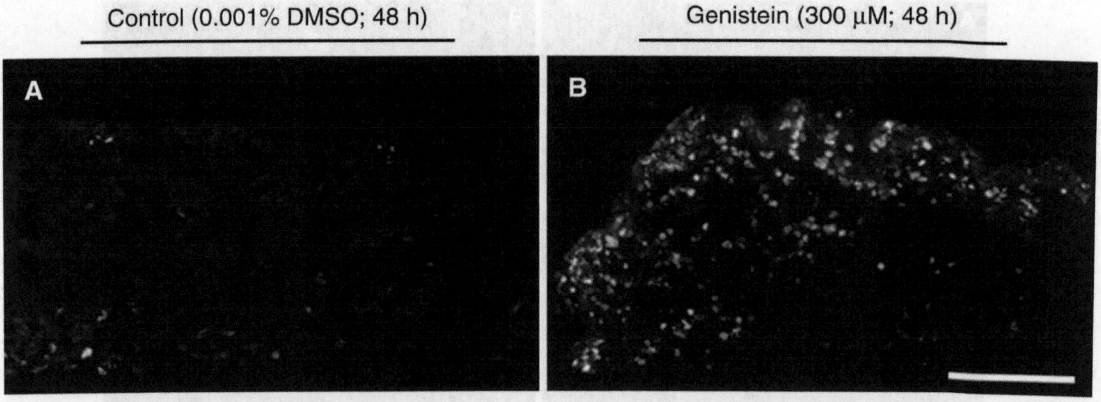

Fig. 2 Ex vivo detection of apoptosis in 18-week-old (postfertilization) human fetal colon under organotypic culture. Representative micrographs of indirect immunofluorescence ISEL following 48 h treatments of explants in L-15 medium with either (**a**) 0.001% DMSO (control), or (**b**) 300 μM genistein ($n \geq 5$). Bar = 25 μM

3.1.2 18 Weeks-Old Human Fetal Colon Explants

1. Set up two organ culture dishes (each with 4–12, 3 mm × 7 mm, explants [47, 48], with one set of explants to be used as a control group and the other as the experimental group.
2. After stabilization and 48 h culture of explants [47, 48], remove medium and replace with medium containing either 0.001% (v/v) DMSO (control group; Fig. 2a), or 300 μM genistein (using the 300 mM genistein-DMSO stock aliquots; experimental group; Fig. 2b) (*see* **Note 34**). Incubate for a further 48 h, under normal culture conditions.
3. Wash explants in PBS, and then OCT-embed grouped explants separately (control vs. experimental) for cryo-sectioning.
4. One microscope slide each for control and experimental, already holding at least two, 4–6 μM-thick explant transverse cryosections grouped together at both their left and right sides (thus, at least four cryosections in total/slide/group), were used. Sections on the left side of each slide were used as negative reaction controls (i.e., no TdT) and those on the right side of the slides were used as experimental (i.e., with TdT).
5. Follow **steps 2–17** of Subheading 3.1.1 above (*see* Fig. 2).

3.1.3 Cell Cultures

1. In a 12-well culture plate, place eight, sterilized 12 mm coverslips (one coverslip/well, two rows of four wells) (*see* **Note 34**).
2. To each coverslip, add 1 mL/well of 0.1 μg/mL poly-L-lysine in autoclaved, bidistilled water (*see* **Notes 4** and **34**).
3. Incubate for 5 min at RT (*see* **Note 34**).
4. Remove the poly-L-lysine solution (*see* **Notes 34** and **35**).
5. Let dry openly for 90 min at RT (*see* **Notes 34** and **36**).
6. Seed HIEC-6 (first row; *see* Fig. 3a–d) and Caco-2/15 (second row; *see* Fig. 3e–h) cells (*see* **Note 34**) and grow them until ~70% confluence under normal culture conditions.

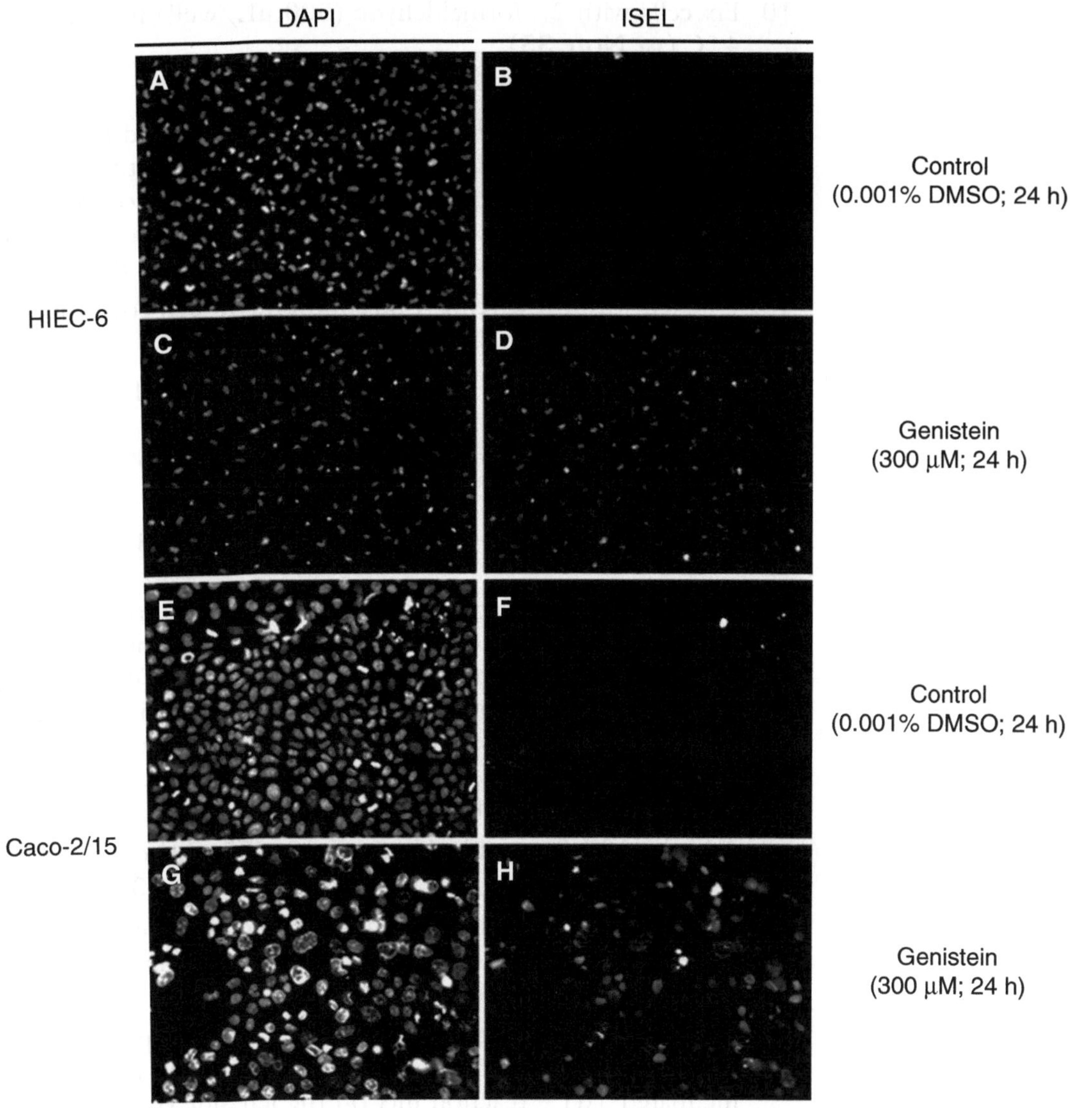

Fig. 3 In cellulo detection of apoptosis in HIEC-6 (**a–d**) and Caco-2/15 (**e–h**) cells. Representative micrographs of nuclei staining (DAPI; **a**, **c**, **e**, **g**) and indirect immunofluorescence ISEL (**b**, **d**, **f**, **h**) following 24 h treatment of cells in serum-free medium with 0.001% DMSO (control; **a–b**, **e–f**), or 300 μM genistein (**c–d**, **g–h**) ($n \geq 6$). Original magnifications: 40× (**a–d**), 20× (**e–h**)

7. Remove medium and wash twice with serum-free medium (*see* **Notes 34** and **35**).
8. For each row, add serum-free medium with 0.001% DMSO to the first two wells (controls; *see* Fig. 3a–b and e–f), and serum-free medium with 300 μM genistein to the last two wells (experimental; *see* Fig. 3c–d and g–h) (*see* **Notes 34** and **35**). Incubate for a further 24 h, under normal culture conditions.
9. Remove medium and wash once with PBS (*see* **Note 35**).

10. Fix cells with 2% formaldehyde (500 μL/well) for 45 min at 4 °C (*see* **Note 35**).
11. Wash 2 × 5 min with PBS, at RT (*see* **Note 35**).
12. With a pincer, carefully remove the coverslips and place them upright onto microscope slides (one coverslip on the right and one on the left) as follows: slide 1, HIEC control; slide 2, HIEC experimental; slide 3, Caco-2/15 control; slide four, Caco-2/15 experimental (*see* **Notes 30** and **37**).
13. Quench with the glycine–PBS solution (50 μL/coverslip), for 15 min at 4 °C (*see* **Notes 30** and **38**).
14. Wash 1 × 5 min with PBS, at RT (75 μL/coverslip) (*see* **Notes 30**, **35**, and **38**).
15. Permeabilize cells with Triton™-PBS solution (50 μL/coverslip), for 3 min at RT (*see* **Notes 30**, **35**, and **38**).
16. Wash 2 × 5 min with PBS, at RT (75 μL/coverslip) (*see* **Notes 30**, **35**, and **38**).
17. Prepare the ApopTag® TdT+ reaction mix (50 μL/coverslip, for each HIEC-6, Caco-2/15 cell coverslip on the right sides of the slides; therefore 200 μL total: 83.32 μL TdT added to 116.68 μL of reaction buffer; vortex gently). In parallel, set aside 200 μL of the reaction buffer alone (TdT−reaction mix, for the left-side coverslips). Preincubate both TdT+ and TdT−reaction mixes for 15 min at 37 °C.
18. Add the 10% Blotto blocking solution (75 μL/coverslip) and incubate for 5 min at RT (*see* **Notes 30**, **35**, and **38**).
19. Remove blocking solution, add the ApopTag® equilibration buffer (50 μL/coverslip) and incubate for 5 min, at RT (*see* **Notes 30**, **35**, and **38**).
20. Remove the equilibration buffer, then add the preincubated TdT+ reaction mix on the right-side coverslips and the preincubated TdT− reaction mix on the left-side ones. Incubate for 1 h at 37 °C (*see* **Notes 30**, **35**, and **38**).
21. Remove the TdT+ and TdT− reaction mixes and wash once, for 10 min at RT, with the ApopTag® stop-wash buffer (50 μL/coverslip; stock solution diluted 1/34 in autoclaved bidistilled water as working solution) (*see* **Notes 30**, **35**, and **38**).
22. Block potential reactive sites again by incubation with 10% Blotto for 15 min at RT (*see* **Notes 30**, **31**, **35**, and **38**).
23. Prepare the anti-DIG antibody reaction mix (again, 50 μL/coverslip is required, thus 400 μL total: 187.68 μL of the anti-DIG antibody added to 212.32 μL of the 10% Blotto solution; vortex gently). Incubate for 45 min at RT (*see* **Notes 30**, **35**, and **38**).

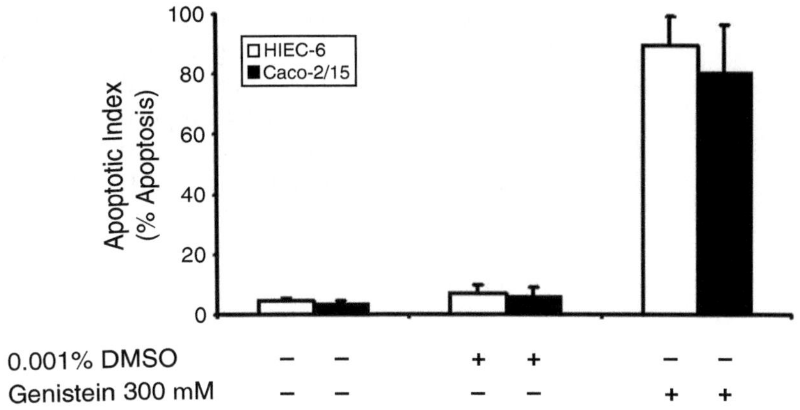

Fig. 4 Apoptotic indices from HIEC-6 (white columns) and Caco-2/15 (black columns) cells following 24 h treatment in serum-free medium alone, or in serum-free medium with either 0.001% DMSO or 300 μM genistein. Nuclei staining (DAPI) and indirect immunofluorescence ISEL were performed, and thereafter apoptotic indices were established by the ratio of ISEL-positive cells over that of total DAPI-stained nuclei counted, ×100 (expressed as "% Apoptosis"), with at least 500 cells counted (±SEM; $n \geq 6$)

24. Wash 3 × 5 min in PBS, at RT (75 μL/coverslip) (*see* **Notes 30**, **35**, and **38**).
25. Stain nuclei with the DAPI stock solution diluted 1/50,000 in PBS, for 5 min at RT (*see* Fig. 3a, c, e, and g; *see* **Notes 30**, **35**, and **38**).
26. Remove DAPI solution and stain cells with working Evans Blue–PBS solution for 30 s at RT.
27. Wash 2 × 5 min in PBS, at RT (75 μL/coverslip).
28. Place a drop (~5 μL) of mounting medium onto the round coverslips and then cover with square coverslips.
29. View cells under a microscope equipped for epifluorescence (*see* Fig. 3).
30. Ascertain apoptotic indices by establishing the ratio of ISEL-positive cells over that of total DAPI-stained nuclei counted (with at least 500 nuclei counted in total over 3–5 different areas of the stained, coverslip-cell cultures; expressed as "% Apoptosis") (*see* Fig. 4) (*see* **Notes 39** and **40**). Alternately, apoptotic indices may be compared to those of controls and expressed as "% of Control" (as examples, *see* [46, 48–54].

3.2 Detection of Apoptosis-Associated Phosphatidylserine (PS) Translocation to Cell Surface

During apoptosis, PS translocates from the cytoplasmic face of the plasma membrane to the cell surface [3, 4, 9, 55]. Since Annexin V has an affinity for binding to PS, it can therefore be used as a probe for staining apoptotic cells. However, there is increasing evidence that the translocation of PS to the external face of the plasma membrane not only occurs in caspase-dependent apoptosis, but also in other forms of RCD [55]. Hence, as in the case of ISEL, it is recommended [3, 4, 9] that at least one or more additional means of detecting/evidencing/measuring caspase-dependent apoptosis be undertaken alongside this approach. Another caveat to this method is that it can not be used with permeabilized cells (if only through fixation) or transverse sections of tissues/explants—for obvious reasons. Mostly devised for use with cells put in suspension (via trypsinization) for subsequent fluorescence-activated cell sorting (FACS) analyses, we have adapted this approach for use with adhering cell cultures.

3.2.1 Cell Cultures

1. Follow **steps 1–9** of Subheading 3.1.3 above.
2. For each row, add serum-free medium with 0.001% DMSO to the first two wells (control), and serum-free medium with 300 μM genistein to the last two wells (experimental) (*see* **Notes 34** and **35**). Incubate for a further 24 h, under normal culture conditions.
3. Remove medium and wash once with PBS (*see* **Note 35**).
4. With a pincer, carefully remove the coverslips and place them upright onto microscope slides (one coverslip on the right and one on the left) as follows: slide 1, HIEC control; slide 2, HIEC experimental; slide 3, Caco-2/15 control (*see* Fig. 5a–b); slide four, Caco-2/15 experimental (*see* Fig. 5c–d) (*see* **Notes 30** and **37**).

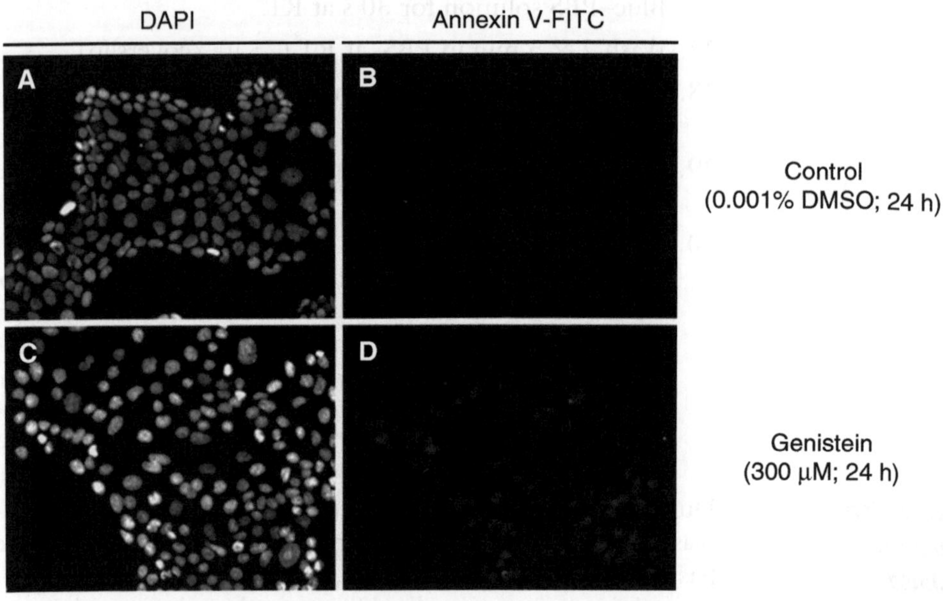

Fig. 5 In cellulo detection of apoptosis-associated PS cell surface exposure in Caco-2/15 cells. Representative nuclei staining (DAPI; **a**, **c**) and direct immunofluorescence Annexin V binding (**b**, **d**) following 24 h treatment of cells in serum-free medium with 0.001% DMSO (control; **a–b**), or 300 μM genistein (**c–d**) ($n = 3$). Original magnification: 40×

5. Add the 10% Blotto blocking solution (75 μL/coverslip) and incubate for 5 min at RT (*see* **Notes 30**, **35**, and **38**).
6. Remove blocking solution and incubate with the kit-supplied binding buffer (diluted 1/10 in PBS; 75 μL/coverslip) for 5 min, RT.
7. Prepare the kit-supplied FITC-coupled recombinant Annexin V+ mix (50 μL/coverslip, for each HIEC-6, Caco-2/15 cell coverslip on the right sides of the slides; therefore 200 μL total: 2 μL FITC-coupled Annexin V stock solution added to 98 μL of binding buffer diluted 1/10 in PBS; vortex gently). In parallel, set aside 200 μL of the binding buffer alone, diluted 1/10 in PBS (Annexin V− mix, for the left-side coverslips) (*see* **Notes 41** and **42**).
8. Remove binding buffer, then add the Annexin V+ mix on the right-side coverslips and the Annexin V− mix on the left-side ones. Incubate for 5 min at RT (*see* **Notes 30**, **35**, **38**, and **41**).
9. Wash 2 × 5 min in PBS, at RT (75 μL/coverslip).
10. Fix cells with 2% formaldehyde (50 μL/coverslip) for 15 min at 4 °C (*see* **Notes 30**, **35**, **38**, and **41**).
11. Wash 2 × 5 min with PBS, at RT.
12. Quench with the glycine–PBS solution (50 μL/coverslip), for 10 min at 4 °C.
13. Wash 1 × 5 min with PBS, at RT (75 μL/coverslip).
14. Permeabilize cells with Triton™-PBS solution (50 μL/coverslip), for 3 min at RT (*see* **Notes 30**, **35**, **38**, and **41**).
15. Wash 2 × 5 min with PBS, at RT (75 μL/coverslip) (*see* **Notes 30**, **35**, **38**, and **41**).
16. Stain nuclei with the DAPI stock solution diluted 1/50,000 in PBS, for 5 min at RT (*see* Fig. 5a and c).
17. Remove DAPI solution and stain cells with working Evans Blue–PBS solution for 30 s at RT (*see* **Notes 30**, **32**, **35**, **38**, and **41**).
18. Place a drop (~5 μL) of mounting medium onto the round coverslips and then cover with square coverslips.
19. View cells under a microscope equipped for epifluorescence (*see* Fig. 5; *see* **Note 43**).
20. Ascertain apoptotic indices by establishing the ratio of Annexin V-positive cells over that of total DAPI-stained nuclei counted (with at least 500 nuclei counted in total over 3–5 different areas of the stained, coverslip-cell cultures) (*see* Fig. 6; *see* **Notes 40** and **44**).

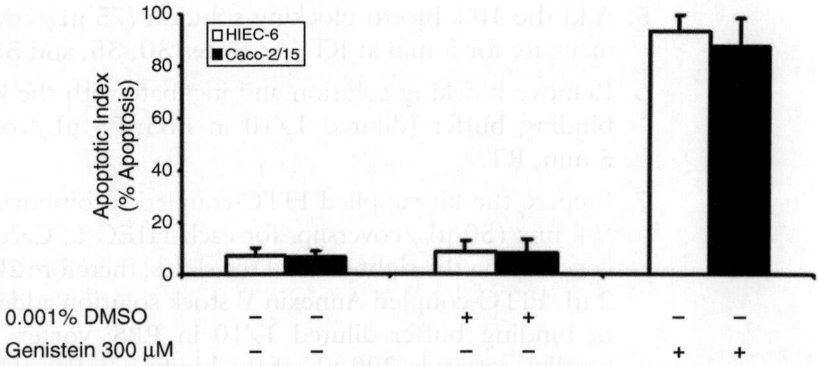

Fig. 6 Apoptotic indices from HIEC-6 (white columns) and Caco-2/15 (black columns) cells following 24 h treatment in serum-free medium alone, or in serum-free medium with either 0.001% DMSO or 300 μM genistein. Nuclei staining (DAPI) and direct immunofluorescence Annexin V binding were performed, and thereafter apoptotic indices were established by the ratio of Annexin V-positive cells over that of total DAPI-stained nuclei counted, ×100 (expressed as "% Apoptosis"), with at least 500 cells counted (±SEM; $n = 3$)

3.3 Visualization of Caspase-Dependent Internucleosomal DNA Fragmentation ("DNA Laddering")

Once CASP-3 is activated, one of its many roles is to go to the nucleus and cleave iCAD (inhibitor of CAD), subsequently freeing CAD (Caspase-Activated DNase) to perform its specialized function of digesting internucleosomal DNA. Consequently, this results in one of the hallmarks of caspase-dependent apoptosis, namely a DNA laddering of ~200 bp fragments and multiples thereof [3, 4, 9, 56]. The DNA laddering assay method described below is meant for use with cell cultures (whether treated for induction of apoptosis or anoikis), since the latter undergoing caspase-dependent apoptosis/anoikis constitute an abundant source of DNA laddering that can be visualized by EtBr-stained DNA agarose gel electrophoresis. However, in the case of biopsies of pathologies, or even explant cultures, with the proportion of apoptotic cells within tissue samples being relatively quite low, a classic nick-end labeling approach (DNA extraction, use of ^{32}P–labeled nucleotides and autoradiography [57] should instead be applied to evidence DNA laddering. Lastly, the method described herein allows for the isolation of fragmented DNA predominantly, with little (if any) non-fragmented/intact DNA (*see* Fig. 7) (for additional examples, *see* [46, 49–54]).

3.3.1 Apoptosis Induction

1. Seed HIEC-6 cells in eight, and Caco-2/15 cells in four, 100 mm standard tissue culture dishes (*see* **Note 45**). Grow the cultures until ~70% confluence under normal culture conditions.
2. Remove medium and wash twice with serum-free medium (*see* **Note 34**).
3. For HIEC-6 cells, add serum-free medium with 0.001% DMSO to the first four dishes (control), and serum-free

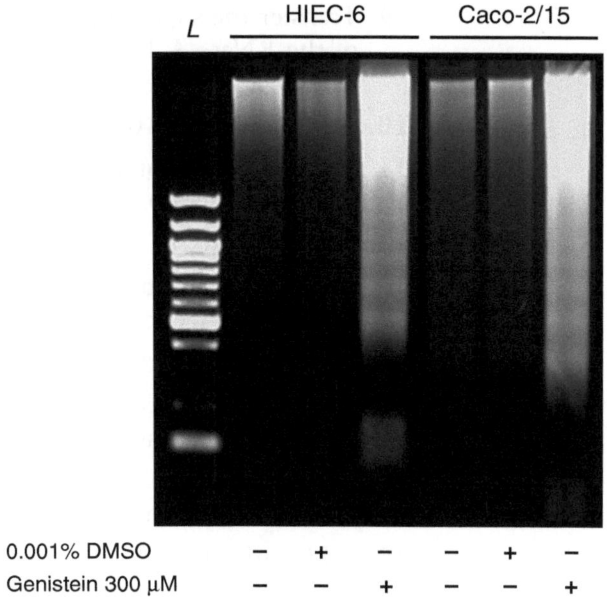

Fig. 7 Internucleosomal DNA fragmentation following induction of caspase-dependent apoptosis. Representative DNA laddering assays of HIEC-6 and Caco-2/15 cells following 24 h treatment in serum-free medium alone, or in serum-free medium with either 0.001% DMSO or 300 μM genistein ($n \geq 6$). *L*, 1 kb DNA ladder

medium with 300 μM genistein to the last four dishes (experimental). For Caco-2/15 cells, do the same for the first two dishes and the last two dishes, respectively (*see* **Notes 34** and **35**). Incubate for a further 24 h, under normal culture conditions.

4. For each set of dishes (HIEC-6, Caco-2/15; controls, experimental), recuperate 6/10 of the culture medium and put in sterile 15 mL Falcon™ conical centrifuge tubes, accordingly (*see* **Note 46**). Scrape cells off of dishes in the remaining medium, collect and pool with their proper previously recuperated medium.
5. Centrifuge at 2250 RPM for 5 min, at RT.
6. Remove the medium (*see* **Note 47**) and wash once cell pellets with 3 mL PBS (*see* **Notes 3** and **47**) at RT.
7. Remove PBS (*see* **Note 47**) and resuspend cells in 300 μL of the TE/Triton buffer. Transfer into a 1.5 mL Eppendorf™ microcentrifuge tubes and incubate on ice for 10 min with occasional, gentle swirling.
8. Centrifuge at 11,800 RPM for 15 min, at 4 °C.

9. Transfer the supernatants to fresh microfuge tubes, add 18 μL of the RNase A 1 mg/mL (*see* **Note 48**). Incubate for 1 h at 37 °C.
10. Add 15.9 μL of 10% SDS (*see* **Note 49**) and vortex gently.
11. Add 5 μL of Proteinase K 10 mg/mL (*see* **Note 50**), vortex gently, and incubate for 1 h at 50 °C.
12. Add 33.89 μL of 5 M NaCl.
13. Add 372.8 μL of −20 °C isopropanol. Vortex gently and incubate on ice for 10 min.
14. Centrifuge at 11,800 RPM for 15 min, at 4 °C.
15. Decant the supernatant by inverting the microfuge tube on a drying paper/tissue.
16. Resuspend the DNA pellet in 20 μL of TE buffer (can be stored at 4 °C for a month).
17. Add 2 μL of the loading buffer stock solution and 1 μL of a 1 μg/mL EtBr working solution (*see* **Note 51**). Keep in the dark.
18. Prepare a horizontal 2% agarose separating gel. Once gel has solidified, place in an horizontal electrophoresis chamber containing the TAE running buffer.
19. Load the samples (20 μL/well, of all of each sample depending on size of the gel) and a 1 kb DNA reference ladder. Run the gel for 1–2 h at 100 V.
20. View/photograph the gel under UV illumination (*see* **Note 52**) (*see* Fig. 7).

3.3.2 Anoikis Induction

The following method describes the procedure for establishing a time-course kinetic of DNA laddering emergence following induction of anoikis, by seeding Caco2/15 cells in polyHEMA-coated dishes (time points: 0, 4, 8, 12 and 24 h) (*see* Fig. 8, left). PolyHEMA is a non-cell adhesive polymer, thus ensuring that cells remain in suspension in culture and, therefore, undergo anoikis. If only seeking to compare adhering cells to cells kept in suspension (usually for 24 h; *see* Fig. 8, right), then the number of cell cultures and polyHEMA-coated dishes should be reduced accordingly. In any event, the number of cultures and polyHEMA-coated dishes should be properly adjusted if using HIEC-6 cells (*see* **Note 45**) (for additional examples, *see* [46, 49–54].

1. Prepare a working solution of polyHEMA 10 mg/mL in ethanol 100% (*see* **Note 53**).
2. Put the polyHEMA solution (6 mL/dish) into eight, 100 mm standard tissue culture dishes (*see* **Notes 34** and **54**).
3. Let dry openly for 1.5 h at RT (*see* **Notes 34** and **36**).

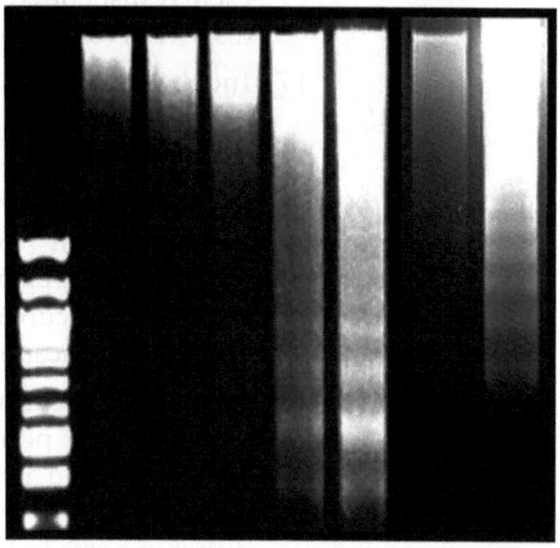

Fig. 8 Time-course kinetics of internucleosomal DNA fragmentation following induction of anoikis. Representative DNA laddering assays of (left) Caco-2/15 cells maintained in suspension 0–24 h in serum-free medium, or (right) HIEC-6 cells maintained 24 h in serum-free medium while still adhering (0 h) or in suspension (24 h) ($n \geq 3$). *L*, 1 kb DNA ladder. Adapted in part from [46]

4. Add another 6 mL/dish of polyHEMA (*see* **Note 34**).
5. Let dry openly again for 1.5 h at RT (*see* **Notes 34** and **36**).
6. Wash twice with sterile PBS (*see* **Notes 3** and **34**).
7. Put covers back on culture dishes and seal with Parafilm (*see* **Notes 34** and **54**).
8. Seed Caco-2/15 cells in ten 100 mm standard tissue culture dishes (*see* **Note 45**). Grow the cultures until ~70% confluence under normal culture conditions.
9. Remove medium and wash once with 5 mL sterile PBS (*see* **Notes 3** and **34**).
10. Trypsinize eight of the ten cultures with 1 mL trypsin–EDTA solution for 5 min, at 37 °C.
11. To the remaining two, nontrypsinized cultures, add serum-free medium (*see* **Note 34**).
12. Resuspend trypsinized cells (do not pool, keep separate) in 5 mL of medium with serum and transfer in individual sterile 15 mL Falcon™ conical centrifuge tubes.
13. Centrifuge at 1500 RPM for 5 min, at RT.
14. In the meantime, rinse the polyHEMA-coated dishes once with 5 mL serum-free medium (*see* **Notes 34** and **55**).
15. Resuspend each cell pellet in 5 mL serum-free medium.

16. Remove medium from polyHEMA-coated dishes and reseed each resuspended cell pellet into its own polyHEMA-coated dish (*see* **Note 34**).
17. Incubate polyHEMA-seeded ("suspension"; experimental) cultures under normal conditions.
18. For the two, nontrypsinized ("adhering"; controls; time point: 0 h), recuperate 4/5 of the culture medium and pool in a sterile 15 mL Falcon™ conical centrifuge tube. Scrape cells off of dishes in the remaining medium, collect and pool with their previously recuperated medium. Then proceed with **steps 5–16** of Subheading 3.3.1 above.
19. For the incubating eight suspension cultures, remove two dishes at time points 4, 8, 12 and 24 h. For each time point, recuperate and pool all of the medium (which includes the suspended cells, dying-by-anoikis or otherwise) from the two dishes in a sterile 15 mL Falcon™ conical centrifuge tube, then proceed with **steps 5–16** of Subheading 3.3.1 above.
20. For all time points (0–24 h), proceed thereafter with **steps 17–19** of Subheading 3.3.1 above.
21. View/photograph the gel with a detector/imager under UV illumination (*see* **Note 52**) (*see* Fig. 8).

3.4 Assessment of CASP-3 Activation/ Activity by Western Blotting

One of the main executioner caspases during apoptosis and/or anoikis, CASP-3 is expressed as an inactive, pro-CASP-3 form (32 kDa). Upon its activation (either via initiator caspases CASP-8 or CASP-9, or by already activated CASP-3), the long (17/19 kDa) and short (12 kDa) subunits are released from the 32 kDa proform, in order to subsequently associate, with other released CASP-3 long and short subunits, as active CASP-3 hetero-tretramers [58]. Hence, CASP-3 activation can be observed by Western blotting with the help of commercially available antibodies that specifically recognize the released long, or short, subunits (*see* **Notes 56** and **57**). An alternate means of evidencing CASP-3 activation, as well as its activity (indirectly), is to probe by Western blotting for the cleavage of protein substrates that are targets of CASP-3, such as PARP [58]. The most commonly used target to evidence CASP-3 activation/activity in studies dealing with apoptosis/anoikis, antibodies that recognize native PARP (116 kDa) along with its CASP-3-generated 89 kDa fragment are likewise available commercially. However, it should be kept in mind that CASP-7, as well as cathepsin B, D, and G (which are involved in caspase-independent apoptosis, autophagic cell death and/or necroptosis), not only cleave PARP as well, but likewise produce the 89 kDa fragment [59, 60]—hence, as in the case of ISEL and

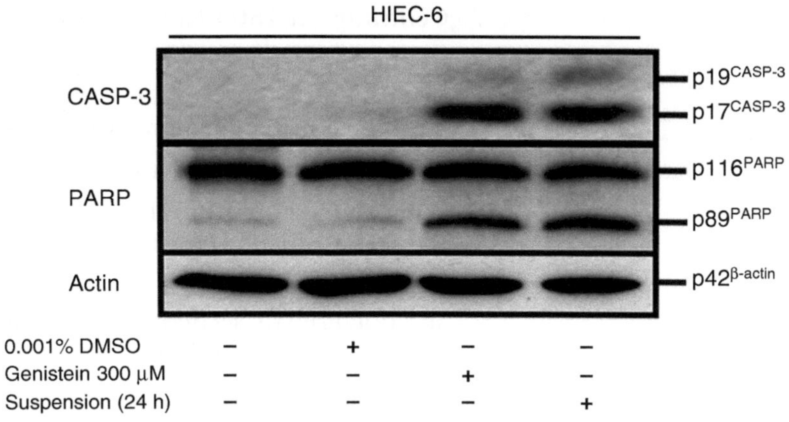

Fig. 9 CASP-3 activation/activity following induction of apoptosis, anoikis. Representative Western blot analyses of the activation of CASP-3 (emergence of its long 17/p19 kDa subunit released from its inactive, procaspase form) and the cleavage of PARP (116 kDa) by CASP-3 (releasing an 89 kDa PARP fragment), from HIEC-6 cells maintained 24 h in serum-free medium alone, in serum-free medium with either 0.001% DMSO or 300 μM genistein, or maintained in suspension for 24 h in serum-free medium. Antibodies which recognize specifically the p17/p19 subunit of activated CASP-3, or both native PARP and its cleaved p89 fragment, were used. The detection of β-actin (42 kDa) was used as reference ($n \geq 3$)

Annexin V, it is recommended that at least one or more additional means of detecting/evidencing/measuring caspase-dependent apoptosis be undertaken alongside the probing for PARP cleavage. The following method describes the application of using antibodies directed to activated CASP-3 and cleaved PARP, following the induction of apoptosis and/or anoikis (*see* Fig. 9; *see* also [58, 61, 62] as examples).

3.4.1 Apoptosis, Anoikis Induction

1. Seed HIEC-6 cells in four, 100 mm standard tissue culture dishes. Grow the cultures until ~70% confluence under normal culture conditions (*see* **Note 58**).
2. Process two of the dishes as indicated in **steps 2–3** of Subheading 3.3.1 above, for induction of apoptosis (DMSO as control, genistein as experimental). Incubate for 24 h under normal culture conditions.
3. For the remaining two dishes, remove medium and wash once with 5 mL sterile PBS (*see* **Notes 3** and **34**).
4. Trypsinize one of the cultures with 1 mL trypsin–EDTA solution for 5 min, at 37 °C.
5. To the remaining nontrypsinized culture, add serum-free medium (*see* **Note 34**).
6. Resuspend trypsinized cells in 5 mL of medium with serum and transfer to a sterile 15 mL Falcon™ conical centrifuge tube.

7. Centrifuge at 1500 RPM for 5 min, at RT.
8. In the meantime, rinse a polyHEMA-coated dish (prepared according to **steps 1–7** of Subheading 3.3.2 above) once with 5 mL serum-free medium (*see* **Notes 34** and **55**).
9. Resuspend the cell pellet in 5 mL serum-free medium.
10. Remove medium from the polyHEMA-coated dish and reseed the resuspended cell pellet into it (*see* **Note 34**).
11. Incubate for 24 h both nontrypsinized ("adhering"; control) and polyHEMA-seeded ("suspension"; experimental) cultures under normal conditions.
12. For each of the three non-polyHEMA-coated dishes, remove 6/10 of the culture medium and put in sterile 15 mL Falcon™ conical centrifuge tubes, accordingly (*see* **Note 46**). Scrape cells off of dishes in the remaining medium, collect and pool with their proper previously recuperated medium.
13. Centrifuge at 1500 RPM for 5 min, at RT.
14. Remove the medium (*see* **Note 47**) and resuspend cell pellets with 5 mL cold PBS (*see* **Note 3**).
15. Centrifuge at 1500 RPM for 5 min, at RT.
16. Remove PBS, resuspend cell pellets again with 5 mL cold PBS (*see* **Note 3**), and centrifuge again at 1500 RPM for 5 min, at RT.
17. Remove PBS (*see* **Note 47**) and resuspend cell pellets in 200 μL of Laemmli solubilization buffer with 5% β-mercaptoethanol (*see* **Note 59**). Transfer each cell lysate to its own 1.5 mL Eppendorf™ microcentrifuge tube, vortex vigorously, then heat for 5 min at 105 °C (*see* **Note 60**).
18. For the polyHEMA-seeded culture, recuperate all of the medium (which includes the suspended cells, dying-by-anoikis or otherwise) in a sterile 15 mL Falcon™ conical centrifuge tube and then follow previous **steps 13–17** herein.
19. Cool the samples then sonicate (2 × 15 s) and centrifuge at 12,500 RPM for 5 min, at RT.
20. Transfer the supernatants in new microfuge tubes (*see* **Note 61**).

3.4.2 SDS-PAGE and Western Blotting

1. The following steps are based on the use of the Mini-Protean® (Bio-Rad) handcast, electrophoresis, and trans-blot, systems; however, they are nonetheless adaptable to other formats/ systems, including large gels.
2. Prepare the 12% separating gel mix as described in Subheading 2.5.4 (*see* **Note 62**). Mix gently and pour the solution slowly into the Mini-Protean® handcast gel-frame, leaving space for the stacking gel.

3. Overlay the separating gel with 100% isopropanol and allow the separating gel to polymerize for 1 h, at RT (*see* **Note 21**).
4. Prepare the 4% stacking gel mix as described in Subheading 2.5.4 (*see* **Note 62**).
5. Remove the overlay (*see* **Note 21**) and pour the stacking gel mix. Insert comb. Allow to polymerize for 30–45 min, at RT.
6. Assemble the Mini-Protean® electrophoresis apparatus. Fill the top chamber with running buffer, remove the comb and wash the wells with running buffer. Fill the bottom chamber with remaining running buffer and remove any accumulated bubbles from the lower edge of the gel.
7. Prepare samples containing 50 μg protein per well (normalize final loading volumes to 35 μL with Laemmli buffer +5% β-mercaptoethanol).
8. Heat samples for 5 min at 105 °C (*see* **Note 60**).
9. Centrifuge at 12,500 RPM for 5 min, at RT.
10. Load samples along with an appropriate protein marker. Run the gel at 70 V for 15 min to allow the proteins to enter the gel. Thereafter, raise voltage to 100 V and continue running the gel for a subsequent 90–120 min.
11. After migration, remove gel and equilibrate by immersion in a small amount of chilled transfer buffer for 15 min.
12. Prepare the Mini-Protean® electro-transfer cassette/sandwich as typically described for any electro-transfer protocol [40].
13. Mount the Mini-Protean® electro-transfer chamber (already containing chilled transfer buffer) with the sandwich. Run the electro-transfer of separated proteins onto the nitrocellulose membrane at 100 V (*see* **Note 63** for time of running).
14. Disassemble the cassette/sandwich, peel off nitrocellulose from the gel, mark it for orientation and wash in distilled H_2O for 10 min, at RT.
15. Stain transferred proteins by soaking the nitrocellulose membrane in Ponceau S solution for 15–30 s, then wash twice with distilled H_2O (*see* **Note 64**). The protein molecular weight markers can be labeled with a pencil.
16. Wash the membrane twice with PBS for 5 min at RT, to remove the Ponceau S staining (*see* **Note 65**), and then incubate in blocking solution overnight at RT (*see* **Note 66**).
17. Place the blocked membrane in a plastic bag, add the appropriate antibody diluted in the blocking solution, and then seal the bag. Incubate overnight at 4 °C.
18. Wash the membrane 4 × 10 min, RT, with the washing buffer.

19. Block again the membrane for 1 h, RT, and this time with the blocking solution minus sodium azide (*see* **Note 24**).
20. Incubate with the secondary antibody (*see* **Note 24**), 1 h at RT.
21. Wash the membrane 2 × 10 min, RT, with the washing buffer.
22. Wash the membrane 2 × 10 min, RT, with PBS.
23. ECL Immobilon™ reaction mix is prepared according to the manufacturer's instructions and placed on the membrane, between the leaves of a plastic sheet (*see* **Note 67**).
24. View/photograph protein bands with a detector/imager (*see* **Note 68**) (*see* Fig. 9).

3.5 Direct Assessment of Caspase Activity during Apoptosis, Anoikis

Not unlike DNA laddering visualization, the assessment of caspase catalytic activity constitutes a high-confidence means of evidencing caspase-dependent apoptosis/anoikis (*see* **Note 69**). Fluorogenic caspase activity assays are based on the detection of the cleavage of caspase-specific, synthetic peptide substrates, which are coupled to the fluorescent dye AFC at their C-terminal. When liberated from the peptide by cleavage, AFC undergoes a fluorescence shift that is read/measured in comparison with its nonreleased state. The method outlined below describes the application of fluorogenic caspase assays following the induction of apoptosis and/or anoikis (*see* Fig. 10), including within the context of the experimental establishment of a time-course kinetic of caspase activity (*see* Fig. 11a), as well as for evidencing/verifying the resistance to anoikis (if any) displayed by CRC cells (*see* Fig. 11b).

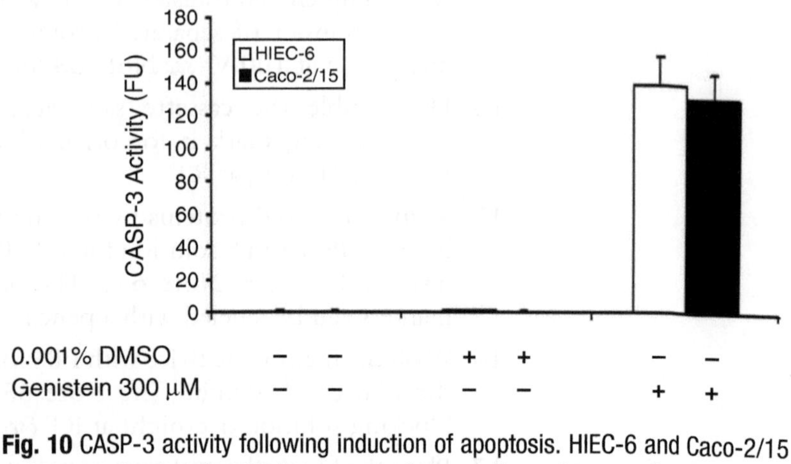

Fig. 10 CASP-3 activity following induction of apoptosis. HIEC-6 and Caco-2/15 cells were treated for 24 h in serum-free medium alone, or in serum-free medium with either 0.001% DMSO or 300 µM genistein. Fluorogenic caspase activity assays (using the CASP-3-specific substrate Ac-DEVD-AFC) were subsequently performed and data was expressed as "CASP-3 Activity (FU)" (±SEM; $n = 3$)

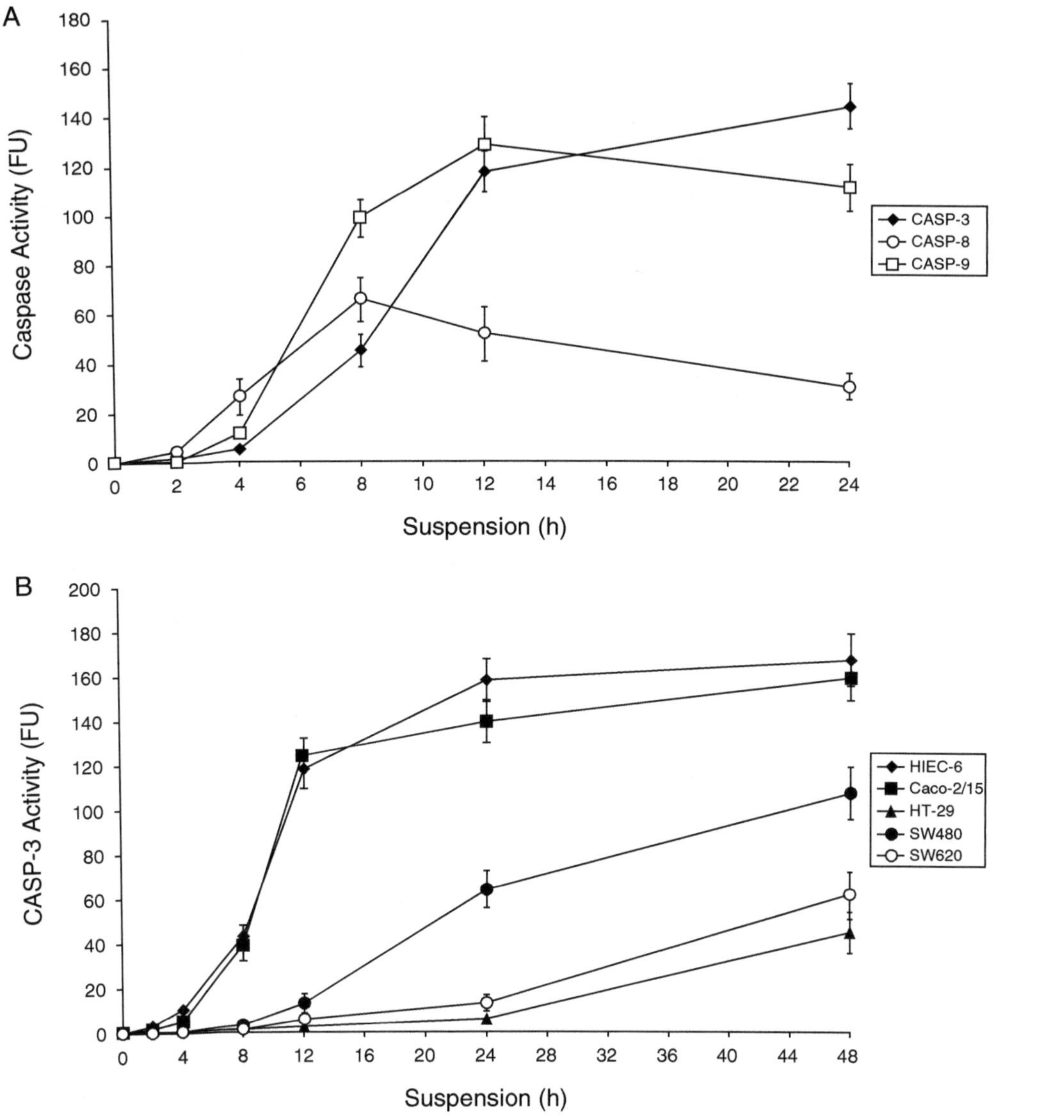

Fig. 11 (**a**) Time-course kinetics of CASP-3, CASP-8, CASP-9 activities following induction of anoikis. Caco-2/15 cells were maintained in suspension 0–24 h in serum-free medium. Fluorogenic caspase activity assays for CASP-3, CASP-8, and CASP-9 (using the specific substrates Ac-DEVD-AFC, Ac-LETD-AFC, or Ac-LEHD-AFC, respectively) were subsequently performed and data was expressed as "Caspase Activity (FU)" (±SEM; $n \geq 3$) (adapted from ref. 46). (**b**) Time-course kinetics of CASP-3 activity following induction of anoikis in normal intestinal epithelial cells and CRC cells. HIEC-6, Caco-2/15, HT-29, SW480, and SW620 cells were maintained in suspension 0–48 h in serum-free medium. Fluorogenic caspase activity assays for CASP-3 (using the specific substrate Ac-DEVD-AFC) were subsequently performed and data was expressed as "CASP-3 Activity (FU)" (±SEM; $n \geq 3$)

3.5.1 Apoptosis Induction

1. For apoptosis induction, seed two 100 mm culture dishes each for HIEC-6 and Caco-2/15 cells. Grow until ~70% confluence.
2. Remove medium and wash twice with serum-free medium (*see* **Note 34**).
3. Add serum-free medium with 0.001% DMSO to the first dish (control), and serum-free medium with 300 μM genistein to the second dishes (experimental) (*see* **Note 34**). Incubate for a further 24 h, under normal culture conditions.
4. For each dish, remove 6/10 of the culture medium and put in sterile 15 mL Falcon™ conical centrifuge tubes, accordingly (*see* **Notes 46** and **70**). Scrape cells off of dishes in the remaining medium, collect and pool with their proper previously recuperated medium (*see* **Note 71**).
5. Centrifuge at 1500 RPM for 5 min, at 4 °C.
6. Remove the medium (*see* **Note 47**) and resuspend cell pellets with 5 mL cold PBS (*see* **Note 3**).
7. Centrifuge at 1500 RPM for 5 min, at 4 °C.
8. Remove PBS, resuspend cell pellets again with 5 mL cold PBS (*see* **Note 3**), and centrifuge again at 1500 RPM for 5 min, at 4 °C.
9. Remove PBS (*see* **Note 47**) and resuspend cell pellets in 200 μL of the lysis buffer (*see* **Note 59**). Transfer each cell lysate to its own 1.5 mL Eppendorf™ microcentrifuge tube and vortex vigorously.
10. Incubate in ice for 30 min; vortex every 5 min.
11. Centrifuge at 15,000 RPM for 5 min, at 4 °C.
12. Transfer the supernatants in new microfuge tubes (*see* **Note 61**).
13. In a sterile 15 mL Falcon™ conical centrifuge tube, mix 1.5 mL of the reaction buffer (*see* **Note 26**), 1.5 mL of the lysis buffer, and 30 μL of 1 M DTT.
14. From the mix, take 7 × 250 μL and put in seven microfuge tubes labeled #1–#7; take 490 μL and put in an eighth microfuge tube, labeled #8.
15. Prepare the AFC standard concentration samples (from microfuge tubes #1–8: 0, 0.3, 0.6, 1.3, 2.5, 5.0, 10.0 and 20.0 μM AFC) as follows: add 10 μL of the 1 mM AFC stock solution to tube #8. Vortex vigorously. Take 250 μL from tube #8 and put it in tube #7. Vortex again. Take 250 μL from tube #7 and put in tube #6, vortex, and so on and so forth, up to tube #2. Leave tube #1 as is (background control).
16. In a 96-well black-bottom microplate, aliquots (105 μL/well) the AFC standard samples #1–8, in duplicate. Keep the microplate on ice and in the dark.

17. Mix 980 μL of the reaction buffer with 20 μL of 1 M DTT (*see* **Note 71**).
18. For each HIEC-6, Caco-2/15 cell sample (in lysis buffer): take 80–100 μg proteins and complete to a volume of 50 μL with lysis buffer (*see* **Note 71**).
19. Retrieve the microplate (with standard curve AFC samples) and transfer the 50 μL-prepared HIEC-6, Caco-2/15 cell samples in their own wells (*see* **Notes 71** and **72**).
20. To each HIEC-6, Caco-2/15 cell sample-containing well, add 50 μL of the reaction buffer + DTT and 5 μL of 1 mM Ac-DEVD-AFC (CASP-3 substrate stock solution) (*see* **Notes 71** and **72**).
21. At the same time, fill two other wells with 50 μL of the lysis buffer, 50 μL of the reaction buffer + DTT, and 5 μL of 1 mM Ac-DEVD-AFC (these are duplicate "nontemplate controls" [NTCs], used for subtracting background from the substrate) (*see* **Notes 71** and **72**).
22. Incubate the microplate in a plate reader spectrophotometer for 60 min, at 37 °C.
23. Read fluorescence every 10 min (λexcitation = 405 nm, λemission = 510 nm) for tested samples and NTCs. Read fluorescence of AFC concentration standards only at the 60 min mark.
24. With the plate reader spectrophotometer's software, process values of tested samples against the averaged AFC standard curve from duplicate standard samples (with averaged values of background "0 μM AFC" and NTC duplicates subtracted). Values are given as "fluorescence units" (FU); express CASP-3 activity as "CASP-3 activity (FU)" (*see* **Note 73**) (*see* Fig. 10) (*see* [46, 49] as additional examples).

3.5.2 Time-Course Kinetic of CASP-8, CASP-9 and CASP-3 Activity Following Anoikis Induction

The following describes the procedure for establishing a time-course kinetic of CASP-8, CASP-9 and CASP-3 activity following induction of anoikis by maintaining Caco2/15 cells in suspension in polyHEMA-coated dishes (time points: 0, 2, 4, 8, 12 and 24 h). Herein, we find that initiator caspase CASP-8 activity emerges before that of initiator caspase CASP-9 which, subsequently, leads to a sharp increase in executioner caspase CASP-3 activity over time—as expected in the case of anoikis [19, 36, 63] (*see* Fig. 11a).

1. Prepare polyHEMA-coated dishes according to **steps 1**–7 of Subheading 3.3.2 above.
2. Seed Caco-2/15 cells in six 100 mm standard tissue culture dishes (*see* **Note 45**). Grow the cultures until ~70% confluence under normal culture conditions.

3. Remove medium and wash once with 5 mL sterile PBS (*see* **Notes 3** and **34**).
4. Trypsinize five of the six cultures with 1 mL trypsin–EDTA solution for 5 min, at 37 °C.
5. To the remaining nontrypsinized culture, add serum-free medium (*see* **Note 34**).
6. Resuspend trypsinized cells (do not pool, keep separate) in 5 mL of medium with serum and transfer in individual sterile 15 mL Falcon™ conical centrifuge tubes.
7. Centrifuge at 1500 RPM for 5 min, at RT.
8. In the meantime, rinse the polyHEMA-coated dishes once with 5 mL serum-free medium (*see* **Notes 34** and **55**).
9. Resuspend each cell pellet in 5 mL serum-free medium.
10. Remove medium from polyHEMA-coated dishes and reseed each resuspended cell pellet into its own polyHEMA-coated dish (*see* **Note 34**).
11. Incubate polyHEMA-seeded ("suspension"; experimental) cultures under normal conditions.
12. For the nontrypsinized cells ("adhering; control; time point: 0 h), recuperate 4/5 of the culture medium in a sterile 15 mL Falcon™ conical centrifuge tube (*see* **Notes 46** and **70**). Scrape cells off of dishes in the remaining medium, collect and pool with their previously recuperated medium (*see* **Note 71**). Then proceed with **steps 5–12** of Subheading 3.5.1 above.
13. For the incubating five suspension cultures, remove one dish at time points 2, 4, 8, 12, and 24 h. For each time point, recuperate all of the medium (which includes the suspended cells, dying-by-anoikis, or otherwise) from the dish in a sterile 15 mL Falcon™ conical centrifuge tube (*see* **Note 71**), then proceed with **steps 5–12** of Subheading 3.5.1 above.
14. Follow **steps 13–16** of Subheading 3.5.1 above for the AFC standard curve and microplate preparations.
15. Mix 4.9 mL of the reaction buffer with 100 μL of 1 M DTT (*see* **Note 71**).
16. For each 0–24 h time point (in lysis buffer): take 80–100 μg proteins and complete to a volume of 50 μL with lysis buffer. Perform this in triplicate for each time point (*see* **Note 71**).
17. Retrieve the microplate (with standard curve AFC samples) and transfer the 50 μL-prepared 0–24 h time point sample triplicates in their own "0–24 h" row of wells (*see* **Notes 71** and **72**).
18. To each row of 0–24 h time point sample-containing wells, add 50 μL of the reaction buffer + DTT, and (1) 5 μL of 1 mM Ac-

DEVD-AFC (CASP-3 substrate; first row), (2) 5 μL of 1 mM Ac-LETD-AFC (CASP-8 substrate; second row), or (3) 5 μL of 1 mM Ac-LEHD-AFC (CASP-9 substrate; third row) (*see* **Notes 71** and **72**).

19. At the same time, fill six other wells with 50 μL of the lysis buffer, 50 μL of the reaction buffer + DTT, and (1) 5 μL of 1 mM Ac-DEVD-AFC (two wells), (2) 5 μL of 1 mM Ac-LETD-AFC (two wells), or (3) 5 μL of 1 mM Ac-LEHD-AFC (two wells) (*see* **Notes 71** and **72**). These are duplicate NTCs for each substrate.
20. Incubate the microplate in a plate reader spectrophotometer for 60 min, at 37 °C.
21. Read fluorescence every 10 min (λexcitation = 405 nm, λemission = 510 nm) for tested samples and NTCs. Read fluorescence of AFC concentration standards only at the 60 min mark.
22. With the plate reader spectrophotometer's software, process values of tested samples against the averaged AFC standard curve from duplicate standard samples (with averaged values of background "0 μM AFC" and NTC duplicates for each substrate subtracted). Values are given as "fluorescence units" (FU); express CASP-3, CASP-8, and/or CASP-9 activity as "Caspase activity (FU)" (*see* **Note 73**) (*see* Fig. 11a) (*see* [46] as additional example).

3.5.3 Time-Course Kinetic of CASP-3 Activity for Evidence of Anoikis Resistance Displayed by CRC Cells

The following describes the procedure for establishing a time-course kinetic of anoikis susceptibility/resistance by maintaining HIEC, as well as CRC Caco2/15, HT-29, SW480, and SW620 cells, in suspension in polyHEMA-coated dishes (time points: 0, 2, 4, 8, 12, 24 and 48 h). Herein, we observe a high anoikis resistance displayed by HT-29 and SW620 CRC cells, a moderate anoikis resistance displayed by SW480 CRC cells, and a "baseline normal" susceptibility to anoikis displayed by HIEC-6 cells, as well as by CRC Caco-2/15 cells (*see* Fig. 11b).

1. Prepare polyHEMA-coated dishes according to **steps 1–7** of Subheading 3.3.2 above.
2. Seed HIEC, Caco-2/15, HT-29, SW480, and SW620 cells each in their own set of seven 100 mm standard tissue culture dishes (*see* **Note 45**). Grow the cultures until ~70% confluence under normal culture conditions.
3. Remove medium and wash once with 5 mL sterile PBS (*see* **Notes 3** and **34**).
4. For HIEC, Caco-2/15, HT-29, SW480, and SW620 cells, trypsinize six of the seven cultures with 1 mL trypsin–EDTA solution for 5 min, at 37 °C.

5. To the remaining nontrypsinized cultures, add serum-free medium (*see* **Note 34**).
6. Resuspend trypsinized cells (do not pool, keep separate) in 5 mL of medium with serum and transfer in individual sterile 15 mL Falcon™ conical centrifuge tubes.
7. Centrifuge at 1500 RPM for 5 min, at RT.
8. In the meantime, rinse the polyHEMA-coated dishes once with 5 mL serum-free medium (*see* **Notes 34** and **55**).
9. Resuspend each cell pellet in 5 mL serum-free medium.
10. Remove medium from polyHEMA-coated dishes and reseed each resuspended cell pellet into its own polyHEMA-coated dish (*see* **Note 34**). Incubate polyHEMA-seeded ("suspension"; experimentals) cultures under normal conditions.
11. For the nontrypsinized ("adhering; control; time point: 0 h), individually recuperate 4/5 of the culture medium in a sterile 15 mL Falcon™ conical centrifuge tube (*see* **Notes 46** and **70**). Scrape cells off of dishes in the remaining medium, collect and pool with their previously recuperated medium (*see* **Note 71**). Then proceed with **steps 5–12** of Subheading 3.5.1 above.
12. For the incubating six suspension cultures for each of HIEC, Caco-2/15, HT-29, SW480 and SW620 cells, remove one dish at time points 2, 4, 8, 12, 24, and 48 h. For each time point for each cell line, recuperate all of the medium (which includes the suspended cells, dying-by-anoikis or otherwise) from the dish in a sterile 15 mL Falcon™ conical centrifuge tube (*see* **Note 71**), then proceed with **steps 5–12** of Subheading 3.5.1 above.
13. Follow **steps 13–16** of Subheading 3.5.1 above for the AFC standard curve and microplate preparations.
14. Mix 9.8 mL of the reaction buffer with 200 μL of 1 M DTT (*see* **Note 71**).
15. For each 0–48 h time point (in lysis buffer) of each cell line: take 80–100 μg proteins and complete to a volume of 50 μL with lysis buffer (*see* **Note 71**).
16. Retrieve the microplate (with standard curve AFC samples) and transfer the 50 μL-prepared 0–48 h time point samples of each cell line in their own "0–48 h" row of wells (*see* **Notes 71** and **72**).
17. To each row of 0–48 h time point sample-containing wells of each cell line, add 50 μL of the reaction buffer + DTT, and 5 μL of 1 mM Ac-DEVD-AFC (CASP-3 substrate) (*see* **Notes 71** and **72**).
18. Then follow **steps 21–23** of Subheading 3.5.1 above.

19. With the plate reader spectrophotometer's software, process values of tested samples against the averaged AFC standard curve from duplicate standard samples (with averaged values of background "0 μM AFC" and NTC duplicates for the substrate subtracted). Values are given as "fluorescence units" (FU); express CASP-3 activity as "Caspase activity (FU)" (*see* **Note 73**) (*see* Fig. 11b).

4 Notes

1. This medium is used for Caco-2/15, HT-29, SW480, and SW620 cells.
2. This medium is used for HIEC-6 cells.
3. Stock solution is autoclaved and thereafter stored at 4 °C (for a maximum of 6 months).
4. Prepare a stock solution of 5 mg/mL poly-L-lysine hydrobromide in autoclaved PBS within a culture hood, divide the stock solution into 60 μL in autoclaved 0.5 mL Eppendorf™ snap-cap microcentrifuge tubes (Sigma-Aldrich), and then store at −20 °C (for a maximum of 3 months). The working solution stipulated in the item consists of further diluting aliquots of the stock solution in autoclaved, bidistilled H_2O.
5. The processing of obtained tissues for OCT-embedding and subsequent cryostat sectioning has been described elsewhere [32, 64]. Because this method falls out of scope of the crux of the present chapter (i.e., apoptosis, anoikis detection methods), only the materials are listed herein.
6. The processing and subsequent organotypic/explant culture of obtained tissues, as well as their OCT-embedding and cryostat sectioning, has been described elsewhere [47, 48]. Because this method falls out of scope of the crux of the present chapter (i.e., apoptosis, anoikis detection methods), only the materials are listed herein.
7. Aluminum holders containing OCT and specimens are set on aluminum cups that float over the liquid nitrogen—nitrogen vapors are responsible for the cryo-freezing of embedded specimens. Cryo-embedded specimens are thereafter stored at −80 °C.
8. Genistein is a pan-inhibitor of protein tyrosine kinase activity [65]. For the purpose of the present chapter, this pharmacological compound was used to induce caspase-dependent apoptosis. Incidentally, genistein exposure (of cell, explant cultures) is useful as a positive control for caspase-dependent apoptosis.

9. Divide stock solution into 10 μL aliquots and store at −20 °C (for a maximum of 6 months).
10. Stock solution is stored at 4 °C (for a maximum of 6 months).
11. Always freshly prepared.
12. Stock solution is stored at RT.
13. Divide stock solution into 1 mL aliquots in 1.5 mL Eppendorf™ snap-cap microcentrifuge tubes (Sigma-Aldrich). Centrifuge aliquots 10,000 RPM, 5 min, RT. Store supernatants at 4 °C (for a maximum of 2 weeks).
14. DAPI is light sensitive. Stock solution is divided into 5 μL aliquots and thereafter stored at −20 °C (for a maximum of 1 year) in an aluminum foil-covered container.
15. Prepare an Evans Blue 1% (w/v) in PBS (pH 7.4) stock solution, filter it through a Whatman® Grade 4 filter paper (Sigma-Aldrich), and thereafter store at RT in an opaque container (for a maximum of 1 year). The working solution stipulated in the item consists of diluting the 1% stock solution into a 0.01% one, still in PBS (pH 7.4).
16. Paraphenylenediamine is light sensitive. Divide stock solution into 50 μL aliquots and store at −80 °C (for a maximum of 1 year) in an aluminum foil-covered container.
17. Prepare a stock solution of 2% (w/v) Triton™ X-100 in autoclaved, bidistilled H_2O and store at 4 °C (for a maximum of 1 month). The working solution stipulated in the item consists of diluting the 2% stock solution into a 0.2% one in TE buffer. The working solution is always freshly prepared and kept on ice before use.
18. A stock solution of 5 M NaCl (Thermo Fisher Scientific) in autoclaved, bidistilled H_2O is prepared. The working solution stipulated in the item consists of diluting the 5 M stock solution into a 50 mM one in TE buffer.
19. This is the 1× working solution. Prepare a 10× stock solution and store at RT. The working solution is freshly prepared by diluting the stock solution to 1× with bidistilled H_2O.
20. This is the 1× working solution. Prepare a 50× stock solution, sterilize it by autoclave and thereafter store at 4 °C. The working solution is freshly prepared by diluting the stock solution to 1× with bidistilled H_2O.
21. A thin layer of isopropanol is laid over the already-poured separating gel mixture (between the glass plates). This allows the separating gel to polymerize while preventing its dehydration. Once polymerization is completed, the isopropanol is carefully removed and the top of the polymerized separating

gel is gently washed with bidistilled H_2O, before the overlaying of the stacking gel mixture.

22. Buffer solution is chilled to 4 °C prior to usage.
23. Primary antibodies are diluted in the same solution as the blocking solution.
24. Secondary antibodies are diluted 1/5000 in the same solution as the blocking solution, minus the sodium azide.
25. Solution is chilled to 4 °C and kept on ice, prior to usage.
26. Prepare in advance the reaction buffer and store it at 4 °C (for a maximum of 3 months).
27. AFC is light sensitive. Stock solution is divided into 50 μL aliquots and thereafter stored at −20 °C (for a maximum of 6 months) in an aluminum foil-covered container.
28. The 10 mM storage stock solutions are divided into 10 μl aliquots and stored at −80 °C (for a maximum of 1 year) in an aluminum foil-covered container. Working-stock solutions consist in diluting 10 mM storage-stock solution aliquots to 1 mM in DMSO, in turn divided into 25 μl aliquots and stored at −20 °C (for a maximum of 6 months), again in an aluminum foil-covered container.
29. The in vivo use of ISEL outlined herein can be applied also for cryo-embedded adult intestine/colon tissue specimens, including biopsies of physiopathologies (e.g., CRC). When dealing with small intestinal samples, one must keep in mind that the embedding process invariably results in transverse sections bearing villi that are often cut at various angles, with their apex (where exfoliation by normally anoikis occurs for 1–3 cells at this location; *see* Fig. 1b as example) not available for ISEL staining—thus giving the false impression that only a few villi are positive for ISEL.
30. This is performed in a humidity chamber.
31. Although the ApopTag® kit supplies its own blocking solution for this specific step, we found that 10% Blotto works better for the anti-DIG antibody.
32. Evans Blue staining reduces background appreciatively when viewing fluorescence with an FITC filter.
33. Prior to this step, nuclei staining with DAPI may be performed, if desired.
34. This is performed under a culture hood.
35. Use extreme care of not causing the coverslips to move/displace and/or to accidentally aspirate cells.
36. Turn on the hood's UV lights to ensure preservation of sterility.

37. The coverslips should easily adhere to the microscope slides via capillarity, thanks to their humid undersides.
38. Extreme care must be taken to cover the coverslip with the solution without: (1) spilling the solution over the coverslip, which will leave it unstably set, if not floating/moving, on the microscope slide, in addition to diminishing the effect of the solution by loss of volume exposure to the cells; and (2) causing a fluid shear stress that will displace/wash away the cells.
39. All shades of ISEL-positive staining (from weak to blindingly bright) must be counted, as these represent various stages of advancement into the apoptotic process following its induction.
40. Normal, healthy cell cultures will display apoptotic indices between 0 and 9%. Greater indices means that the cell culture has become unhealthy (e.g., too many passages) and, therefore, fresh cells must be thawed from cryogenized stocks to restart cultures from younger passages.
41. The FITC-coupled Annexin V is light sensitive. All steps must be performed in the dark.
42. The kit-supplied propidium iodide (PI) dye may be added to the mix if desired (equal volume as that of FITC-coupled Annexin V). Cells that have lost plasma membrane integrity (i.e., death by something other than apoptosis) will take up the dye and consequently display red fluorescence staining under a lissamine rhodamine filter (however, if PI staining is used, then a subsequent Evans Blue staining must be avoided, since the latter likewise fluoresces under a lissamine rhodamine filter).
43. When cells are spread and nonpolarized, Annexin V binding tends to predominate overwhelmingly around/about the position of the nuclei of cells.
44. Staining with Annexin V is generally rather weak and diffuse, and typically lacking any sharpness to it. Nonetheless, all shades of Annexin V-positive staining must be counted, as these represent various stages of advancement into the apoptotic process following its induction.
45. Typically, two 100 mm culture dishes of CRC cells (such as Caco-2/15 cells which, in this case, are hypertetraploid) are required per treatment (and controls), in order to obtain sufficient DNA laddering to visualize. However, HIEC-6 being normal and diploid, the number of dishes must be doubled.
46. The medium invariably contains apoptotic cells and apoptotic bodies (*see* Fig. 12 as example).
47. Extreme care must be given to not disturb/dissociate the pellet.
48. The final concentration of RNase A should be 60–70 μg/mL.

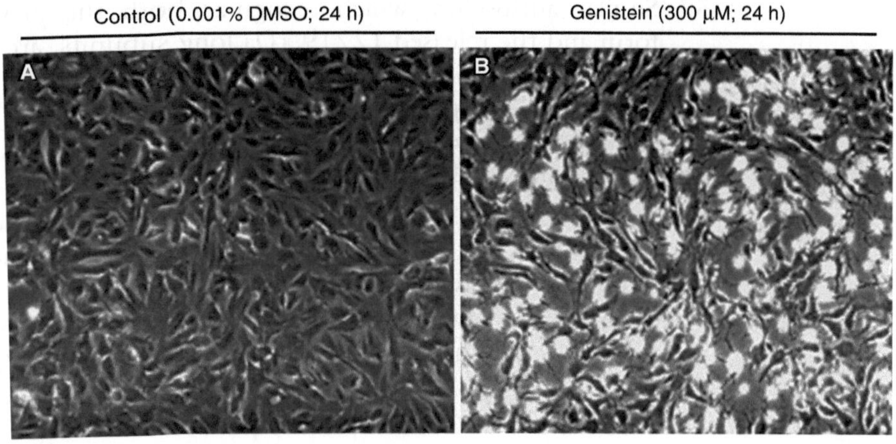

Fig. 12 Cell cultures undergoing apoptosis exhibit numerous, floating apoptotic cells and apoptotic bodies. Representative phase contrast micrographs of HIEC-6 cells following 24 h treatment in serum-free medium with either (**a**) 0.001% DMSO, or (**b**) 300 μM genistein ($n \geq 3$). Floating apoptotic cells and bodies are refractory to light under phase contrast (*see* also ref. 54 for additional examples). Original magnification: 20×

49. The final concentration of SDS should be 0.5%.
50. The final concentration of Proteinase K should be 150 μg/mL.
51. Adding EtBr at this step allows for a "prebinding" of EtBr to the isolated DNA, subsequently increasing the staining signal under UV following DNA agarose gel electrophoresis.
52. When the apoptotic process is sufficiently advanced, the degradation of genomic DNA (by DNases other than CAD) will have already well begun. Hence, the CAD-produced DNA laddering will appear smeared/diffuse (*see* Fig. 7 as example).
53. Use an opaque container with a lid. PolyHEMA is sensitive to air humidity, so extreme care must be given to avoid hydration. Dissolve overnight in 100% ethanol with lid on opaque container. If dissolution appears incomplete after that time, add minimum heat to help the dissolution process to complete.
54. Numerous polyHEMA-coated culture dishes may be prepared in advance. After sealing with Parafilm, store coated dishes at 4 °C (for a maximum of 1 month).
55. If using polyHEMA-coated dishes prepared in advance and stored (*see* **Note 54**), coated dishes should be taken out and kept under the culture hood to allow them to return to RT before use.
56. Some of such commercially available anti-activated CASP-3 antibodies are also usable for indirect immunofluorescence studies in cell cultures and/or tissues, thus adding to the arsenal of tools to evidence caspase-dependent apoptosis in situ, ex vivo, or in cellulo.

57. Similar antibodies, which recognize both the pro-CASP-3 form and the released 17/19 kDa long subunits, are available commercially [61]. Furthermore, other antibodies that are directed to the proform and/or released long and/or short subunits for other caspases (CASP-8, CASP-9, etc.), are likewise commercially available.
58. In contrast to DNA laddering assays, only one 100 mm dish is needed here per control or apoptosis-inducing treatment. The same goes with regard to maintaining cells in suspension (poly-HEMA). This applies to HIEC-6 as well as to CRC cells.
59. For HIEC-6 cells only, it is 200 μL. For Caco-2/15 cells, 350 μL is required. For other CRC cell lines such as HT-29, SW480, or SW620, 550 μL is required instead.
60. Cut ends of pipette tips for wider openings, as the lysates are viscous at this stage. During heating, vortex samples regularly every minute or so.
61. Samples may be stored at −80 °C for long-term storage. However, too many freeze–thaw cycles should be avoided.
62. Apply vacuum for 5 min to reduce solubilized oxygen, then add the APS and TEMED.
63. Typically, for the Mini-Protean® electrotransfer system, the time required for the transfer is 30–45 min for ≥45 kDa proteins, 60 min for 50–85 kDa proteins, and 75 min for 85–125 kDa proteins.
64. This allows the verification of the success of the electrotransfer. To this effect, pay attention to the molecular weight area (with help from the protein molecular weight markers) of your protein(s) of interest that are to be probed subsequently by Western blotting.
65. All Ponceau S staining must be neutralized/washed away. Add one or two, additional 5 min PBS washes if needed.
66. Either in a sealed plastic bag or in a covered container (to prevent dehydration).
67. Alternately, place a plastic sheet-covered membrane in an X-ray film cassette in a darkroom, place a film over it and expose suitably (usually a few seconds to a 1–5 min).
68. Semiquantitative, densitometric analyses may be performed, especially when a reference protein (e.g., β-actin; *see* Fig. 9) is used.
69. Pan and/or specific caspase inhibitors may also be used [66]. However, caution with regard to the timing of their use, following induction of apoptosis/anoikis, must be taken into consideration [3, 4, 9, 19].
70. Keep in ice.

71. This must be performed on ice.
72. Work as fast as possible to avoid as much light-driven AFC fluorescence quenching as possible.
73. Alternately, the software allows for the calculation of the release of AFC from the caspase substrate as "μM AFC/μg protein" (which can be done manually as well), given the slope of the averaged AFC standard curve with the averaged background/NTC values subtracted appropriately. Yet another means of expressing the data is by comparing experimental to their respective control, ×100 (expressed as "Relative Caspase Activity (% of Control").

Acknowledgments

The author thanks Rona K. Graham (Département de pharmacologie-physiologie, FMSS, U. de Sherbrooke), for access to the LI-Cor Odyssey Fc imaging system and the VICTOR X multilabel plate reader spectrophotometer, and Jean-François Beaulieu (Département d'anatomie et de biologie cellulaire, FMSS, U. de Sherbrooke) for the generous gift of the HIEC-6, Caco-2/15, and HT-29 cell lines. This work was supported in part by a grant from the Natural Sciences and Engineering Research Council (NSERC) of Canada (RGPIN 227935-2013). The author is a Researcher of the Canadian Foundation for Innovation (CFI) and a member of the FRQS-funded Centre de Recherche du CHUS.

References

1. Edinger AL, Thompson CB (2004) Death by design: apoptosis, necrosis and autophagy. Curr Opin Cell Biol 16:663–669
2. Eroglu M, Derry WB (2016) Your neighbours matter - non-autonomous control of apoptosis in development and disease. Cell Death Differ 23:1110–1118
3. Galluzzi L, Bravo-San Pedro JM, Vitale I et al (2015) Essential versus accessory aspects of cell death: recommendations of the NCCD 2015. Cell Death Differ 22:58–73
4. Galluzzi L, Vitale I, Abrams JM et al (2012) Molecular definitions of cell death subroutines: recommendations of the Nomenclature Committee on Cell Death 2012. Cell Death Differ 19:107–120
5. Penaloza C, Orlanski S, Ye Y et al (2008) Cell death in mammalian development. Curr Pharm Des 14:184–196
6. Tait SW, Ichim G, Green DR (2014) Die another way--non-apoptotic mechanisms of cell death. J Cell Sci 127:2135–2144
7. Berghe TV, Linkermann A, Jouan-Lanhouet S et al (2014) Regulated necrosis: the expanding network of non-apoptotic cell death pathways. Nat Rev Mol Cell Biol 15:135–147
8. Eisenberg-Lerner A, Bialik S, Simon HU et al (2009) Life and death partners: apoptosis, autophagy and the cross-talk between them. Cell Death Differ 16:966–975
9. Kroemer G, Galluzzi L, Vandenabeele P et al (2009) Classification of cell death: recommendations of the Nomenclature Committee on Cell Death 2009. Cell Death Differ 16:3–11
10. Kroemer G, Martin SJ (2005) Caspase-independent cell death. Nat Med 11:725–730
11. Srivastava R (ed) (2007) Apoptosis, cell signaling and human diseases (molecular mechanisms, Vol. 1). Humana Press, Totowa
12. Srivastava R (ed) (2007) Apoptosis, cell signaling and human diseases (molecular mechanisms, Vol. 2). Humana Press, Totowa
13. Bertrand K (2011) Survival of exfoliated epithelial cells: a delicate balance between anoikis

and apoptosis. J Biomed Biotechnol 2011:534139
14. Gilmore AP (2005) Anoikis. Cell Death Differ 12:1473–1477
15. Gilmore AP, Owens TW, Foster FM et al (2009) How adhesion signals reach a mitochondrial conclusion - ECM regulation of apoptosis. Curr Opin Cell Biol 21:654–661
16. Horbinski C, Mojesky C, Kyprianou N (2010) Live free or die: tales of homeless (cells) in cancer. Am J Pathol 177:1044–1052
17. Ma Z, Liu Z, Myers DP et al (2008) Mechanotransduction and anoikis: death and the homeless cell. Cell Cycle 7:2462–2465
18. Taddei ML, Giannoni E, Fiaschi T et al (2012) Anoikis: an emerging hallmark in health and diseases. J Pathol 226:380–393
19. Vachon PH (2011) Integrin signalling, cell survival, and anoikis: distinctions, differences, and differentiation. J Signal Transduct 2011:738137
20. Vaux DL, Korsmeyer SJ (1999) Cell death in development. Cell 96:245–254
21. Marastoni S, Ligresti G, Lorenzon E et al (2008) Extracellular matrix: a matter of life and death. Connect Tissue Res 49:203–206
22. Murray P, Edgar D (2000) Regulation of programmed cell death by basement membranes in embryonic development. J Cell Biol 150:1215–1221
23. Chiarugi P, Giannoni E (2008) Anoikis: a necessary death program for anchorage-dependent cells. Biochem Pharmacol 76:1352–1364
24. Dagenais M, Douglas T, Saleh M (2014) Role of programmed necrosis and cell death in intestinal inflammation. Curr Opin Gastroenterol 30:566–575
25. Edelblum KL, Yan F, Yamaoka T, Polk PB (2006) Regulation of apoptosis during homeostasis and disease in the intestinal epithelium. Inflamm Bowel Dis 12:413–424
26. Günther C, Buchen B, Neurath MF et al (2014) Regulation and pathophysiological role of epithelial turnover in the gut. Semin Cell Dev Biol 35:40–50
27. Günther C, Neumann H, Neurath MF et al (2013) Apoptosis, necrosis and necroptosis: cell death regulation in the intestinal epithelium. Gut 62:1062–1071
28. Ménard D, Beaulieu JF, Boudreau F et al (2005) Gastrointestinal tract (GI tract). In: Unsicker K, Krieglstein K (eds) Cell signalling and growth factors in development - part II. - Wiley-VCH, Verlag
29. Negroni A, Cucchiara S, Stronati L (2015) Apoptosis, necrosis, and necroptosis in the gut and intestinal homeostasis. Mediat Inflamm 2015:250762
30. Potten CS (1997) Epithelial cell growth and differentiation. II. Intestinal apoptosis. Am J Phys 273:G253–G2577
31. Tarnawski AS, Szabo I (2001) Apoptosis-programmed cell death and its relevance to gastrointestinal epithelium: survival signal from the matrix. Gastroenterology 120:294–299
32. Vachon PH, Cardin E, Harnois C et al (2000) Early establishment of epithelial apoptosis in the developing human small intestine. Int J Dev Biol 44:891–898
33. West NJ, Courtney ED, Poullis AP et al (2009) Apoptosis in the colonic crypt, colorectal adenomata, and manipulation by chemoprevention. Cancer Epidemiol Biomark Prev 18:1680–1687
34. Shanmugathasan M, Jothy S (2000) Apoptosis, anoikis and their relevance to the pathobiology of colon cancer. Pathol Int 50:273–279
35. Buchheit CL, Weigel KJ, Schafer ZT (2014) Cancer cell survival during detachment from the ECM: multiple barriers to tumour progression. Nat Rev Cancer 14:632–641
36. Frisch SM, Schaller M, Cieply B (2013) Mechanisms that link the oncogenic epithelial-mesenchymal transition to suppression of anoikis. J Cell Sci 126:21–29
37. Guadamillas MC, Cerezo C, del Pozo MA (2011) Overcoming anoikis - pathways to anchorage independent growth in cancer. J Cell Sci 124:3189–3197
38. Paoli P, Giannoni E, Chiarugi P (2013) Anoikis molecular pathways and its role in cancer progression. Biochim Biophys Acta 1833:3481–3498
39. Crotti S, Piccoli M, Rizzolio F et al (2017) Extracellular matrix and colorectal cancer: how surrounding microenvironment affects cancer cell behavior? J Cell Physiol 232:967–975
40. Beaulieu J-F, Ménard D (2012) Isolation, characterization, and culture of normal human intestinal crypt and villus cells. Methods Mol Biol 806:157–173
41. Perreault N, Beaulieu J-F (1996) A novel method for the establishment of a pure population of nontransformed human intestinal primary epithelial cell (HIPEC) lines in long term culture. Exp Cell Res 224:354–364
42. Perreault N, Beaulieu J-F (1998) Primary cultures of fully differentiated and pure human intestinal epithelial cells. Exp Cell Res 245:34–42

43. Beaulieu J-F, Quaroni A (1991) Clonal analysis of sucrase-isomaltase expression in the human colon adenocarcinoma Caco-2 cells. Biochem J 280:599–608
44. Pageot LP, Perreault N, Basora N et al (2000) Human cell models to study small intestinal functions: recapitulation of the crypt-villus axis. Microsc Res Tech 49:394–406
45. Gavrieli Y, Sherman Y, Ben-Sasson SA (1992) Identification of programmed cell death in situ via specific labeling of nuclear DNA fragmentation. J Cell Biol 119:493–501
46. Beauséjour M, Thibodeau S, Demers MJ et al (2013) Suppression of anoikis in human intestinal epithelial cells: differentiation state-selective roles of α2β1, α3β1, α5β1, and α6β4 integrins. BMC Cell Biol 14:53
47. Lévy E, Delvin E, Ménard D et al (2009) Functional development of human fetal gastrointestinal tract. Methods Mol Biol 550:205–224
48. Gauthier R, Laprise P, Cardin E et al (2001) Differential sensitivity to apoptosis between the human small and large intestinal mucosae: linkage with segment-specific regulation of BCL-2 homologs and involvement of signaling pathways. J Cell Biochem 82:339–355
49. Beauséjour M, Noël D, Thibodeau S et al (2012) Integrin/Fak/Src-mediated regulation of cell survival and anoikis in human intestinal epithelial crypt cells: selective engagement and roles of PI3-K isoform complexes. Apoptosis 17:566–578
50. Bouchard V, Demers MJ, Thibodeau S et al (2007) Fak/Src signaling in human intestinal epithelial cell survival and anoikis: differentiation state-specific uncoupling with the PI3-K/Akt-1 and MEK/Erk pathways. J Cell Physiol 212:717–728
51. Bouchard V, Harnois C, Demers MJ (2008) β1 integrin/Fak/Src signaling in intestinal epithelial crypt cell survival: integration of complex regulatory mechanisms. Apoptosis 13:531–542
52. Demers MJ, Thibodeau S, Noël D et al (2009) Intestinal epithelial cancer cell anoikis resistance: EGFR-mediated sustained activation of Src overrides Fak-dependent signaling to MEK/Erk and/or PI3-K/Akt-1. J Cell Biochem 107:639–654
53. Gauthier R, Harnois C, Drolet JF et al (2001) Human intestinal epithelial cell survival: differentiation state-specific control mechanisms. Am J Physiol Cell Physiol 280:C1540–C1554
54. Harnois C, Demers MJ, Bouchard V et al (2004) Human intestinal epithelial crypt cell survival and death: complex modulations of Bcl-2 homologs by Fak, PI3-K/Akt-1, MEK/Erk, and p38 signaling pathways. J Cell Physiol 198(2):209–222
55. Klöditz K, Chen YZ, Xue D et al (2017) Programmed cell clearance: from nematodes to humans. Biochem Biophys Res Commun 482:491–497
56. Frisch SM (2000) Anoikis. Methods Enzymol 322:472–479
57. Bursch W, Kleine L, Tenniswood M (1990) The biochemistry of cell death. Biochem Cell Biol 68:1071–1074
58. Benoit YD, Larrivée JF, Groulx JF et al (2010) Integrin alpha8beta1 confers anoikis susceptibility to human intestinal epithelial crypt cells. Biochem Biophys Res Commun 399:434–439
59. Julien O, Wells JA (2017) Caspases and their substrates. Cell Death Differ 24 (8):1380–1389. https://doi.org/10.1038/cdd.2017.44
60. Chaitanya GV, Alexander JS, Babu PP (2010) PARP-1 cleavage fragments: signatures of cell-death proteases in neurodegeneration. Cell Commun Signal 8:31
61. Dufour G, Demers MJ, Gagné D et al (2004) Human intestinal epithelial cell survival and anoikis. Differentiation state-distinct regulation and roles of protein kinase B/Akt isoforms. J Biol Chem 279:44113–44122
62. Vachon PH, Harnois C, Grenier A et al (2002) Differentiation state-selective roles of p38 isoforms in human intestinal epithelial cell anoikis. Gastroenterology 123:1980–1991
63. Fiandalo MV, Kyprianou N (2012) Caspase control: protagonists of cancer cell apoptosis. Exp Oncol 34:165–175
64. Vachon PH, Cardin E, Harnois C et al (2001) Early acquisition of bowel segment-specific Bcl-2 expression profiles during the development of the human ileum and colon. Histol Histopathol 16:497–510
65. Anderson P (1997) Kinase cascades regulating entry into apoptosis. Microbiol Mol Biol Rev 61:33–46
66. Francoeur C, Escaffit F, Vachon PH et al (2004) Proinflammatory cytokines TNF-alpha and IFN-gamma alter laminin expression under an apoptosis-independent mechanism in human intestinal epithelial cells. Am J Physiol Gastrointest Liver Physiol 287:G592–G598

Check for updates

Chapter 8

Molecular Analysis of the Microbiome in Colorectal Cancer

Fiona Clegg, Susan H. Berry, Richard Hansen, and Georgina L. Hold

Abstract

The human gut microbiota plays a major role in the development of colorectal cancer (CRC). Many studies have attempted to define links between microbiota residents, their function and disease development. We now have incredible molecular tools to allow us to study the gut microbiome however in order to make best use of these sophisticated approaches we need to ensure that samples are collected and processed using standardized and reproducible protocols. Here we provide an overview of molecular analysis methods and describe protocols for collecting and processing clinical samples for subsequent microbiome analysis.

Key words Colorectal cancer, Microbiome, Microbial diversity, Clinical samples, Stool, Biopsy, DNA, RNA, Bacteria, Fungi, Molecular microbiology

1 Introduction

Early attempts at microbial research which linked the gut microbiota with CRC were published by Weisburger in 1975 [1]. Subsequently links between the gut microbiota and CRC have focussed around the understanding that in difference to other cancers where a single causative agent has been defined, such as the case of *Helicobacter pylori* induced gastric cancer, the contribution of gut microbes to CRC is explained as due to the presence of dysbiosis, an altered gut microbial community which exhibits pro-carcinogenic features leading to cancer [2–4]. Studies have also identified links between pathogenic bacteria and CRC including *Streptococcus gallolyticus* [5], *Fusobacterium nucleatum* [6], enterotoxigenic *Bacteroides fragilis* [7], and *E. coli* [8–10].

Culture work was the mainstay of microbial research until the advent of culture-independent, molecular methods. The main strength of culture studies remains the ability to work with an isolate of a single organism rather than inferred data from a pool of organisms. Although hampered by important biases, culture studies still have an important role in CRC research and we now more than ever realize the necessity of having

Jean-François Beaulieu (ed.), *Colorectal Cancer: Methods and Protocols*, Methods in Molecular Biology, vol. 1765, https://doi.org/10.1007/978-1-4939-7765-9_8,

cultured gut isolates to allow us to validate the findings from molecular-based analyses.

1.1 Molecular-Based Assessment of the Microbiota

The study of microbial diversity should involve the examination of all microbes within an ecosystem. Nevertheless, studies are generally confined to a single kingdom such as bacteria or fungi with the study of the gut virome lagging behind due to lack of established techniques and reference databases. Molecular assessment of bacterial and fungal diversity generally interrogates ribosomal genes which contain both highly conserved and highly variably DNA region [11]. Conventionally, bacterial diversity is based on the 16S ribosomal RNA gene and the 18S or ITS region for fungal diversity. The conserved regions allow the design of polymerase chain reaction (PCR) primers that will align with all known sequences. The variable regions allow phylogenetic identification of an organism based on interspecies variability in the corresponding sequence. These are generated through comprehensive database searches against known organisms, using publically accessible databases. An important caveat of PCR-based identification of organisms is that positive results reflect detection of DNA only, and this could theoretically be present as a result of environmental contamination or foodborne DNA. Therefore combining PCR-based studies with other approaches that allow direct visualization of organisms in situ such as fluorescent hybridization can offer reassurance that potentially viable whole organisms are also present in the sample [12].

Pattern-based assessment methods are perhaps the easiest and least expensive modalities for bacterial diversity assessment. Generally, these studies utilize PCR-amplified DNA—focused on a suitable gene for diversity studies. Such approaches can allow differences in microbial communities, reflected as microbial DNA fingerprints, within individuals or samples, without providing sufficient detail to be able to attribute identity of microbial constituents. As sequencing technologies have become more financially accessible, the use of pattern-based assessment has diminished. Nevertheless, for a while the approach was used frequently to visualize biogeography studies or sequential/time course microbial profiles [13, 14].

1.2 Sequencing Based Approaches to Assessing Microbial Diversity

Applying formal identification methods to a diverse microbial community remains challenging, but with recent technological advances, it is becoming increasingly straightforward, automated, and affordable. Now the main consideration when embarking on such approaches needs to be whether sufficient bioinformatics support exists to handle the vast amounts of data that are inevitably generated. This is a huge step away from the traditional clinical sample laboratory setup with effective setups now requiring state of the art wet-labs and a corresponding computational facility to be most effective.

The conventional approach to microbial diversity analysis utilizes PCR to amplify an appropriate gene (16S rRNA for bacteria or 18S/ITS for fungal diversity). For the purposes of explanation, we will discuss this in relation to 16S rRNA gene studies, which remain the most common approach. When applied to a mixed pool of DNA from a complex microbial community, a 16S rRNA PCR will amplify the corresponding gene region from all bacteria present [15]. Key assumptions that are conventionally made, but which may be of importance, are, firstly, that the DNA from all bacteria are fully extracted and available for PCR within the sample, and, secondly, that bacterial DNA will be amplified in an unbiased manner in the resultant reaction. The resultant PCR product will therefore theoretically contain a mixture of DNA that correspond broadly to the mixture of organisms present in the original sample.

Until the early 2000s the approach to assessing microbial diversity from PCR amplified samples was by inserting PCR amplicons into a competent bacterial host cell by use of a vector, then utilizing bacterial culture to clonally expand the original DNA strand which could then be subjected to sequence analysis and phylogenetic assignation [16, 17]. Next-generation sequencing (NGS) has essentially replaced cloning based approaches to studying microbial diversity and are now affordable considerations for most laboratories. NGS utilises the same approach of PCR amplification of the 16S rRNA gene; however, the primers used contain sequences that allow the binding of single strands of DNA to beads during sequencing. These beads then drop into physically separated reservoirs on the sequencer and are subjected to independent PCR and sequencing thereafter [18]. This technology was initially hampered by short sequence reads, but can now comfortably sequence 500+bp products with further increases beyond 1 Kbp already predicted.

The main limitation of large-scale NGS and its predecessors however is that they provide a qualitative viewpoint on microbial diversity and there is now much more consideration for quantitative information on microbial composition. Customized phylogenetic microarrays have been designed for the identification and importantly quantification of microbes from a sample, but the caveat to these methods is that they rely on existing knowledge to design probe sequences. Essentially you need to know what you are looking to measure before you start. Approaches to quantitative measurement of gut microbe communities include the human intestinal tract chip (HITchip) [19]. This approach has compared favourably with next-generation sequencing [20]. Finally, real-time quantitative PCR is another method of performing microbial identification in combination with quantification. Again, this method requires primers directed against specific bacteria or groupings of bacteria and hence is perhaps best used to provide supportive quantitative data in conjunction with a broader diversity approach [21, 22].

1.3 Looking Beyond Who Is There: What Are They Doing

In recent years, the understanding that microbial function capabilities is actually more important to assess rather than just knowing what microorganisms are present has become apparent. The advent of metagenomics and metatranscriptomics now offers the reality of unraveling the functional capabilities of the microbiota in relation to CRC. Metagenomics describes the sequencing of all genomic content within a given sample and is a DNA-based methodology. The drawback of metagenomics is that redundant, evolutionarily conserved but functionally unimportant/inactive genes are weighted based on abundance alone as for all other genes. Metatranscriptomics addresses this issue by describing only transcribed genes within a given population and is thus based on RNA rather than DNA. Both techniques require very broad sequencing and generally use a "shotgun" approach to next-generation sequencing where the original sample DNA (or RNA converted back to DNA) is randomly broken into short sequences that are then directly sequenced without any selective PCR amplification [23, 24]. This approach helps add confidence to the breadth and nonselective nature of these methods, but results in a fundamental difficulty when examining a diverse ecosystem such as the colonic mucosa or human faeces. In either of these samples, there will be a mixture of human, bacterial, fungal, viral, and possibly foodborne nucleotide sequences. If we were to assume a metagenomic study of the mucosally adherent bacteria in CRC, we would have no option but to sequence all of the DNA present from each of these potential sources, some of which (particularly the human constituent) may heavily outweigh our DNA of interest within the sample. Any attempt to physically separate the DNA of interest, for example by microdissection of the mucosal layer may introduce a potential bias by underestimating intracellular bacteria if these were abundant in the sample. Sufficient sequencing would then have to be applied to our sample to ensure that, after in silico removal of any sequences that were deemed "not of interest", sufficient sequences "of interest" remained with sufficient coverage to answer our original question. The in silico analysis required also builds in a level of assumption that may introduce substantial bias, namely, when sequencing genes from unknown organisms, how can we correctly identify them as such in silico to enable us to include/exclude them from subsequent analysis?

In summary, the application of molecular analysis tools to study the gut microbiota in CRC is hugely exciting and offers tremendous scope in terms of further understanding CRC initiation and pathogenesis. Nevertheless there will always be a strong reliance on ensuring the robustness of sample integrity in terms of collection and processing to guarantee the data from such molecular approaches is as true to the clinical situation as possible.

2 Materials

Unless specified otherwise, prepare and store all reagents at room temperature.

2.1 Sample Collection: Biopsies

1. Equipment required: Eppendorf tubes (1.5 mL), liquid nitrogen, ice or appropriate sample buffer for example RNA later.

2.2 Sample Collection: Stool

1. Faecal collection kit.
2. Phase-change refrigerant gel packs. Alternative options include commercially available stool stabilization buffer systems which are amenable to room temperature storage.

2.3 Biopsy DNA Extraction

1. QIAamp® DNA Mini and Blood Mini (Qiagen, Manchester, UK). This kit includes the spin columns, collection tubes, Buffer AL, Buffer ATL, Buffer AW1 concentrate, Buffer AW2 concentrate, Buffer AE, Proteinase K.
2. Equipment required: shaking thermomixer, vortex, microcentrifuge, pipette (30–500 μL), pipette tips with aerosol barrier, microcentrifuge tubes (1.5 and 2.0 mL).
3. Additional reagents required: Molecular grade ethanol (96–100%).

2.3.1 Stool DNA Extraction

1. PSP® Spin Stool DNA Kit/PSP® Spin Stool DNA Plus Kit (STRATEC Molecular GmbH, Berlin, Germany).
   (a) This kit includes the Stool Collection Tubes with DNA stabilizer, Safe-Lock-Tubes, Zirconia Beads II, InviAdsorb Tubes, Receiver Tubes, Proteinase K, Binding Buffer A, Wash Buffers I and II, Elution Buffer, RTA Spin Filter Set, RTA Receiver Tubes.
   (b) Proteinase K should be dissolved in ddH_2O, volumes according to number of planned extractions as per user manual.
   (c) Binding Buffer, Proteinase K, Wash Buffers I and II require dilution as described in Table 1.
   (d) Elution Buffer should be preheated to 70 °C in a thermomixer.
2. Equipment required: shaking thermomixer, ice, vortex, microcentrifuge, pipettes (25–1500 μL), microcentrifuge tubes (1.5 and 2.0 mL).
3. Additional reagents required: ddH_2O, 70% isopropanol, molecular grade ethanol.

Table 1
Reagent dilutions for Stratec PSP® Spin Stool DNA Plus kit

Solution	Addition for a 50 kit	Addition for a 250 kit
Binding Buffer A	Add 21 mL 99.7% isopropanol to 9 mL Binding Buffer A	Add 84 mL 99.7% isopropanol to 36 mL Binding Buffer A
Proteinase K	Add 1.5 mL ddH_2O to each vial (make up as needed and store in fridge between batches)	Add 1.5 mL ddH_2O to each vial (make up as needed and store in fridge between batches)
Wash Buffer I	Add 30 mL molecular ethanol to 30 mL Wash Buffer I	Add 80 mL molecular ethanol to 80 mL Wash Buffer I
Wash Buffer II	Add 42 mL molecular ethanol to 18 mL Wash Buffer II	Add 105 mL molecular ethanol to 45 mL Wash Buffer II

2.3.2 Stool DNA Extraction

1. FastDNA® SPIN Kit for Soil (MP Biomedicals, Solon, USA).
2. This kit includes Lysing Matrix E, Sodium Phosphate Buffer (SPB), MT Buffer, PPS Solution, Binding Matrix, SPIN Modules, Catch Tubes, Concentrated SEWS-M Buffer, DES Buffer, BBS Gel Loading Dye.
3. Equipment required: Rotator or low-speed vortex, FastPrep bead beater machine, ice, microcentrifuge, microcentrifuge tubes (1.5 and 2.0 mL), Parafilm, pipettes (100–600 μL).
4. Additional reagents required: 100% ethanol.

2.4 Biopsy RNA Extraction

1. Equipment required: sterile micropestles, small spatula, 21G needle and 5 mL syringe, liquid nitrogen, cooling metal block suitable to withstand cooling in a liquid nitrogen container, microcentrifuge, microcentrifuge tubes (1.5 and 2 mL), pipettes (2–500 μL), vortex, ice.
2. Reagents required: RNaseZap, nuclease-free H_2O, TRIzol, chloroform, isopropanol, 75% ethanol.

2.5 RNA Cleanup and Concentration

1. RNeasy® Micro kit ordered from Qiagen includes RNeasy® Mini Spin Columns, Collection Tubes (1.5 and 2 mL), Buffer RLT, Buffer RW1, Buffer RPE concentrate, RNase-free water, carrier RNA, poly-A, RNase-free DNase Set (RNase-free DNase I (lyophilized), Buffer RDD, RNase-free water).
   (a) Buffer RPE concentrate should be diluted as 1:4 with molecular level ethanol.
   (b) 80% ethanol: prepare by diluting 24 mL of molecular level ethanol with 6 mL RNase-free water.
   (c) DNase I stock solution: prepare according to manufacturer's instructions OR keeping the vial closed to prevent loss of DNase I, inject 550 μL of RNase-free water using

an RNase-free needle and syringe directly into the vial and mix by inversion. Do not vortex.

2. Equipment required: microcentrifuge, microcentrifuge tubes (1.5 mL), thermomixer, vortex, pipettes (2–550 μL), vortex, thermomixer.
3. Reagents required: Molecular level ethanol, 70% ethanol.

3 Methods

3.1 Sample Collection: Biopsies

1. Collect mucosal biopsies using standard endoscopic forceps and place directly into sterile 1.5 mL Eppendorf container. Immediately place samples on cooling medium (*see* Subheading 2.1).
2. Store at −80 °C and extract DNA within 1 month of collection.

3.2 Sample Collection: Stool

1. Collect faecal sample using faecal collection kit (e.g., Fisher Faecal Commode Collection Kit) and chill in phase-change refrigerant gel packs for transport.
2. Store at −80 °C and extract DNA within 1 month of collection.

3.3 Biopsy DNA Extraction Using Qiagen miniPrep Kit

1. Without letting the sample thaw add 180 μL of Buffer ATL (*see* **Notes 1–3**).
2. Add 30 μL Proteinase K (*see* **Note 4**), mix by vortex, and incubate at 56 °C in incubator with a shaking plate set at ~700 rpm until the tissue or cells have completely lysed (*see* **Note 5**).
3. Briefly centrifuge the 1.5 mL microcentrifuge tube and add 200 μL Buffer AL to the sample, mix by pulse-vortex for 15 s, and incubate at 70 °C for 30 min.
4. Briefly centrifuge and add 200 μL molecular grade ethanol.
5. Briefly centrifuge the 1.5 mL microcentrifuge tube then carefully apply the mixture from **step 4** (including any precipitate) onto the QIAamp® Spin Column without wetting the rim and touching the filter at the base. Close the cap, and centrifuge at 6000 × *g* for 1 min.
6. Discard collection tube or discard the flow-through.
7. Mix molecular grade ethanol with Buffer AW1 and Buffer AW2 concentrates as per instructions.
8. Wash column by adding 500 μL Buffer AW1 and centrifuge at 6000 × *g* for 1 min. Discard collection tube or discard the flow-through.

9. Wash column by adding 500 μL Buffer AW2 buffer and centrifuge at full speed 20,000 × *g* for 3 min. Discard collection tube or discard the flow-through.
10. Place the QIAamp® Spin Column in a NEW 2 mL collection tube, centrifuge at 20,000 × *g* for 3 min to dry column. Discard collection tube.
11. Place the QIAamp® Spin Column in a clean 1.5 mL microcentrifuge tube; add 50 μL sterile ddH_2O or Buffer AE. Incubate at room temperature for 1–5 min, and then centrifuge at 6000 × *g* for 1 min.

3.4 Stool DNA Extractions

There are a number of DNA extraction kits available that are suitable for stool DNA extraction. The two used routinely in our laboratory are described below.

3.4.1 Using the Stratec PSP® Spin Stool DNA Plus Kit

1. Transfer approximately 1 g of stool into the Stool Collection Tube and mix by shaking for a 1–2 min. If stool is not in Stool DNA Stabilizer freeze on arrival and on extraction add 1.4 amount of Stool DNA Stabilizer and mix well.
2. Remove 1.4 mL of the stool sample into a 2.0 Safe-Lock Tube and incubate for 10 min at 95 °C on a shaking thermomixer set at 900 rpm. This is followed by incubation for 3 min on ice then samples are returned to the shaking thermomixer for a further 3 min.
3. Add 5 Zirconia Beads to the sample mixture and vortex for 2 min, then centrifuge at 11,000 × *g* for 1 min.
4. Transfer the supernatant into an InviAdsorb tube and mix by vortexing for 15 s. Incubate at room temperature for 1 min and then centrifuge at 14,000 × *g* for 3 min.
5. Transfer the supernatant into a new 1.5 mL receiver tube and centrifuge at 14,000 × *g* for 3 min.
6. Mix 800 μL of supernatant with 25 μL of Proteinase K (provided in the kit, *see* **Note 4**) and vortex to mix for 15 s.
7. Incubate for 10 min at 70 °C on a shaking thermomixer set at 900 × *g*.
8. Add 400 μL Binding Buffer A and mix either by vortex or by pipetting up and down.
9. Add 700 μL of mixture to the provided RTA Spin Filter and incubate for 1 min at room temperature. Centrifuge at 11,000 × *g* for 2 min. Discard the filtrate and repeat for the second part of the sample.
10. Discard the filtrate and transfer the Spin Filter into a new RTA tube and add 500 μL Wash buffer I. Centrifuge at 11,000 × *g* for 1 min.

11. Repeat using 700 μL Wash buffer II and centrifuge at 11,000 × *g* for 1 min.
12. Discard the flow-through tube containing filtrate. Centrifuge at 14,000 × *g* for 4 min to remove all traces of ethanol.
13. Transfer the spin filter to a new tube, pipette 100–200 μL of preheated Elution Buffer, directly onto the membrane of the RTA Spin Filter and incubate at room temperature for 1 min before centrifuging at 11,000 × *g* for 1 min.
14. Discard the RTA-Spin Filter. Quantify the DNA and store the extracted DNA immediately at −20 °C until required for further analysis.

3.4.2 Using the FastDNA® SPIN Kit for Soil

1. Weigh 500 mg of stool sample straight into the Lysing Matrix E Tube and add 489 μL of SPB and 122 μL MT Buffer, vortex well to mix.
2. Add a further 489 μL of SPB (*see* **Note 6**), mix using vortex and seal the tubes with Parafilm.
3. Homogenize on the FastPrep bead beater machine for 30 s at full speed (20,000 × *g* or 14,000 rpm) and place directly on ice.
4. Centrifuge sample at 14,000 × *g* for 5 min and transfer supernatant to a clean tube before adding 250 μL PPS reagent. Mix by hand inversion 10 times.
5. Centrifuge at 14,000 × *g* for 5 min. Transfer supernatant to a clean 1.5 mL tube alongside 1 mL of resuspended binding matrix (*see* **Note** 7). Mix by hand for 2 min and allow to stand for 3 min.
6. Discard the top 500 μL of solution from each tube and mix the remaining contents.
7. Load 600 μL onto the spin column at a time and centrifuge at full speed (20,000 × *g*) for 1 min. Discard flow-through and repeat until all the sample has been loaded onto spin column, gently resuspending the pellet with the pipette tip each time.
8. Dilute 12 mL of Concentrated SEWS-M Wash Solution with 100 mL of 100% ethanol.
9. Wash the binding matrix by adding 0.5 mL SEWS-M buffer (*see* **Note 8**) and centrifuging at 14,000 × *g* for 1 min discarding the flow-through. Return to the spin column to the collection tube and spin at 14,000 × *g* for a further 2 min to remove any ethanol left behind on the column and leave to stand for 5 min to dry.
10. Transfer to a new 1.5 mL collection tube add 100 μL DES buffer mix carefully then spin at 14,000 × *g* for 1 min.
11. Incubate the tubes at 65 °C for 10 min, then 95 °C for 10 min before storing at −80 °C.

3.5 Biopsy RNA Extraction

This should be carried out in a fume hood.

3.5.1 RNA Extraction Procedure

1. Clean micropestle and small spatula with RNaseZap, then nuclease-free water.
2. Add 0.5 mL of TRIzol to 1.5 mL RNase-free tubes and place them in extraction block and place in Dewar along with tissue grinder. Cool in liquid nitrogen for approximately 15 min, the TRIzol will freeze giving you a flat surface.
3. Collect samples from −80 °C and transport in liquid nitrogen. Tip the sample onto the frozen TRIzol.
4. Using the cooled tissue grinder smash the tissue to form a powder.
5. Extract 0.5 mL of TRIzol into a pipette tip, remove the ground tissue, place a few drops of TRIzol on top of the tissue then use the rest to wash the end of the grinder. This will freeze so chip off into the tube using the spatula. Allow to thaw while processing other samples.
6. Pass the tissue–TRIzol through a 21G needle gently 3–4 times to further break up tissue.
7. Centrifuge at 12,000 × *g* for 10 min at 2–8 °C and transfer supernatant to clean RNase-free 1.5 mL tube and discard cell debris. The supernatant can now be stored at −80 °C for up to 1 month.
8. Incubate at room temp for 5 min, add 0.2 mL chloroform to 1 mL TRIzol, invert for 15 s then allow to stand at room temperature for 2–3 min.
9. Centrifuge at 12,000 × *g* for 15 min at 2–8 °C. This will give you three phases, a pink phase (TRIzol), a white phase (organic phase) which can be kept for other analysis, and a clear aqueous layer which contains the nucleic acids.
10. Carefully remove the clear layer, without disturbing the white layer, and place into a fresh nuclease-free 1.5 mL tube.
11. Add 0.5 mL isopropanol to the tube, invert to mix then leave at room temp for 10 min. Centrifuge at 12,000 × *g* for 10 min at 2–8 °C. Discard the supernatant.
12. Wash the pellet by adding 1 mL of 75% ethanol vortex and centrifuge at 10,000 × *g* for 10 min at 2–8 °C. Discard the supernatant. Leave to air-dry for 10 min (do not let it dry out completely).
13. Add 34 μL nuclease-free water and allow RNA to dissolve for 15 min on ice.
14. Remove 2×2 μL aliquots and retain them on ice for nucleic acid quantity/quality analysis. Store RNA at −80 °C or proceed to RNA cleanup.

3.5.2 RNA Cleanup and Concentration

1. Adjust the RNA sample volume to 100 μL (by adding nuclease-free water) and add 250 μL RLT buffer and mix well. Add 250 μL molecular ethanol and mix by pipetting.
2. Load the total sample onto the MinElute spin column, centrifuge at 8000 × *g* for 15 s and discard the flow-through.
3. Wash column with 350 μL RW1, centrifuge at 8000 × *g* for 15 s and discard the flow-through.
4. Add 40 μL DNase (*see* **Note 9**) in RDD directly onto the white center of the column (do not touch the center with the tip), and incubate at room temperature for 15 min.
5. Wash column with 350 μL RW1, centrifuge at 8000 × *g* for 15 s and discard the flow-through.
6. Place columns in clean 2 mL collection tubes, add 500 μL RPE buffer, centrifuge at 8000 × *g* for 15 s and discard the flow-through.
7. Add 500 μL 80% ethanol, centrifuge at 8000 × *g* for 2 min and discard the flow-through.
8. Place columns in clean 2 mL collection tubes, centrifuge at full speed for 5 min to dry the column.
9. Place columns in RNase-free 1.5 mL tubes add 18 μL nuclease-free water and centrifuge at full speed for 1 min.
10. Remove 2×2 μL aliquots and retain on ice for nucleic acid quantity/quality analysis. Store RNA at −80 °C or proceed to RNA cleanup.

3.6 Nucleic Acid Quantity/Quality Assessment

There are numerous ways to assess nucleic acid quantity/quality and depending on the purpose of the assessment, we utilize different approaches. For most day-to-day sample assessment we rely on spectrophotometric readings from a Thermo NanoDrop 1000 spectrophotometer. For accurate assessment, for example sequencing library preps (DNA or RNA) we use Agilent Technologies 2100 Bioanalyzer Instrument. The basis of such approaches is to define the integrity of nucleic acids while defining the level of potential contamination such as proteins or organic contaminants introduced during sample extraction. Typically the spectrophotometric output is given as 260/280 and 260/230 ratios. Absorbance readings at 260 nm should fall between 0.15 and 1.0. Note that absorbance measurements at 260 nm cannot discriminate between DNA and RNA. Depending on the method used for template preparation, the purified DNA may be contaminated with RNA, or the purified RNA may be contaminated with DNA. If this is the case, the A260 value will be too high, leading to inaccurate quantification. A ratio of approximately 1.8 is generally accepted as "pure" for DNA and approximately 2.0 is generally accepted as "pure" for RNA. If the ratio is appreciably lower in either case, it may indicate the presence of protein, phenol, or other contaminants that absorb strongly at or near 280 nm.

For "pure" nucleic acid: 260/230 values higher than the respective 260/280 values.

260/230 values are commonly in the range of 1.8–2.2. If the ratio is appreciably lower, this may indicate the presence of copurified contaminants, (carbohydrates, peptides, phenols, or aromatic compounds) (*see* **Note 10**).

3.7 PCR Approaches to Assess Microbial Diversity Within Samples

Following on from DNA quantity/quality analysis, the reading gives you no idea still of microbial DNA content as the majority of DNA signal will be from the host. This is obviously dependent on sample type—tissue samples will be almost exclusively host DNA (>99%) while stool samples will have a higher percentage of microbial DNA. The next step is to perform PCR analysis to confirm the presence of microbial DNA. We routinely assess the presence of bacterial and fungal DNA using the primers described in Table 2. The 27F/1492r primer pair amplifies almost the entire 16S rRNA gene, which is a ubiquitous bacterial gene. This primer pair is used widely in the literature. If you are wishing to consider microbial fingerprinting techniques such as denaturing gradient gel electrophoresis (DGGE), which was very popular in the 1990s and early 2000s then there are two primer pairs that give good results. The 968f/1401r pair generate ~450 bp product within the V8/V9 region of the 16S rRNA gene. The 357f/538r pair generate ~180 bp product within the V3/V4 region of the same gene. Both pairs have been used extensively to define microbial community profiles.

Primers which are used to look for the presence of fungal DNA within samples rely generally on exploiting the 18S rRNA gene or the ITS (internal transcribed spacer) regions. 18S analysis was the

Table 2
Primer sequences for confirmation of bacterial and fungal DNA

Primer name	Sequence	Use	Reference
27f/1492r	5′-AGAGTTTGATCMTGGCTCAG-3′ 5′-TACCTTGTTACGACTT-3′	Bacteria	[25]
Bacterial DGGE 968f/1401r	5′-AACGCGAAGAACCTTAC-3′ 5′-GCGTGTGTACAAGACCC-3′	Bacteria	[14]
Bacterial DGGE 357f/538r	5′-CCTACGGGAGGCAGCAG-3′ 5′-ATTACCGCGGCTGCTGG-3′	Bacteria	[13]
18S rRNA	5′-ACTTTCGATGGTAGGATAG-3′ 5′-TACGGCGGTCCTAGAAAC-3′	Fungi	[26]
ITS1F/ITS2	5′-CTTGGTCATTTAGAGGAAGTAA-3′ 5′-GCTGCGTTCTTCATCGATGC-3′	Fungi	[27]

initial gene of choice however was shown to lack sensitivity in discriminating between fungal species. Various ITS primer pairs have been proposed, the pair we use targets the ITS4 region.

4 Notes

1. Ensure that all equipment and required tubes are ready in advance and check that the ethanol has been added to the appropriate buffers.
2. If the tissue is not at the bottom, briefly spin the tubes.
3. If the samples are frozen, prepare a master mix of ATL buffer and proteinase K in advance and add to the samples while they are still frozen. Also ensure that ATL buffer has not precipitated out, if it has warm at 37 °C until the SDS has gone back into solution.
4. Check that proteinase K has been prepared according to instructions and avoid repeated freeze–thaw cycles; freeze by storing in appropriately sized aliquots.
5. Lysis time for tissue varies and may need an overnight incubation.
6. For FastPrep kit, it is easier to add the SPB buffer in two lots.
7. Check ethanol has been added to the SAWS-M buffer.
8. Ensure the binding matrix is fully suspended.
9. Check RNAse free DNAse has been prepared according to instructions and avoid repeated freeze–thaw cycles.
10. Absorbance readings characteristics: A230: Organic contaminants like phenol; thiocyanate, TRIzol, and some reagents used in RNA extraction absorb light at 230 nm. A260: Nucleic acids only absorb light that has a wavelength of 260 nm. A280: Proteins especially aromatic amino acids absorb light at 280 nm. 260/280: used to assess the purity of DNA and RNA. 260/230: a secondary measure of nucleic acid purity.

Acknowledgments

This work was supported by grants from The Chief Scientist Office, Friends of Anchor, NHS Grampian Endowments, NHS Grampian Gastroenterology Endowment funds as well as donations from CRC patients.

References

1. Weisburger JH, Reddy BS, Narisawa T et al (1975) Germ-free status and colon tumor induction by N-methyl-N′-nitro-N-nitrosoguanidine. Proc Soc Exp Biol Med 148 (4):1119–1121
2. Louis P, Hold GL, Flint HJ (2014) The gut microbiota, bacterial metabolites and colorectal cancer. Nat Rev Microbiol 12(10):661–672
3. Hold GL, Garrett WS (2015) Gut microbiota: microbiota organisation a key to understanding CRC development. Nat Rev Gastroenterol Hepatol 12(3):128–129
4. Wang T, Cai G, Qiu Y et al (2012) Structural segregation of gut microbiota between colorectal cancer patients and healthy volunteers. ISME J 6(2):320–329
5. Boleij A, van Gelder MM, Swinkels DW et al (2011) Clinical Importance of *Streptococcus gallolyticus* infection among colorectal cancer patients: systematic review and meta-analysis. Clin Infect Dis 53(9):870–878
6. Kostic AD, Chun E, Robertson L et al (2013) *Fusobacterium nucleatum* potentiates intestinal tumorigenesis and modulates the tumor-immune microenvironment. Cell Host Microbe 14(2):207–215
7. Sears CL (2009) Enterotoxigenic *Bacteroides fragilis*: a rogue among symbiotes. Clin Microbiol Rev 22(2):349–369
8. Martin HM, Campbell BJ, Hart CA et al (2004) Enhanced *Escherichia coli* adherence and invasion in Crohn's disease and colon cancer. Gastroenterology 127(1):80–93
9. Swidsinski A, Khilkin M, Kerjaschki D et al (1998) Association between intraepithelial *Escherichia coli* and colorectal cancer. Gastroenterology 115(2):281–286
10. Arthur JC, Perez-Chanona E, Mühlbauer M et al (2012) Intestinal inflammation targets cancer-inducing activity of the microbiota. Science 338(6103):120–123
11. Olsen GJ, Lane DJ, Giovannoni SJ et al (1986) Microbial ecology and evolution: a ribosomal RNA approach. Annu Rev Microbiol 40 (1):337–365
12. Thomson J, Hansen R, Berry S et al (2011) Enterohepatic *helicobacter* in ulcerative colitis: potential pathogenic entities? PLoS One 6(2): e17184
13. Muyzer G, de Waal EC, Uitterlinden AG (1993) Profiling of complex microbial populations by denaturing gradient gel electrophoresis analysis of polymerase chain reaction-amplified genes coding for 16S rRNA. Appl Environ Microbiol 59 (3):695–700
14. Zoetendal EG, Akkermans AD, De Vos WM (1998) Temperature gradient gel electrophoresis analysis of 16S rRNA from human fecal samples reveals stable and host-specific communities of active bacteria. Appl Environ Microbiol 64(10):3854–3859
15. Weisburg WG, Barns SM, Pelletier DA et al (1991) 16S ribosomal DNA amplification for phylogenetic study. J Bacteriol 173 (2):697–703
16. Giovannoni SJ, Britschgi TB, Moyer CL et al (1990) Genetic diversity in Sargasso Sea bacterioplankton. Nature 345(6270):60
17. Hold GL, Pryde SE, Russell VJ et al (2002) Assessment of microbial diversity in human colonic samples by 16S rDNA sequence analysis. FEMS Microbiol Ecol 39(1):33–39
18. Margulies M, Egholm M, Altman WE et al (2005) Genome sequencing in microfabricated high-density picolitre reactors. Nature 437 (7057):376–380
19. Rajilić-Stojanović M, Heilig HG, Molenaar D et al (2009) Development and application of the human intestinal tract chip, a phylogenetic microarray: analysis of universally conserved phylotypes in the abundant microbiota of young and elderly adults. Environ Microbiol 11(7):1736–1751
20. Claesson MJ, O'Sullivan O, Wang Q et al (2009) Comparative analysis of pyrosequencing and a phylogenetic microarray for exploring microbial community structures in the human distal intestine. PLoS One 4(8):e6669
21. Hansen R, Russell RK, Reiff C et al (2012) Microbiota of de-novo pediatric IBD: increased Faecalibacterium Prausnitzii and reduced bacterial diversity in Crohn's but not in ulcerative colitis. Am J Gastroenterol 107 (12):1913–1922
22. Watt E, Gemmell MR, Berry S et al (2016) Extending colonic mucosal microbiome analysis—assessment of colonic lavage as a proxy for endoscopic colonic biopsies. Microbiome 4 (1):61
23. Wheeler DA, Srinivasan M, Egholm M et al (2008) The complete genome of an individual by massively parallel DNA sequencing. Nature 452(7189):872–876

24. Qin J, Li R, Raes J et al (2010) A human gut microbial gene catalogue established by metagenomic sequencing. Nature 464 (7285):59–65
25. Frank JA, Reich CI, Sharma S et al (2008) Critical evaluation of two primers commonly used for amplification of bacterial 16S rRNA genes. Appl Environ Microbiol 74(8):2461–2470
26. Mukhopadhya I, Hansen R, Meharg C et al (2015) The fungal microbiota of de-novo paediatric inflammatory bowel disease. Microbes Infect 17(4):304–310
27. Ghannoum MA, Jurevic RJ, Mukherjee PK et al (2010) Characterization of the oral fungal microbiome (mycobiome) in healthy individuals. PLoS Pathog 6(1):e1000713

Chapter 9

Proteomics Analysis of Colorectal Cancer Cells

Anaïs Chauvin and François-Michel Boisvert

Abstract

Proteomics allows the simultaneous detection and identification of thousands of proteins within a sample. Here, we describe a quantitative method to compare protein expression and subcellular localization of different cell lines representative of different stages of colorectal cancer using stable isotope labeling with amino acids in culture, or SILAC. We also describe a biochemical fractionation approach to separate different cellular compartments and the necessary steps to obtain a specific proteomic profile of each cell line. This technique enables a comprehensive proteomic analysis of cancer cell lines and the identification of pathways that are deregulated in different cancer cell lines.

Key words Proteomics, Colorectal cancer, SILAC, Subcellular fractionation, Mass spectrometry

1 Introduction

"Proteomics" is a recent term used for the first time in 1997 in a paper from James P. titled "Protein identification in the post-genome era: the rapid rise of proteomics" [1]. Proteomics is the study of the proteome aiming to characterize all the proteins constituting a living organism, a tissue, a cell or a cell compartment [2]. The proteomic approach also aims to establish the identity, quantity, and function of these proteins and to determine their expression according to different conditions [3]. Herein, we demonstrate an approach to compare colorectal cancer cells.

Stable isotope labeling with amino acids in cell culture (SILAC) is a simple in vivo labeling strategy for mass spectrometry-based quantitative proteomics using nonradioactive isotopic labeling allowing the detection of global protein expression changes between different samples [4]. Biochemical fractionation coupled to mass spectrometry-based identification permits the characterization of subcellular organization [5, 6]. Finally, study of the cellular protein expression and localization will provide information on their contribution in the mechanisms involved in the initiation and evolution of cancer [7].

Jean-François Beaulieu (ed.), *Colorectal Cancer: Methods and Protocols*, Methods in Molecular Biology, vol. 1765, https://doi.org/10.1007/978-1-4939-7765-9_9, © Springer Science+Business Media, LLC, part of Springer Nature 2018

Thus, we have combined these different techniques (colorectal cancer cell lines, SILAC culture, subcellular fractionation, mass spectrometry analysis, and quantification) to identify changes in protein expression and localization in colorectal cancer cells [8].

2 Materials

Prepare all solutions using mass spectrometry grade solvents (water, acetonitrile, and methanol) and analytical grade reagents. Whenever possible, use low protein binding tubes and vials to minimize loss in samples of low concentration. Most solutions are prepared fresh, unless otherwise indicated.

2.1 Cell Culture

1. Colorectal cancer cell lines: HCT-116, CCL-233, HT-29, CCL-228, CCL-227 [9], DLD-1, Caco-2/15 [10] (Table 1).
2. Normal colon fibroblast cell line: CRL-1459 (Table 1).
3. SILAC medium: Dulbecco's modified Eagle's medium (DMEM) depleted of arginine and lysine, 10% dialyzed fetal bovine serum (FBS) (*see* **Note 1**), 100 U/mL penicillin/streptomycin, 2 mM GlutaMAX, 10 μg/mL L-proline (*see* **Note 2**) [11], 28 μg/mL arginine (R) and 49 μg/mL lysine (K), with either light or medium or heavy isotopes of carbon and nitrogen (*see* **Note 3**):
   (a) Light (i.e., $^{12}C^{14}N$) = R0K0;
   (b) Medium (L-arginine-$^{13}C_6{}^{14}N_4$ and L-lysine-$^{2}H_4$) = R6K4;
   (c) Heavy (L-arginine-$^{13}C_6$-$^{15}N_4$ and L-lysine-$^{13}C_6$-$^{15}N_2$) = R10K8.
4. Human intestinal epithelial crypt-like cells (HIEC-6) [12].
5. Opti-MEM medium: Opti-MEM, 2.4 g/L sodium bicarbonate, 2 mM GlutaMAX, 10 mM HEPES, 5% FBS, 5 ng/mL Epidermal Growth Factor (EGF).

2.2 Subcellular Fractionation and Validation

1. EDTA-based cell dissociation buffer, enzyme free (*see* **Note 4**).
2. 70% ethanol.
3. PBS 1×.
4. QProteome Cell Compartment kit (*see* **Note 5**).
5. Antibodies: anti-GAPDH (rabbit monoclonal antibody, Cell Signaling #2118), anti-claudin-1 (rabbit polyclonal antibody, Invitrogen #51-9000), anti-H2AX (rabbit polyclonal antibody, Santa Cruz Biotechnology #sc-101696), anti-cytokeratin (mouse monoclonal antibody, Sigma-Aldrich #C8541).

2.3 Protein Dosage

1. Bovine serum albumin fraction V (BSA) 2 mg/mL stock solution.

Table 1
The table lists the name of the different cell lines used in this study, the Duke's stage, the genetic profile, and the associated mutations

Cells	HCT-116	CCL-233	HT-29	CCL-228	CCL-227	DLD-1	Caco-2/15	HIEC-6	CRL-1459
Type	Colorectal carcinoma							Human intestinal epithelial cells	Normal colon fibroblasts
Duke's stage	A	A	B	B	C	C	Unknown	Normal	Normal
Genetic profile and mutations									
CIN		+	+	+	+		+		
MSI	+					+			
CIMP	+		+			+			
KRAS	G13D	G12A		G12V	G12V	G13D			
BRAF			V600E						
PIK3CA	H104R		P449T			E545K;D549N			
TP53		A159D	R273H	R273H;P309S	R273H;P309S	S241F	E204X		

The (+) sign indicates the presence of the phenotype/mutation

2. Prepare the following dilutions from the stock solution: 0, 0.1, 0.2, 0.4, 0.8, 1.2, 1.6, and 2 mg/mL BSA.
3. Pierce bicinchoninic acid (BCA) protein assay.
4. Prepare a 2 mg/mL solution of BSA in PBS (stock solution) from bovine serum albumin fraction V (Roche, Basel, Switzerland).

2.4 Reduction and Alkylation

1. 1.4-dithiothreitol (DTT): prepare a 1M stock solution by dissolving 1.55 g DTT in 10 mL MS water (*see* **Note 6**).
2. Iodoacetamide (IAA). Prepare a 1M stock solution by dissolving 0.18 g IAA in 1 mL MS water (*see* **Note 7**).

2.5 Gel Electrophoresis and Coloration

1. NuPAGE® LDS Sample Buffer (4×).
2. Running buffer, MOPS 1×. Prepare a 1 L stock solution of MOPS 20× and keep it in the dark by dissolving 83.8 g 3-(N-morpholino) propanesulfonic acid (MOPS), 16.4 g sodium acetate, and 7.44 g EDTA in H_2O.
3. One-dimensional Novex™ 4–12% Tris-Glycine Mini Gels, WedgeWell™ format, 10-well.
4. SimplyBlue SafeStain (Invitrogen).

2.6 Gel Discoloration

1. 100% acetonitrile (CH_3CN) (*see* **Note 8**).
2. 1 M ammonium bicarbonate (NH_4HCO_3) stock solution: 0.79 g NH_4HCO_3 in 10 mL distilled water (*see* **Note 9**).

2.7 In-Gel Trypsin Digestion

1. 1 μg/μL Trypsin Gold: dissolve 100 μg Trypsin Gold in 100 μL 50 mM acetic acid (*see* **Note 10**).
2. 20 mM NH_4HCO_3.
3. 12.5 ng/μL modified trypsin: mix a 10 μL Trypsin Gold aliquot with 800 μL 20 mM NH_4HCO_3 (*see* **Note 11**).

2.8 Peptides Extraction

1. 100% CH_3CN.
2. 1% formic acid (FA) (*see* **Note 12**) (diluted in MS water).
3. 0.1% trifluoroacetic acid (TFA) (diluted in MS water).

2.9 Peptides Purification

1. Wetting solution: 100% CH_3CN.
2. Equilibration and wash solution: 0.1% TFA.
3. Elution solution: 1% FA/50% CH_3CN.

2.10 LC-MS/MS

1. 1% FA.
2. Solvent A: 0.1% FA.
3. Solvent B: 80% CH_3CN, 0.1% FA.

3 Methods

For an overview of the protocol, *see* Fig. 1.

3.1 Cell Culture

1. Grow the colorectal cancer cell lines and the normal colon fibroblast cell line in either light (L), or medium (M) or heavy (H) SILAC medium at 80–95% confluence for at least 5 or 6 passages (*see* **Note 13**).
2. Grow the HIEC-6 cells in Opti-MEM medium at 80–95% confluence.

3.2 Subcellular Fractionation and Validation

1. Harvest the cells (*see* **Note 14**) by scraping from the petri dishes with the enzyme free dissociation buffer (*see* **Note 15**).
2. Follow the protocol of Qiagen website "QProteome® Cell Compartment Kit" using a 100 μL cell pellet (*see* **Note 16**) (Fig. 2).
3. Validate the subcellular fractionation by western blot with the antibodies previously mentioned (Fig. 1).

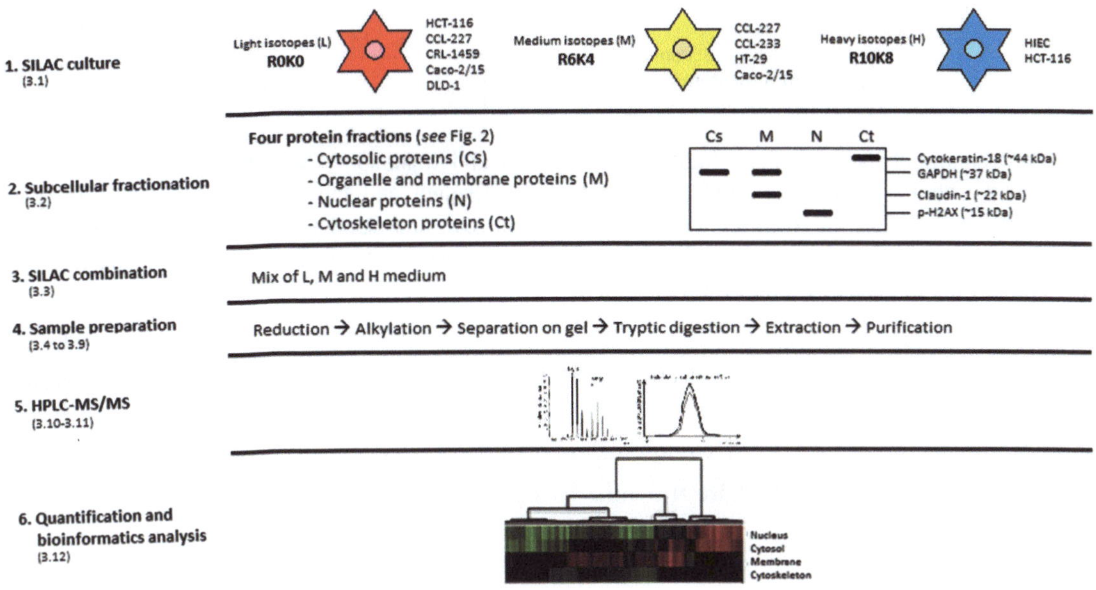

Fig. 1 Experimental SILAC approach to label and combine different fractions isolated from various colorectal cancer cell lines or normal cell lines for protein identification and quantification. Nine cell lines were grown in light (L), medium (M), or heavy (H) SILAC medium (Step 1). The protein content of each cell line is fractionated in four fractions (Step 2) before being combined in different mixes (Step 3). Samples are prepared (Step 4) and peptides are analyzed by high performance liquid chromatography (HPLC) coupled with mass spectrometry (MS) (Step 5). Quantification with MaxQuant software and bioinformatics analyses with Perseus software are performed on the data (Step 6)

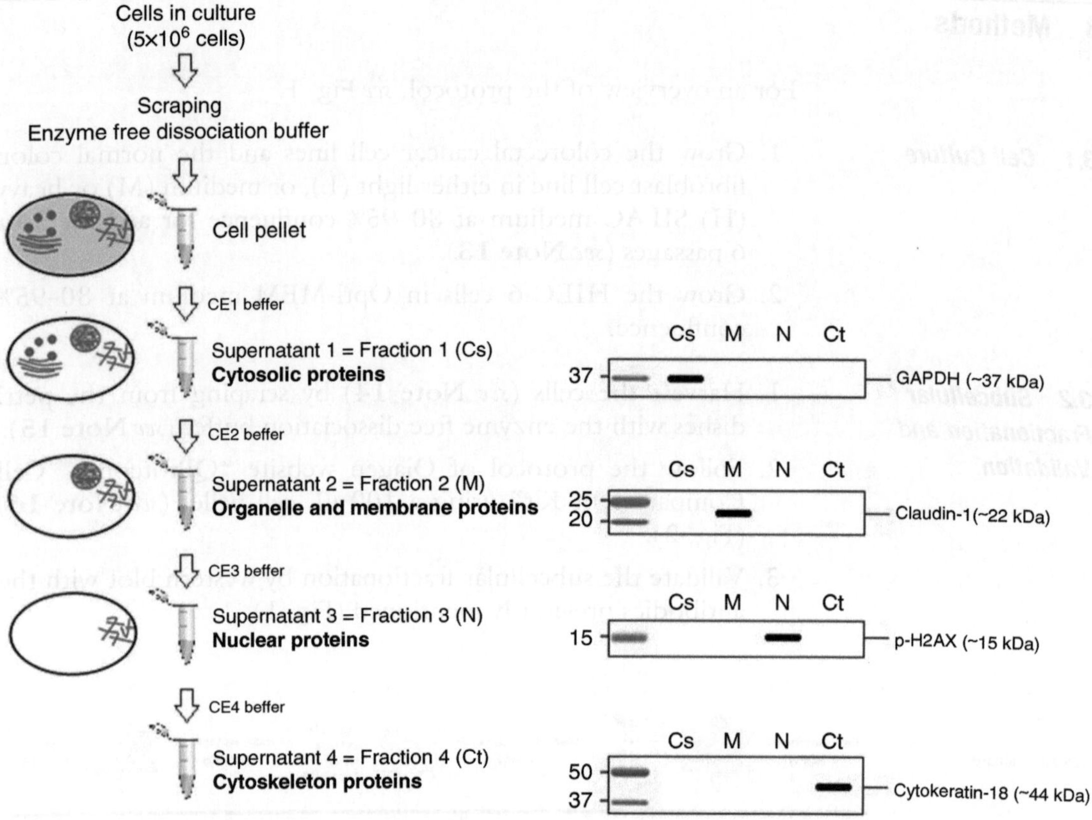

Fig. 2 Overview of the subcellular fractionation protocol and validation. The subcellular fractionation is performed with the QProteome® Cell Compartment Kit (Qiagen) and the validation with the following antibodies: anti-GAPDH (37 kDa) for the cytosolic fraction (Cs); anti-claudin-1 (22 kDa) for organelle and membrane fraction (M); anti-phospho-H2AX (15 kDa) for the nuclear fraction (N); and anti-cytokeratin-18 (44 kDa) for the cytoskeleton fraction (Ct)

3.3 SILAC Combination and Protein Dosage

1. Different SILAC combinations should be arranged (*see* Note 17).
2. Mix reagents A and B (50:1) of the BCA protein assay.
3. Add the mix to each sample and to the 0–2 mg/mL BSA dilutions and incubate for 30 min to 37 °C.
4. Read the absorbance at 562 nm.
5. Define a standard curve with the concentration and absorbance of each BSA dilution to estimate the protein concentration of the samples.

3.4 Reduction and Alkylation

1. Reduce with a final concentration of 10 mM DTT.
2. Boil for 5 min.
3. Alkylate with a final concentration of 50 mM IAA.
4. Incubate for 30 min in the dark.

3.5 Gel Electrophoresis

1. Add NuPAGE LDS sample buffer 4× in each sample and load the gel.
2. Migrate in running buffer (200 V, 120 mA, 35 min).
3. Wash the gel three times in distilled water.
4. Color the gel with SimplyBlue SafeStain for an hour under agitation.
5. Let the gel discolor in distilled water under light agitation changing water several times, then overnight (*see* **Note 18**).

3.6 Gel Discoloration

1. Excise the protein gel lane with a razor blade (*see* **Note 19**).
2. Cut each lane into eight slices (*see* **Note 20**).
3. Cut each slice into small cubes (*see* **Note 21**) of about 2 × 2 mm (*see* **Note 22**) and put them in low protein binding tubes.
4. Wash with 300 μL MS water for 15 min (*see* **Note 23**).
5. Wash with 300 μL 50% CH_3CN for 15 min.
6. Wash with 300 μL 20 mM NH_4HCO_3 for 15 min.
7. Wash with 300 μL (v:v) 20 mM NH_4HCO_3: 100% CH_3CN for 15 min.
8. Repeat **steps 6** and 7.
9. Dehydrate with 300 μL 100% CH_3CN for 5 min.
10. Repeat **step 9** until the pieces of gel being white and solid.
11. Lyophilize by speed vacuum centrifugation to 60 °C (*see* **Note 24**).

3.7 In-Gel Trypsin Digestion

1. Rehydrate with 100 μL per slice of 12.5 ng/μL modified trypsin in 20 mM NH_4HCO_3 for 30 min to 30 °C.
2. Recover with 20 mM NH_4HCO_3.
3. Note the digestion volume.
4. Incubate at 30 °C overnight.

3.8 Peptides Extraction

1. Add 100% CH_3CN to equal volume to digestion for 30 min (see **Note 25**).
2. Harvest the medium in a new low-binding tube (see **Note 26**).
3. Add 1% FA to equal volume to digestion for 20 min.
4. Harvest the medium in the same low-binding tube at **step 2**.
5. Repeat **steps 3** and **4**.
6. Add 100% CH_3CN to equal volume to digestion for 10 min.
7. Harvest the medium in the same low-binding tube at **step 2**.
8. Repeat **steps 6** and 7 until the pieces of gel being white and solid.
9. Lyophilize all pooled media by speed vacuum centrifugation to 60 °C (*see* **Notes 27–29**).

3.9 Peptides Purification

1. Resuspend the lyophilized pellet in 30 μL 0.1% TFA.
2. Prepare the 96-well plate (*see* **Note 30**):
   - Wetting solution in the wells on line A.
   - Equilibration solution in the wells on line B.
   - Wash solution in the wells on line D.
   - Elution solution in the wells on line E (*see* **Note 31**).
3. Place ZipTip C18 column on a P10 pipet (*see* **Note 32**).
4. Aspirate 10 μL of the wetting solution and discard it in the solvent bin (line G) three times.
5. Aspirate 10 μL of the equilibration solution and discard it in the solvent bin (line G) three times.
6. Aspirate 10 μL of the sample and perform ten up and downs in the loading well (line C), then discard it in the sample bin three times (*see* **Note 33**).
7. Aspirate 10 μL of the wash solution and discard it in the solvent bin (line G) three times.
8. Aspirate 10 μL of the elution solution and perform ten up and downs in a new low binding tube until there is no more sample.
9. Lyophilize the sample containing the peptides by speed vacuum centrifugation to 60 °C (*see* **Note 34**).
10. Resuspend in 25 μL 1% formic acid.
11. Peptides dosage: deposit 1 μL of the sample on the base of a NanoDrop 2000C spectrophotometer (*see* **Note 35**).

3.10 High Performance Liquid Chromatography (HPLC) Separation, Coupled to Mass Spectrometry

1. Trypsin-digested purified peptides are separated using a Dionex Ultimate 3000 nanoHPLC system.
2. Load 2 μg of the sample in 1% formic acid (v:v) with a constant flow of 4 μL/min on an Acclaim PepMap100 C18 column (0.3 mm id × 5 mm).
3. After trap enrichment, peptides are eluted in a PepMap C18 nanocolumn (75 μm × 50 cm) with a linear gradient of 95%:5% to 65%:35% solvent A–solvent B over 240 min with a constant flow of 200 nL/min.

3.11 Mass Spectrometry Analysis

1. The HPLC system is coupled to an OrbiTrap QExactive mass spectrometer (Thermo Fisher Scientific Inc) via an EasySpray source.
2. The spray voltage is set to 2.0 kV and the temperature of the column is set to 40 °C.
3. Full scan MS survey spectra (*m/z* 350–1600) in profile mode are acquired in the Orbitrap with a resolution of 70,000 after accumulation of 1,000,000 ions. The ten most intense peptide ions from the preview scan in the Orbitrap are fragmented by

collision induced dissociation (normalized collision energy 35% and resolution of 17,500) after the accumulation of 50,000 ions. Maximal filling times are 250 ms for the full scans and 60 ms for the MS/MS scans.

4. Precursor ion charge state screening is enabled and all unassigned charge states as well as singly, 7, and 8 charged species are rejected. The dynamic exclusion list is restricted to a maximum of 500 entries with a maximum retention period of 40 seconds and a relative mass window of 10 ppm.
5. The lock mass option was enabled for survey scans to improve mass accuracy.

3.12 Quantification and Bioinformatics Analysis (Fig. 3)

1. Process, search and quantified the data using the MaxQuant software package [13, 14] employing the Human Uniprot database.

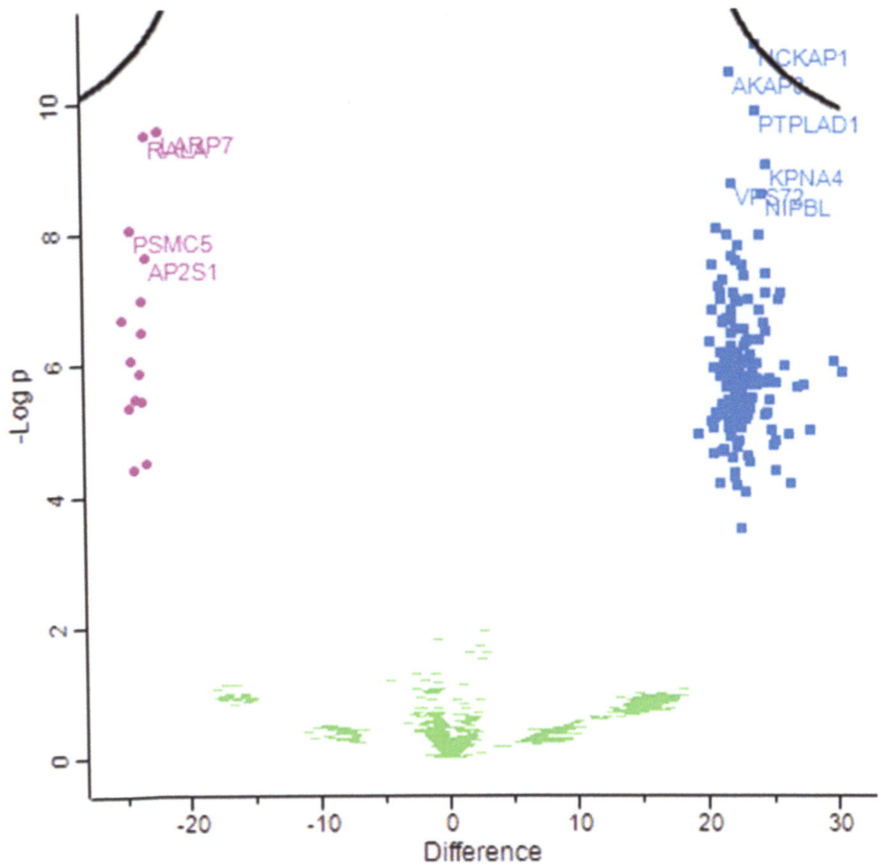

Fig. 3 Example of results obtained with the Perseus software. Here, the example shows the comparison between the protein compositions of the nuclear fractions of the Caco-2/15 and HIEC cells. The proteins overexpressed in the HIEC cells nucleus are represented with purple circles and those overexpressed in the Caco-2/15 cell nucleus with blue squares

2. Use these settings for the MaxQuant analysis: two miscleavages allowed; fixed modification is carbamidomethylation on cysteine; enzyme is trypsin (K/R not before P); variable modifications included in the analysis are methionine oxidation and protein *N*-terminal acetylation; mass tolerance of 7 ppm for precursor ions and 20 ppm for fragment ions; requantify option selected to calculate the ratio for isotopic patterns not assembled in SILAC pairs as often observed during pulldown experiments [8].

4 Notes

1. Because the serum is dialyzed, it is possible that some growth factor will be missing.
2. Recent studies using SILAC in quantitative proteomics have made mention of the problematic conversion of isotope-coded arginine to proline in cells. The resulting converted proline peptide divides the heavy peptide ion signal causing inaccuracy when compared with the light peptide ion signal. It was demonstrated that by adding an additional 200 mg/L of proline, it is possible to prevent this conversion, thus allowing correct interpretation of light and heavy peptide ratios [11].
3. We use isotopically incorporated amino acids from Cambridge Isotopes Laboratories, Inc. for this purpose.
4. We use Cell Dissociation Buffer, enzyme-free, PBS from ThermoFisher Scientific for this purpose.
5. We use QProteome Cell Compartment kit from Qiagen for this purpose.
6. Store 500 μL aliquots at −20 °C.
7. Store 25 μL aliquots at −20 °C.
8. Work under the chemical hood using CH_3CN because it is very volatile and toxic.
9. Store 1 mL aliquots at −20 °C.
10. Trypsin is very sensitive so it is better to keep it in the form of 10 μL aliquots to −80 °C.
11. Trypsin is not stable so the stock solution of trypsin gold is diluted in NH_4HCO_3 only before use.
12. Work under the chemical hood diluting FA in MS water because concentrated vapors are corrosive and prepare the solution only before use.
13. It is recommended to grow your cells for at least six populations doubling to ensure near 100% incorporation of the isotopic amino acids before you can do your experiment. We

normally dilute cells that are 80% confluent 1/3 into a new plate, and let it grow back to 80%. This constitutes one passage. We recommend performing these passages initially using a small volume to save costs.

14. It is recommended to work with 5×10^6 cells for this step.
15. Thoroughly clean the scraper with 70% ethanol before scraping.
16. Add protease inhibitors in each buffer before use.
17. Each cell line must be represented at least three times and the HCT-116 cell line is used in every combination for normalization and internal calibration.
18. Only parts of the gel containing proteins will remain blue.
19. Change the razor blade for each sample.
20. Cut the lane in a new petri dish for each lane.
21. Leave water at the bottom of the petri dish to prevent pieces of gel from leaping.
22. The size of the cubes is important because if they are too small, you risk losing material in the next steps and if they are too big, you may have an incomplete extraction of the gel proteins.
23. Proteins are contained in the gel so after each wash, do a quick spin and discard the supernatant with P1000 + P10 tips montage. Each wash is under strong agitation (about 1500 rpm) to ambient temperature.
24. It is possible to store the sample to −80 °C at the end of this step.
25. All the incubations are made to 30 °C under strong agitation (about 1500 rpm).
26. By doing a quick spin before harvest the supernatant with P1000 + P10 tips montage.
27. The volume to be dried is about 1 mL, so the drying will therefore take 3–4 h.
28. At the end of the drying, the peptides remain at the bottom of the low binding tube in the form of an almost invisible pellet.
29. It is possible to store the sample to −80 °C at the end of this step.
30. It is possible to treat 12 samples with a 96-well plate.
31. The elution solution is deposited afterwards because it is very volatile because of the CH_3CN.
32. Avoid introducing air in the column bed.
33. This is the loading step during which the peptides will cling to the column.

34. At the end of the drying, the purified peptides remain at the bottom of the low binding tube in the form of an almost invisible pellet. It is possible to store the sample to −80 °C at the end of this step.

35. Use 1% FA as blank for the dosage.

References

1. James P (1997) Protein identification in the post-genome era: the rapid rise of proteomics. Q Rev Biophys 30(4):279–331
2. Kenyon GL, DeMarini DM, Fuchs E, Galas DJ, Kirsch JF, Leyh TS, Moos WH, Petsko GA, Ringe D, Rubin GM, Sheahan LC, National Research Council Steering Committee (2002) Defining the mandate of proteomics in the post-genomics era: workshop report. Mol Cell Proteomics 1(10):763–780
3. Patterson SD, Aebersold RH (2003) Proteomics: the first decade and beyond. Nat Genet 33(Suppl):311–323
4. Harsha HC, Molina H, Pandey A (2008) Quantitative proteomics using stable isotope labeling with amino acids in cell culture. Nat Protoc 3(3):505–516
5. Boisvert FM, Lam YW, Lamont D, Lamond AI (2010) A quantitative proteomics analysis of subcellular proteome localization and changes induced by DNA damage. Mol Cell Proteomics 9(3):457–470
6. Drissi R, Dubois ML, Boisvert FM (2013) Proteomics methods for subcellular proteome analysis. FEBS J 280:5626–5634
7. Hung MC, Link W (2011) Protein localization in disease and therapy. J Cell Sci 124 (Pt.20):3381–3392
8. Mathieu AA, Ohl-Séguy E, Dubois ML, Jean D, Jones C, Boudreau F, Boisvert FM (2016) Subcellular proteomics analysis of different stages of colorectal cancer cell lines. Proteomics 23:3009–3018
9. Leibovitz A, Stinson JC, McCombs WB, McCoy CE, Mazur KC, Mabry ND (1976) Classification of human colorectal adenocarcinoma cell lines. Cancer Res 36 (12):4562–4569
10. Fogh J, Fogh JM, Orfeo T (1977) One hundred and twenty-seven cultured human tumor cell lines producing tumors in nude mice. J Natl Cancer Inst 59(1):221–226
11. Bendall SC, Hughes C, Stewart MH, Doble B, Bhatia M, Lajoie GA (2008) Prevention of amino acid conversion in SILAC experiments with embryonic stem cells. Mol Cell Proteomics 7(9):1587–1597
12. Perreault N, Beaulieu JF (1996) Use of the dissociating enzyme thermolysin to generate viable human normal intestinal epithelial cell cultures. Exp Cell Res 224(2):354–364
13. Cox J, Mann M (2008) MaxQuant enables high peptide identification rates, individualized p.p.b.-range mass accuracies and proteome-wide protein quantification. Nat Biotechnol 26:1367–1372
14. Cox J, Matic I, Hilger M, Nagaraj N, Selbach M, Olsen JV, Mann M (2009) A practical guide to the MaxQuant computational platform for SILAC-based quantitative proteomics. Nat Protoc 4:698–705

Check for updates

Chapter 10

Autophagic Flux Assessment in Colorectal Cancer Cells

Annie Lauzier and Steve Jean

Abstract

Autophagy protects colorectal cancer cells against therapeutic intervention. Autophagy is a continuous process, and autophagic flux requires both autophagosome synthesis and their subsequent degradation at lysosomes. Hence, cells with elevated autophagic flux display both rapid autophagosome generation and degradation. Here, we describe an immunoblot protocol coupled to pharmaceutical inhibition of autophagosome clearance to monitor autophagic flux levels between colorectal cancer cell lines.

Key words Autophagy, Colorectal cancer cells, Immunoblots, LC3, Bafilomycin A1

1 Introduction

The process of autophagy, defined as the lysosomal degradation and subsequent recycling of cytoplasmic components [1], is an essential homeostatic mechanism of eukaryotic cells [2]. Autophagic dysfunctions has now been involved with various etiologically different diseases. In cancer, autophagy prevents against transformation by eliminating protein aggregates and dysfunctional mitochondria, among others [3]. Therefore, by removing cytotoxic stress agents, autophagy averts cancer formation. However, once cell transformation has occurred, autophagy protects cancer cells from multiple stresses, ranging from nutrient deprivation, to chemotherapeutic or radiation therapies [4]. As such, autophagy inhibition represents a potentially promising way to increase the effectiveness of chemotherapy or radiotherapy [5–8]. Although inhibition of autophagy is now being investigated in clinical settings, there are still a lot of unanswered questions regarding mechanisms by which autophagy protects cancer cells from treatments. Moreover, there is no clear correlation between autophagic levels in cancer cells and their relative sensitivities to treatments or to autophagy inhibition. To better understand the correlation between autophagic levels and cancer cell sensitivity to various treatments, we describe a

Jean-François Beaulieu (ed.), *Colorectal Cancer: Methods and Protocols*, Methods in Molecular Biology, vol. 1765,
https://doi.org/10.1007/978-1-4939-7765-9_10,

simple immunoblot protocol [9] to measure autophagic levels in colorectal cancer cells.

This immunoblot protocol relies on measurements of LC3 lipidation levels, reflected as LC3-II on immunoblots [10]. LC3 (or Atg8 in lower eukaryotes) is an integral autophagosomal protein [11]. LC3 is required for autophagosome membrane expansion and for recruitment of autophagic cargos, mediated via its interaction with p62 (SQSTM1) [12]. LC3 is incorporated on autophagosomes by the action of two protein complexes. Briefly, LC3 is cleaved by Atg4, which exposes a C-terminal glycine on LC3-I [13]. LC3-I is then bound by Atg7, that acts like a ubiquitin-activating enzyme (E1) and recruits Atg3. Atg3 catalyzes the covalent conjugation of phosphatidylethanolamine (PE) on LC3-I, yielding LC3-II. Lipidated LC3 (LC3-II) is then bound by the Atg5/12-16 complex on autophagosome, and as such LC3-II is transferred to inner and outer autophagosomal membranes [14]. During autophagosome maturation and prior to fusion with lysosomes, LC3-II present on outer autophagosomal membranes is cleaved and recycled by Atg4 [15], while internal LC3-II is degraded in the lysosomes after fusion. Given this propriety of LC3-II, it is essential to analyze LC3-II levels at steady states and under an autophagic flux block, usually achieved through the addition of Bafilomycin A1 [9], a V-ATPase and SERCA inhibitor [16]. Hence, high LC3-II level at steady state might reflect both high autophagosome synthesis, or defective autophagosomal clearance. Thus, by blocking autophagosome degradation and integrating LC3-II levels with steady state levels, one can interpret and assess autophagic flux between cell lines.

2 Materials

Prepare all solutions using ultrapure water and analytical grade reagents.

2.1 Protein Extract Preparation

1. Bafilomycin A1: 100 μM stock solution in DMSO.
2. PBS: Mix 8 g of NaCl, 0.2 g of KCl, 1.44 g of Na_2HPO_4, and 0.24 g of KH_2PO_4.

   Add 900 mL of dH_2O. Adjust pH to 7.4. Adjust final volume to 1000 mL.
3. RIPA buffer: 50 mM Tris, pH 7.4, 150 mM NaCl, 0.5% sodium deoxycholate, 4 mM EDTA, SDS 0.1%, 1% IGEPAL CA-630, 1× protease inhibitor (*see* **Note 1**).
4. BCA protein assay kit (Pierce).
5. 96-well flat bottom plate with lid.
6. Absorbance Plate reader with 562 nm filter.

7. Laemmli buffer (5×): 250 mM Tris, pH 6.8, 10% SDS, 50% glycerol, 5% 2-mercaptoethanol, 0.1% bromophenol blue. In 12.5 mL of 1 M Tris, pH 6.8, dissolve 5 g of SDS and 0.05 g of bromophenol blue. Under the chemical hood, add 25 mL of glycerol and 2.5 mL of 2-mercaptoethanol. Complete to 50 mL with water, mix well, aliquot and freeze. Warm to dissolve precipitated SDS before use (*see* **Note 2**).

2.2 SDS-PAGE and Protein Transfer

1. Stacking buffer: 0.5 M Tris, pH 6.8. Dissolve 30 g of Tris in 300 mL of water. Adjust pH to 6.8. Complete to 500 mL with water (*see* **Note 3**).
2. Separating buffer: 1.5 M Tris, pH 8.8. Add 181.5 g of Tris to 500 mL of water. Adjust pH to 8.8 and complete to 1 L with water (*see* **Note 3**).
3. 30% Acrylamide 29:1.
4. Ammonium persulfate: 10% solution in water (*see* **Note 4**).
5. Isopropanol solution: mix 1 part isopropanol to 1 part water.
6. Running buffer (10×): 250 mM Tris, 1.92 M glycine, 0.1% SDS. Mix 30 g Tris, 140 g glycine, and 10 g of SDS in 500 mL of water. Complete to 1 L with water. You do not need to adjust pH, which should be around 8.3.
7. Prestained molecular weight markers.
8. PVDF membrane.
9. Transfer buffer: 48 mM Tris pH 9.2, 39 mM glycine, 20% methanol, 0.8 mM SDS. To prepare a 5× stock solution, dissolve 29.1 g of Tris and 14.65 g of glycine in 500 mL of water. Adjust pH to 9.2. Add 1 g of SDS. Make up to 1 L with water. Store at 4 degrees. Before use, mix 20 mL of transfer buffer solution 5×, 20 mL of ethanol, and 60 mL of water.

2.3 Antibody Probing and Detection

1. PBST: To 1 L of PBS add 1 mL of Tween 20, mix thoroughly.
2. Blocking solution: 5% powdered skim milk in PBST.
3. Anti-LC3 antibody (Cell signaling), anti-GAPDH antibody (HRP conjugate) (Cell signaling), anti-Tubulin antibody (Sigma-Aldrich).
4. Anti-Rabbit-HRP (Jackson ImmunoResearch).
5. Plastic containers.
6. Polythene bags.
7. Heat sealer.
8. ECL western blotting detection reagent.

3 Methods

All steps are carried out at room temperature unless otherwise specified.

3.1 Cell Culture and Protein Extract Preparation

1. Plate colorectal cancer cells in 6-well plates at a density of 5×10^5 per well. Maintain cells at 37 °C in a humidified 95% air and 5% CO incubator in their respective media for a minimum of 16 h to a maximum of 24 h. Change for fresh complete media or starvation media (HBSS, DMEM without FBS and/or without glucose or DMEM without amino acids supplemented with dialyzed FBS) (*see* **Note 5**). Add bafilomycin A1 at a concentration of 0.2 μM (*see* **Note 6**) in half of the wells at a chosen time prior to protein extraction (*see* **Note 7**).
2. Label 2 sets of identified 1.5 mL microcentrifuge tubes. Keep one series on ice or in a −20 °C freezer. Add 15 μL of 5× Laemmli buffer in the second series and keep at room temperature.
3. For protein extraction, keep plates on ice, aspirate culture media and gently wash cells twice with ice-cold 1× PBS. Carefully aspirate all PBS from wells (leaving PBS at this point will reduce the final concentration of protein lysate).
4. Add 70 μL of RIPA buffer per well. Tip plate to distribute evenly and keep on ice 15 min.
5. Using a cell scraper, collect cell lysate and transfer to a cold microcentrifuge tube previously labelled.
6. Pellet cell debris by centrifugation at 13,000 × *g* for 15 min at 4°.
7. Set aside an aliquot of the supernatant for BCA quantification (5 μL) in 8- or 12-strip tubes and keep at −20 °C.
8. Transfer 50 μL of the cleared protein lysate to the microcentrifuge tube containing 5× Laemmli buffer and mix. Store lysates at −20 °C before use (*see* **Note 8**).

3.2 Protein Quantification

1. Calculate the number of samples, standards and blanks and multiply by 200 μL to calculate the amount of BCA reagents required. Prepare the resulting amount + 10% (in μL) of reagent A′, which corresponds to premix reagents A and B at a 50/1 ratio. Add 200 μL of reagent A′ per well of a 96-well plate. Add 5 μL of standard, RIPA (blank) and the saved 5 μL of each protein sample (*see* **Note 9**). Cover plate and incubate at 37 °C for 15 min. Read at 562 nm on a plate reader, subtracting the blank background to all other wells.
2. Use the standard curve to determine the protein concentration of all prepared samples. Calculate the volume of sample needed to obtain the same amount of protein for each condition (based

on the least concentrated sample and the maximal volume that can be loaded in a single well).

3.3 SDS-PAGE Separation of Proteins

1. 15% polyacrylamide gels (*see* **Note 10**): For 4 gels, mix 7.5 mL of separating buffer, 15 mL of acrylamide 29:1 mix, and 6.9 mL water, mix by swirling, avoiding the introduction of air bubbles. Add 300 μL of SDS, 300 μL of ammonium persulfate, and 12 μL of TEMED mix gently and cast gels within 7.25 × 10 cm × 1.5 mm gel cassettes. Allow space for stacking gel and overlay with isopropanol solution.
2. Rinse and drain the polymerized gels.
3. Stacking gel: Mix 2.5 mL of stacking buffer, 3.4 mL of acrylamide mixture, and 13.6 mL water. Add 200 μL of SDS, 200 μL of ammonium persulfate, and 20 μL of TEMED. Insert a 10 or 15-well gel comb promptly, making sure no air bubbles are introduced.
4. Heat protein extracts in Laemmli buffer at 90 °C for 5 min. Centrifuge heated samples to bring down condensate. Load prestained molecular weight marker in one lane and the calculated volume for each sample in subsequent wells. Migrate proteins in gel at 150 V constant. Stop migration when dye front reaches bottom of gel.

3.4 Protein Transfer and Immunoblot

1. Activate PVDF membranes with ethanol for 15 s. Equilibrate membranes and gels in transfer buffer for at least 5 min while preparing transfer apparatus.
2. Assemble the semi-dry transfer cassette following manufacturer's instructions making sure to remove air bubbles trapped between the layers of the transfer montage. Electroblot at 2.5 A for 10 min.
3. Rinse membranes with PBST for 5 min then incubate in blocking buffer for 1 h at RT. Wash in PBST three times (*see* **Note 11**).
4. Dilute primary antibody in blocking buffer (1/4000—anti-LC3; 1/2000—anti-GAPDH; 1/2000—anti-tubulin). Incubate membrane with primary antibody dilution with gentle agitation overnight at 4 °C (*see* **Note 12**).
5. Wash three times for 5 min in PBST. Incubate membrane with species appropriate HRP-conjugated secondary antibody diluted 1/20,000 in blocking buffer for 1 h at RT (*see* **Note 13**). Wash three times for 5 min in PBST. Wash twice for 5 min in PBS without Tween.
6. Drain excess liquid from membrane using a paper towel and place on a smooth surface (plastic wrap on benchtop or a clean glass plate) protein side up. Add enough ECL solution to cover the entire membrane and incubate 5 min. Remove excess

reagent by draining on a paper towel and place membranes between two sheets of polythene.

7. Scan the membranes on a chemiluminescent imager (such as Bio-Rad Chemidoc XR station, *see* **Note 14**).
8. Quantify and normalize LC3-II band intensities to GAPDH (or tubulin) in order to compare various CRC cell lines.
9. At least 3–4 independent biological repeats must be performed to appropriately assess autophagic flux in each cell line.
10. It is the gold standard in the autophagy field to confirm LC3-II immunoblot analysis with other techniques. We suggests to confirm LC3-II immunoblot results with the autophagic flux reporter mCherry:GFP:LC3.

4 Notes

1. The buffer can be kept at 4 °C for up to 1 month or at −20 °C. Add protein inhibitors immediately before use.
2. Adjust pH of Tris before addition of the other constituents. SDS should be dissolved completely prior to addition of glycerol. Solution will be viscous. Anytime this buffer is frozen or kept on ice, SDS will precipitate. Warm the solution in a 37 °C (or more) water bath or heat block to dissolve before pipetting.
3. Check pH of solutions regularly, discard and make fresh buffer if pH changes.
4. The stability of APS in water is limited, therefore solution should be prepared weekly and kept at 4 °C.
5. Cancer cells have inherently high basal autophagic flux [4]. However, if one wants to assess if autophagic flux can still be regulated, nutrient starvation is a strong inducer of autophagy and might highlight differences between cell lines. In our hands, we observed that only a few CRC cells can upregulate their autophagic flux following nutrient starvation.
6. Accumulation of LC3-II in the presence of Bafilomycin is cell line dependent and should be tested in the cell line of interest. We found that for colorectal cancer cell lines (SW480, SW620, LoVo, HCT116, Caco2-15, T84, HT29) treatments with 0.5–1 μM Balifomycin for short incubations (under 4 h) and 0.2 μM for longer incubation time (over 4 h) gave consistent responses (Fig. 1), without affecting cell viability. Accumulation of LC3-II in the presence of Bafilomycin in CRC cell lines is visible in some cells as early as 30 min following treatment but more pronounced after 4 h or more (Fig. 2).

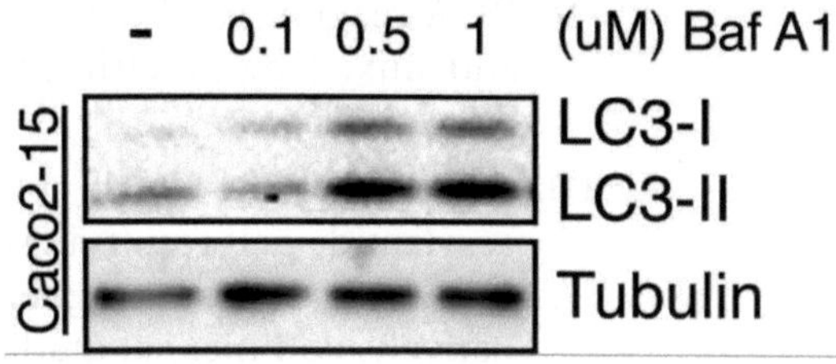

Fig. 1 LC3 immunoblot analysis of Caco2-15 cells treated with increasing concentrations of Bafilomycin A1 for 4 h in complete media

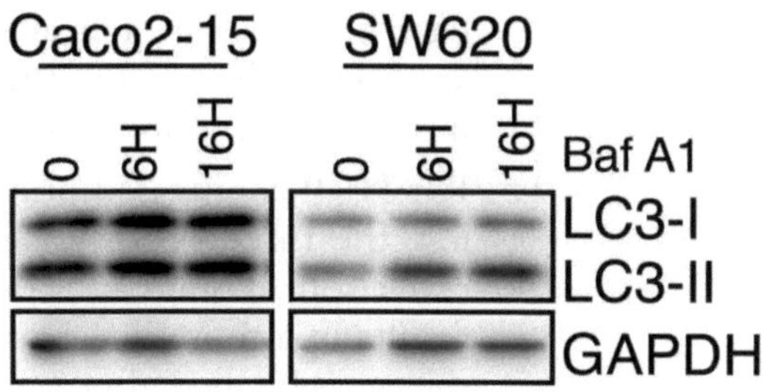

Fig. 2 Comparative autophagic functions measured by LC3 immunoblot analysis of CRC cell lines treated with Bafilomycin A1 (at a concentration of 0.2 μM) for 6 or 16 h in complete media

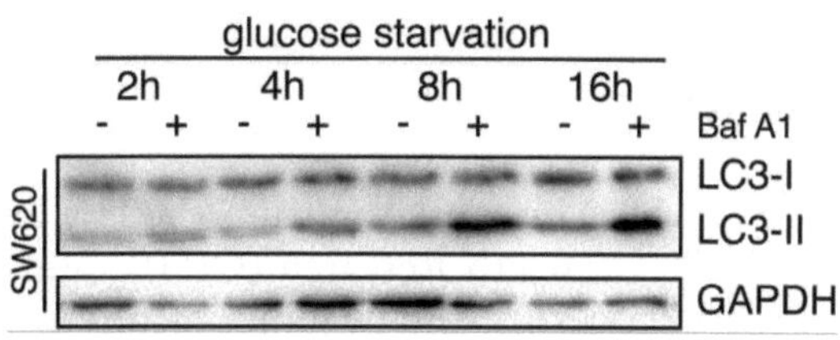

Fig. 3 Immunodetection of LC3-II accumulation at different time points following Bafilomycin induced autophagic blockade (0.2 μM) in SW620 cells under glucose starvation

7. In our experience, CRC cell lines are very sensitive to complete starvation (EBSS or HBSS). By immunofluorescences, changes in cell morphology, reminiscent of apoptosis, are visible 2 h following full starvation. Therefore, depletion of serum and/or glucose, or amino acids is a better option for longer incubation times during autophagic flux measurements (Fig. 3).
8. Changes in western blot output (i.e., presence of LC3-II) are seen after extended storage of extracts (>1 month) due to protein degradation. Therefore, extracts should be run and analyzed by western blot promptly.

9. BCA reagent is added directly to the reserved 5 μL of sample and mixed by pipetting up and down before transfer to the 96-well plate.
10. Because of the small size of LC3, higher concentration of acrylamide gels results in sharper LC3 bands, increased stability in transfer rate and higher western blot reproducibility. Alternatively, commercial gradient gels 4–20% can be used.
11. Membranes can be cut at the height of the 25 kDa molecular weight marker in order to reveal both LC3-II (lower part) and GAPDH (or tubulin) (upper part) simultaneously).
12. We found that incubating one membrane (or two membranes back to back) in a heat-sealed polythene bag with enough antibody solution for the membrane to float freely renders most consistent and reproducible probing signals.
13. For HRP conjugated primary GAPDH antibody, directly follow the three PBST washes with two PBS washes and ECL revelation. Using an HRP conjugated housekeeping gene results in a more linear protein signal, albeit not as strong as the one obtained after secondary antibody amplification.
14. We observed by comparing images acquired on a Chemidoc versus regular films that the linear detection range of the chemiluminescent signal is superior on the Chemidoc, which resulted in better quantification and reproducibility between experiments.

Acknowledgments

This work was supported by grants from the Canadian Institutes of Health Research (CIHR) and the Cancer Research Society (CRS) to S.J. and by junior faculty salary awards from the CIHR and Fond de Recherche du Québec—Santé (FRQS) to S.J.. Steve Jean is a member of the FRSQ-Funded Centre de Recherche du CHUS.

References

1. Mizushima N, Komatsu M (2011) Autophagy: renovation of cells and tissues. Cell 147 (4):728–741. https://doi.org/10.1016/j.cell.2011.10.026
2. Levine B, Kroemer G (2008) Autophagy in the pathogenesis of disease. Cell 132(1):27–42. https://doi.org/10.1016/j.cell.2007.12.018
3. Galluzzi L, Pietrocola F, Bravo-San Pedro JM, Amaravadi RK, Baehrecke EH, Cecconi F, Codogno P, Debnath J, Gewirtz DA, Karantza V, Kimmelman A, Kumar S, Levine B, Maiuri MC, Martin SJ, Penninger J, Piacentini M, Rubinsztein DC, Simon HU, Simonsen A, Thorburn AM, Velasco G, Ryan KM, Kroemer G (2015) Autophagy in malignant transformation and cancer progression. EMBO J 34(7):856–880. https://doi.org/10.15252/embj.201490784
4. Kimmelman AC (2011) The dynamic nature of autophagy in cancer. Genes Dev 25 (19):1999–2010. https://doi.org/10.1101/gad.17558811
5. Burada F, Nicoli ER, Ciurea ME, Uscatu DC, Ioana M, Gheonea DI (2015) Autophagy in

colorectal cancer: an important switch from physiology to pathology. World J Gastrointest Oncol 7(11):271–284. https://doi.org/10.4251/wjgo.v7.i11.271

6. Groulx JF, Khalfaoui T, Benoit YD, Bernatchez G, Carrier JC, Basora N, Beaulieu JF (2012) Autophagy is active in normal colon mucosa. Autophagy 8(6):893–902. https://doi.org/10.4161/auto.19738
7. Sato K, Tsuchihara K, Fujii S, Sugiyama M, Goya T, Atomi Y, Ueno T, Ochiai A, Esumi H (2007) Autophagy is activated in colorectal cancer cells and contributes to the tolerance to nutrient deprivation. Cancer Res 67 (20):9677–9684. https://doi.org/10.1158/0008-5472.CAN-07-1462
8. Zheng HY, Zhang XY, Wang XF, Sun BC (2012) Autophagy enhances the aggressiveness of human colorectal cancer cells and their ability to adapt to apoptotic stimulus. Cancer Biol Med 9(2):105–110. https://doi.org/10.3969/j.issn.2095-3941.2012.02.004
9. Klionsky DJ et al (2016) Guidelines for the use and interpretation of assays for monitoring autophagy (3rd edition). Autophagy 12 (1):1–222. https://doi.org/10.1080/15548627.2015.1100356
10. Mizushima N, Yoshimori T (2007) How to interpret LC3 immunoblotting. Autophagy 3 (6):542–545
11. Nakatogawa H, Ichimura Y, Ohsumi Y (2007) Atg8, a ubiquitin-like protein required for autophagosome formation, mediates membrane tethering and hemifusion. Cell 130(1):165–178. https://doi.org/10.1016/j.cell.2007.05.021
12. Watanabe Y, Tanaka M (2011) p62/SQSTM1 in autophagic clearance of a non-ubiquitylated substrate. J Cell Sci 124(Pt 16):2692–2701. https://doi.org/10.1242/jcs.081232
13. Fujita N, Hayashi-Nishino M, Fukumoto H, Omori H, Yamamoto A, Noda T, Yoshimori T (2008) An Atg4B mutant hampers the lipidation of LC3 paralogues and causes defects in autophagosome closure. Mol Biol Cell 19 (11):4651–4659. https://doi.org/10.1091/mbc.E08-03-0312
14. Chen Y, Klionsky DJ (2011) The regulation of autophagy—unanswered questions. J Cell Sci 124(Pt 2):161–170. https://doi.org/10.1242/jcs.064576
15. Kimura S, Fujita N, Noda T, Yoshimori T (2009) Monitoring autophagy in mammalian cultured cells through the dynamics of LC3. Methods Enzymol 452:1–12. https://doi.org/10.1016/S0076-6879(08)03601-X
16. Mauvezin C, Nagy P, Juhasz G, Neufeld TP (2015) Autophagosome-lysosome fusion is independent of V-ATPase-mediated acidification. Nat Commun 6:7007. https://doi.org/10.1038/ncomms8007

Part II

New Developments in Colorectal Cancer Diagnostics and Screening

Check for updates

Chapter 11

Classification of Colorectal Cancer in Molecular Subtypes by Immunohistochemistry

Sanne ten Hoorn, Anne Trinh, Joan de Jong, Lianne Koens, and Louis Vermeulen

Abstract

Colorectal cancer (CRC) is a heterogeneous disease, which can be categorized into distinct consensus molecular subtypes (CMSs). These subtypes differ in both clinical as well as biological properties. The gold-standard classification strategy relies on genome-wide expression data, which hampers widespread implementation. Here we describe an immunohistochemical (IHC) Mini Classifier, a practical tool that, in combination with microsatellite instability testing, delivers objective and accurate scoring to classify CRC patients into the main molecular disease subtypes. It is a robust immunohistochemical-based assay containing four specific stainings (FRMD6, ZEB1, HTR2B, and CDX2) in combination with cytokeratin. We also describe an online tool for classification of individual samples based on scoring parameters of these stainings.

Key words Colorectal cancer, CRC, Classification, Consensus molecular subtypes, CMS, Immunohistochemistry, IHC, Online classification tool

1 Introduction

Colorectal cancer (CRC) is a heterogeneous disease and patients show a great variation in prognosis and response to therapies [1]. Therefore, in order to tailor therapies to the patient's individual needs, classification of patients in disease subtypes is an intense field of study. In addition to genetic aberrations that have clinical utility, e.g. *RAS* mutations and microsatellite instability (MSI) status, gene expression based classification systems have been proposed over the last few years [2–7]. The initially proposed taxonomies differed in the number of subtypes identified and the properties of the distinct subtypes. In 2015 an international collaborative effort to reconcile differences in these taxonomies by the CRC Subtyping Consortium, resulted in a consensus of the categorization of CRC into four distinct consensus molecular subtypes (CMSs) in a large panel of CRC patients [8]. These subtypes (CMS1-4) are highly distinct

Jean-François Beaulieu (ed.), *Colorectal Cancer: Methods and Protocols*, Methods in Molecular Biology, vol. 1765, https://doi.org/10.1007/978-1-4939-7765-9_11,

CMS1 (14%) MSI Immune	CMS2 (37%) Epithelial	CMS3 (13%)	CMS4 (23%) Mesenchymal
CIN Low Hypermutation Hypermethylation	CIN (SCNA high) MSS No hypermethylation	CIN (SCNA low) Mixed MSI status No hypermethylation	CIN (SCNA high) MSS No hypermethylation
Strong immune activation	Upregulation WNT and MYC downstream targets	Metabolic dysregulation	EMT activation Stromal invasion TGF-β activation
Mutations in BRAF	Mutations in APC, KRAS, TP53		
Good prognosis Poor survival rate after relapse	Relative favorable disease outcome in contrast to CMS4		Often late-stage diagnosis (III and IV) Worse overall and relapse-free survival Higher likelihood of disease recurrence

Fig. 1 CMS Classification of Colorectal Cancer. *CIN* chromosomal instability, *CMS* consensus molecular subtype, *EMT* epithelial–mesenchymal transition, *MSI* microsatellite instability, *MSS* microsatellite stability, *SCNA* somatic copy number alterations

entities that associate with different molecular characteristics and display different biological and clinical presentation. In summary, CMS1 (MSI Immune, 14%) demarcates a hypermutated group with a high proportion of MSI tumors and strong immune activation; CMS2 (Canonical, 37%), the largest subgroup, is associated with chromosomal-instability (CIN) and marked WNT and MYC signaling activation; CMS3 (Metabolic, 13%), a small subset, is an epithelial-like subtype with evident metabolic dysregulation; and CMS4 (Mesenchymal) represents the subtype with the poorest prognosis defined by epithelial–mesenchymal transition (EMT) with stromal invasion and angiogenesis, prominent TGF-β activation and stemness (Fig. 1). A subset of "mixed features or indeterminate" (13%) possibly represent a transition phenotype or intratumoral heterogeneity.

Of note, apart from MSI which is a strong predictor for CMS1 no single genetic defect can be unequivocally assigned to a specific subtype, and all subtypes represent heterogeneous groups with respect to the most commonly found pathogenic mutations in CRC (e.g., KRAS, BRAF, APC). This hampers the allocation of individual samples to molecular subtypes based on a simple genetic test for mutations and currently the gold-standard classification is based on genome wide transcriptional profiles. Evidently in a clinical setting these are not always readily obtainable due to prerequisites for tissue sampling (fresh frozen material) and costs. Therefore, we have previously set out to develop an immunohistochemical (IHC) strategy to identify the key subtypes [3, 9]. Our approach was focused on distinguishing CMS2/3 versus CMS4 due to the clinical implications in separating these classes. The CMS2/3 vs. CMS4 distinction is especially relevant as in early stage cancers (stage I–III) CMS2/3 identifies a group of patients with relative favorable disease outcome in contrast to CMS4 cancers with a higher likelihood of disease recurrence. In addition, we have reported that mesenchymal cancers (CMS4) are resistant to anti-EGFR therapy (e.g., cetuximab, panitumumab), also in the absence of RAS activating mutations [3, 9].

1.1 The IHC Mini Classifier

Here we describe an immunohistochemistry-based (IHC-based) classifier, which adapts the transcriptome-based classification of CMS into a rapid scoring system, which can be used with standard formalin-fixed, paraffin-embedded (FFPE) tissue [9]. We previously reported excellent agreement of the IHC-based classification system with the transcriptome-based classifications [3, 9], and this system is therefore capable to classify the main subtypes of CRC until transcriptomic profiling becomes more widespread available in clinical practice.

To classify patients into their CRC subtype firstly MSI status (MSI-high or MSI-low) has to be obtained to define patients that belong to the CMS1 subtype as it was observed to be almost ubiquitous in these patients. The assessment of MSI status falls beyond the scope of this chapter, but this was described in an earlier edition of Springer Protocols [10, 11]. As demonstrated in these chapters, the detection of MSI can be performed with polymerase chain reaction (PCR) based assays using a panel of different microsatellite loci [11] or using immunohistochemistry with antibodies against mismatch repair (MMR) proteins (MLH1 and MSH2) [10]. Only samples with high-level MSI should be considered instable, and are allocated to CMS1 (MSI).

The IHC-classifier will allocate the remaining patients into "epithelial" (CMS2/3) or "mesenchymal" (CMS4) subtypes using a random forest classifier. The classifier does not distinguish between the two epithelial-like subtypes (CMS2/3), which have similar prognosis. To distinguish between the epithelial-like and mesenchymal subtypes, stainings for four gene product proteins (CDX2, FRMD6, HTR2B, and ZEB1) were selected based on high differential expression between the subtypes [3]. In addition, pan--cytokeratin (KER) was used to normalize for epithelial content. CDX2 is a transcription factor in intestinal epithelial cells, which is expected to be highly expressed in epithelial-like tumors; HTR2B is a serotonin receptor with high expression in mesenchymal like tumors; FRMD6 is an adaptor protein linking plasma membrane associated proteins to actin skeleton and is expressed in colon glandular cells and has a higher expression in mesenchymal-like tumors and ZEB1 is an indicator for epithelial–mesenchymal transition (EMT). To differentiate between the epithelial-like and mesenchymal subtypes the staining intensity and content of the epithelial area of the tissue will be assessed, not the stromal content.

2 Materials

Prepare and store all reagents at room temperature (unless indicated otherwise).

2.1 Preparation of FFPE Sections (See Note 1)

1. Microtome.
2. Microscopy slides.
3. 37 °C incubator.
4. Slide warmer (50–60 °C).
5. Slide holder.
6. Xylene.
7. 70–100% ethanol (*see* **Note 2**).
8. Demineralized water (demi water).
9. Antigen retrieval: 10 mM sodium citrate, pH = 6 (*see* **Note 3**).
10. Heating source for antigen retrieval (90–100 °C) (*see* **Note 4**).

2.2 Staining

1. PBS: 0.137 M NaCl, 0.05 M NaH_2PO_4, pH 7.4.
2. Peroxidase blocking solution (*see* **Note 5**).
3. PAP hydrophobic barrier pen.
4. Normal antibody diluent (*see* **Note 6**).
5. Primary antibodies: (*see* **Note** 7).
   (a) anti-CDX2 (1:200, Novus Biologicals, Rabbit).
   (b) anti-HTR2B (1:100, Sigma, Rabbit).
   (c) anti-FRMD6 (1:500, Sigma, Rabbit).
   (d) anti-ZEB1 (1:500, Sigma, Rabbit).
   (e) anti-cytokeratin (AE1/AE3) (1:500, Dako, Mouse).
6. Secondary antibodies:
   (a) Brightvision poly-HRP anti-Rabbit IgG (Immunologic), store at 4 °C.
   (b) Brightvision poly-HPR anti-Mouse IgG (Immunologic), store at 4 °C.
7. 3,3′-diaminobenzidine (DAB) Solution (*see* **Note 8**).
8. Optional: Hematoxylin.
9. Demineralized water (demi water).
10. 70–100% ethanol (*see* **Note 2**).
11. Xylene.
12. Coverslip.
13. Mounting medium (e.g., Pertex).

2.3 CMS Mini Classifier

1. Online IHC-Mini Classifier available at: https://crcclassifier.shinyapps.io/appTesting/.

3 Methods

At first determine the MSI status of the samples to define patients that belong to the CMS1 subtype. This falls beyond the scope of this chapter, but an excellent description of both the PCR based and the IHC based assay of MSI detection can be found in an earlier edition of Springer Protocols [10, 11]. For the remaining samples follow the instructions below.

3.1 Preparation of FFPE Sections

1. Cut the tissue block into 4–5 μm thick slices on a microtome. Prepare at least five slides from each tissue sample (for each staining). Let the slides dry at 37 °C in the incubator for 4–16 h (until the sections are dry) (*see* **Note 9**). Go to **step 2** or store slides at 4 °C until needed.
2. Incubate slides on a slide warmer at 60 °C for 20–30 min or 50 °C overnight, until the paraffin starts to melt, for optimal adherence of the tissue to the slides. Go to **step 3** or store slides at 4 °C until needed.
3. Deparaffinize sections in xylene, 2 × 5 min (*see* **Note 10**).
4. Rehydrate the slides through a series of ethanol concentrations (*see* **Note 11**): 100% ethanol 2 × 3 min, 96% ethanol 2 × 3 min, 90% ethanol 1 × 3 min, 80% ethanol 2 × 3 min, and 70% ethanol 2 × 3 min.
5. Rinse gently in demi water.
6. Antigen retrieval: to reveal the antigenic epitope masked during the fixation use the heat induced epitope retrieval (HIER) method with citrate buffer (*see* **Note 12**). Boil (95–100 °C) the sections for 15–20 min in 10 mM sodium citrate buffer pH = 6.0, followed by cooling in the same buffer for 10–30 min by putting the glass beaker on ice (*see* **Note 4**).

3.2 Primary Antibody Staining

1. Rinse slides in PBS for 3 × 5 min.
2. Peroxidase blocking: incubate slides in the peroxidase blocking solution for 15 min at room temperature (*see* **Note 13**).
3. Rinse slides in PBS for 3 × 5 min.
4. Draw a circle around your tissue with PAP-pen (*see* **Note 14**).
5. Primary antibody: incubate five slides of each sample with the five primary antibodies at the appropriate dilution (*see* **Note 7**) in antibody diluent for 1 h at room temperature or overnight at 4 °C.

3.3 Secondary Antibody Staining

1. Rinse slides in PBS for 1 × 30 s and 2 × 5 min.
2. Secondary antibody: incubate slides in Brightvision poly-HRP anti-Rabbit IgG (anti-CDX2, anti-HTR2B, anti-FRMD6, and anti-ZEB1) or Brightvision poly-HRP anti-Mouse IgG (anti-cytokeratin) for 30 min at room temperature.
3. Rinse slides in PBS for 4 × 5 min.
4. Incubate slides in DAB solution to cover the entire tissue slide and incubate for 1–3 min in the dark since DAB is light sensitive (*see* **Note 15**).
5. Bring slides in slide holder again and rinse in demi water for 2 × 2 min.
6. Counterstain, if desired, with hematoxylin (*see* **Note 16**), otherwise continue to Step 7.
   (a) Incubate slides for 2–3 min in hematoxylin.
   (b) Rinse slides gently for 2 min with running tap water in slide holder, allowing the water to flow along the sides of the container.
7. Rinse slides in demi water for 2 × 2 min.
8. Dehydrate the slides through a series of ethanol concentrations: 70% ethanol, 2 × 10 sec, 80% ethanol, 2 × 10 sec, 90% ethanol, 1 × 10 sec, 96% ethanol, 2 × 10 sec, 100% ethanol; 2 × 10 sec.
9. Clear slides in xylene for 2 × 5 min.
10. Cover slides using a coverslip with mounting medium (*see* **Note 17**).

3.4 Scoring of the Slides

1. Classify each marker as having low, medium, or high staining intensity, except for Zeb1, which has two classes (absent or present). Make sure to score the epithelial nuclear immunolocalization of ZEB1 as absent or present and not the stromal cell positivity (Fig. 2).
2. Score the stained area fraction for keratin, CDX2, and FRMD6. The keratin area fraction is defined as the fraction of keratin content within a core. The stained area fraction for CDX2 and FRMD6 is the fraction of the epithelium section of the core occupied by positively stained cells (Fig. 3).

3.5 Online IHC Mini Classifier

1. Go to the website providing the mini-IHC-classifier for CRC as a free-to-use online resource (*see* Subheading 2 and Fig. 4).
2. In the left column of the website fill in your obtained scoring intensities and stained area fractions. After scoring all eight variables press apply changes. This will compute the classification of CRC into a probability score to belong to the epithelial-like or the mesenchymal-like subtype (*see* **Note 18**).

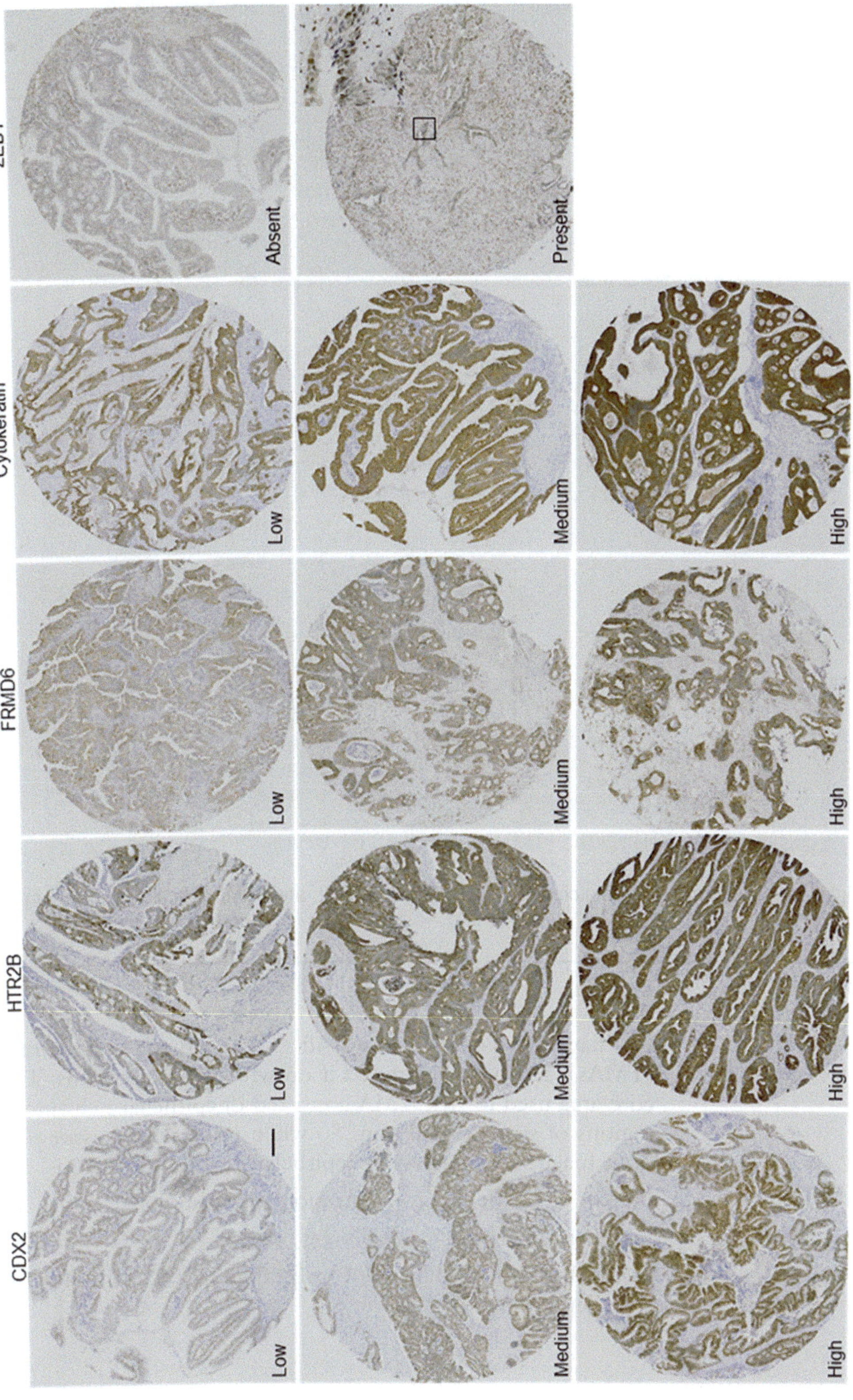

Fig. 2 Examples for scoring of the staining intensity for all five stainings. Scale bar, 200 μm

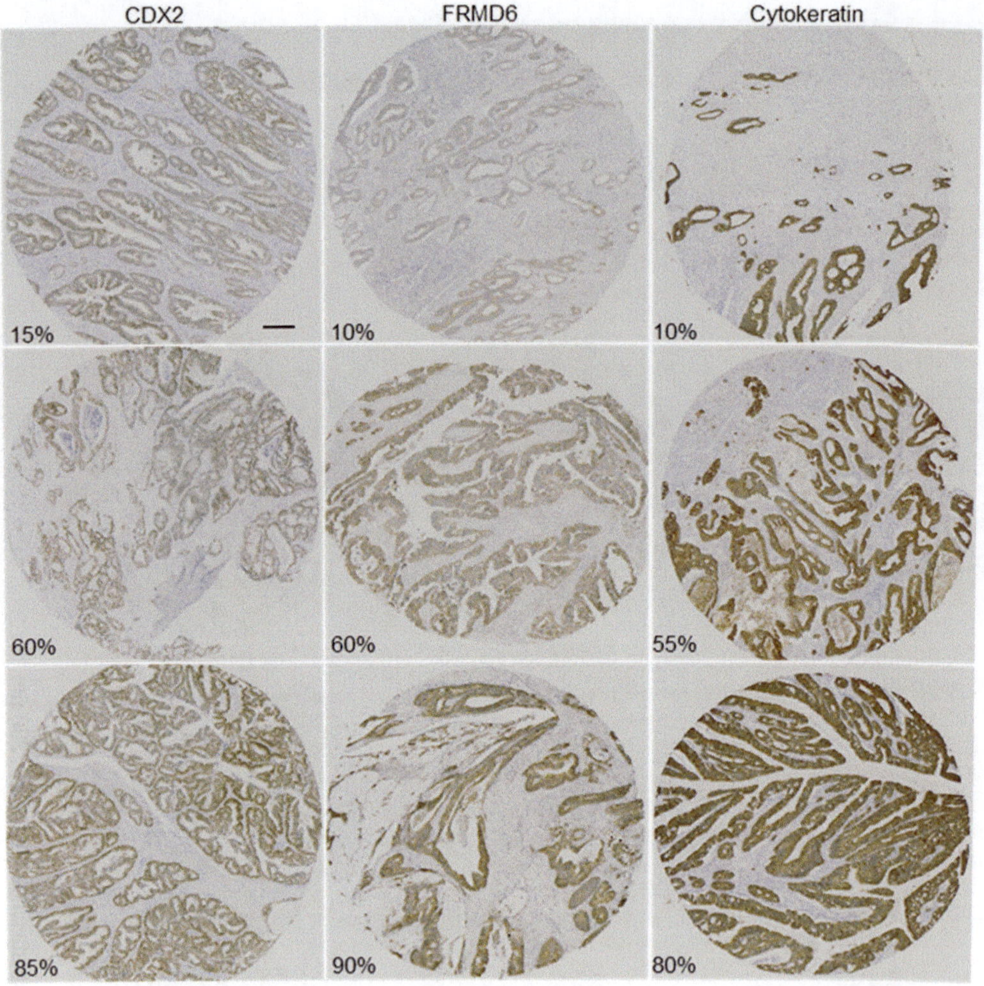

Fig. 3 Examples for the scoring of the staining content of keratin, CDX2, and FRMD6. Scale bar, 200 μm

4 Notes

1. We have developed the classifier using tissue microarrays (TMAs), and have not tested it on whole tissue sections. The core area used for the TMA consisted of epithelial-rich tumor regions of size 0.6–2.0 mm. So when using whole tissue sections make sure to assess the epithelial-rich tumor regions.
2. Prepare five different concentrations of ethanol:
   (a) Ethanol 100%.
   (b) Ethanol 96%: dilute 960 mL ethanol 100% with 40 mL demi water.

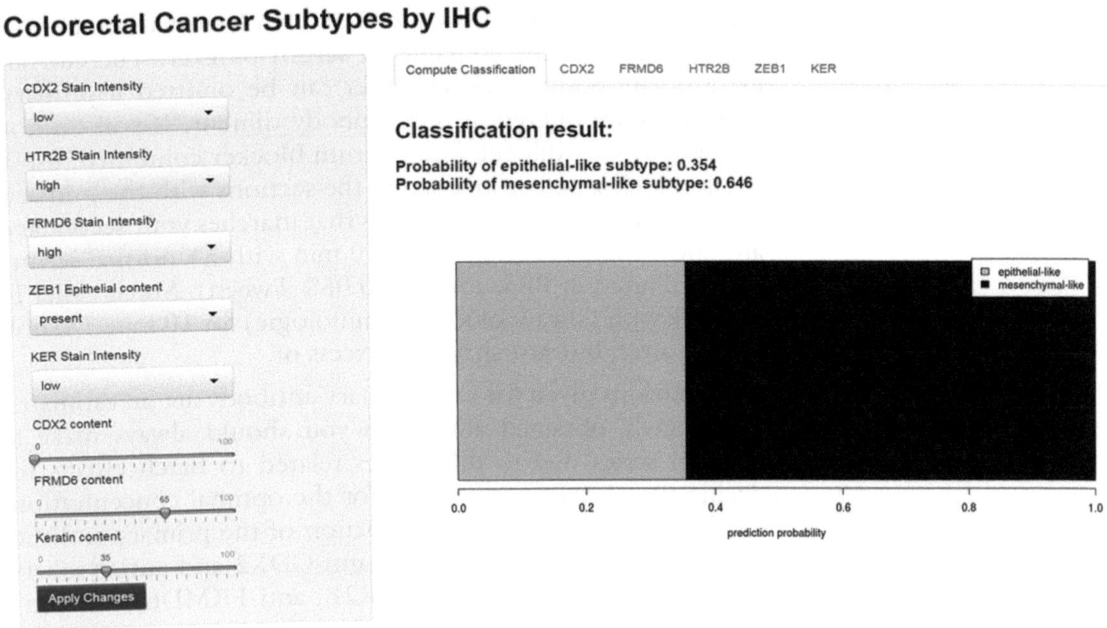

Fig. 4 Online IHC Mini Classifier. Example of a tissue sample classified as mesenchymal subtype of colorectal cancer

(c) Ethanol 90%: dilute 900 mL ethanol 100% with 100 mL demi water.

(d) Ethanol 80%: dilute 800 mL ethanol 100% with 200 mL demi water.

(e) Ethanol 70%: dilute 700 mL ethanol 100% with 300 mL demi water.

3. Dissolve 2.94 g Tri-sodium citrate (dihydrate) with 1000 mL demi water. Ad 1 N HCl to adjust the pH to 6.0. Then add 0.5 mL of Tween 20 and mix well. Store at room temperature for 3 months or at 4 °C for longer storage.
   When using a PT Module™ like we use in our lab (*see* **Note 4**), use a Heat-Induced Epitope Retrieval Solution with Citrate pH 6.0 (PTM Buffer 1). Dilute 100-fold with demi water before use.

4. As a heating source for boiling of the sections one can use a steamer, water bath, microwave, or pressure cooker. As an alternative heating source one can also use the automated Lab Vision™ PT Module.

5. In our lab we experienced the best results for reduction of nonspecific background staining with a ready-to-use Peroxidase-Blocking Solution. Store at 4 °C and protect from sunlight in order to slow its thermal decomposition. For preparing the solution yourself, incubate sections in pure Methanol with 1% H_2O_2 for 15 min at room temperature.

6. We used a Normal antibody diluent (ready-to-use, Immunologic) which already contained a serum blocker. Therefor an extra preantibody blocking buffer can be omitted if primary antibodies are diluted in this antibody diluent. If you do not use an antibody diluent with a serum blocker combined, use a serum blocker before incubating the sections with the primary antibody. Use serum from species that matches your secondary antibody. Incubate sections for 30 min with 5% normal serum block (diluted in PBS, 1% BSA, 0.05% Tween). Much easier is to block with Ultra V block (Immunologic) for 10 min. Do not wash it after, but just shake the excess of.
7. The dilutions given for each primary antibody are an estimate. With newly obtained antibodies you should always make a dilution series due to differences related to batch effects to decide the appropriate dilution for the optimal concentration needed to promote a specific reaction of the primary and the secondary antibodies. Store the anti-CDX2 and anti-cytokeratin at 4 °C; store the anti-HTR2B, anti-FRMD6, and anti-ZEB1 at −20 °C.
8. We used Bright DAB (Klinipath), a ready-to-go DAB two component Kit (DAB Chromogen and DAB Substrate). Store at 4 °C.
9. For optimal adherence of your sections to the slides it is important that you get rid of the water underneath the sections. If you dry the slides horizontal the water is trapped in the middle and the tissue cannot attach to the slide surface.
10. After using the xylene for over 100 slides you need to replace it with fresh stock.
11. Make sure that you use fresh stock of the different concentrations of ethanol and it is not polluted with something like hematoxylin.
12. In general, which antigen retrieval technique is required depends upon the antibody. The most commonly used one seems to be the citrate buffer method which works very well with the antibodies used in this mini classifier. The citrate-based solution is designed to break the protein cross-links, therefore unmask the antigens and epitopes in formalin-fixed and paraffin embedded tissue sections, thus enhancing staining intensity of antibodies.
13. When using HRP conjugated antibodies it is essential to block endogenous peroxidase to prevent nonspecific background staining. We recommend to always incorporate an endogenous peroxidase block step.
14. It is important to prevent your sections from drying while applying the hydrophobic barrier. This can be done by pulling

each slide individually from the slide holder. The other slides can wait in PBS. Tap it gently on a tissue to rapidly remove excess PBS, apply the PAP pen to the dry glass surface and return to the slide holder. Be sure the hydrophobic barrier is dry before submerging in the PBS.

15. Be careful with DAB because it is carcinogenic. Wear gloves, lab coat, and eye protection.
16. This nuclear counterstaining can help you to pinpoint the exact position of the positive cells and obtain crucial insight into the tissue context. Make a dilution series of the Hematoxylin to decide the appropriate dilution for the optimal concentration to provide contrast that helps the primary stain stand out.
17. Cover slides one by one. Be careful that the slides do not dry out, it is not good for your sample and the xylene makes it easier for the mounting medium to spread out. Other slides can wait in xylene.
18. The online mini-IHC-classifier is based on the automated image analysis of Trinh et al. (2016) [9] which uses a random forest classifier to determine patient subtypes. The most common decision rules from 1000 decision trees were extracted and adapted to take semiquantitative scores assigned by pathologist scoring as inputs. Comparison between the automated and (online) semiquantitative classifiers showed strong concordance, highlighting that the simplified classifier is capable of assigning subtype classes in the absence of continuous quantitative information.

    The prediction probability score for each patient sample is the frequency of classification of CMS2/3 compared with CMS4 in the random forest library (random forest of 1000 trees). Probability scores range between 0 and 1, and it is up to the user's discretion on choosing an optimal threshold to categorize their sample of interest. For example, in our previous work, samples with a random forest probability of 60% (prediction threshold 0.6) were scored as "mesenchymal" in a hope to avoid false positives, but may result in false negatives. Samples surrounding 0.5 cannot be assigned with confidence to one of the subtypes.

    Here we described the pathologist scoring online IHC Mini Classifier, but when using TMA cores it is also possible to use the automated computational analysis, for details and code for the image analysis pipeline to develop the CMS-Classifier see Trinh et al. (2016) [9].

Acknowledgment

L.V. is supported by a KWF grant (UVA2014-7245), a Worldwide Cancer Research grant (14-1164), a Maag Lever Darm Stichting grant (MLDS-CDG 14-03), the European Research Council (ERG-StG 638193), The New York Stem Cell Foundation and a Vidi grant (917.15.308) from NWO. L.V. is also a New York Stem Cell Foundation – Robertson Investigator.

References

1. De Sousa EMF, Vermeulen L, Fessler E, Medema JP (2013) Cancer heterogeneity—a multifaceted view. EMBO Rep 14(8):686–695. https://doi.org/10.1038/embor.2013.92
2. Budinska E, Popovici V, Tejpar S, D'Ario G, Lapique N, Sikora KO, Di Narzo AF, Yan P, Hodgson JG, Weinrich S, Bosman F, Roth A, Delorenzi M (2013) Gene expression patterns unveil a new level of molecular heterogeneity in colorectal cancer. J Pathol 231(1):63–76. https://doi.org/10.1002/path.4212
3. De Sousa EMF, Wang X, Jansen M, Fessler E, Trinh A, de Rooij LP, de Jong JH, de Boer OJ, van Leersum R, Bijlsma MF, Rodermond H, van der Heijden M, van Noesel CJ, Tuynman JB, Dekker E, Markowetz F, Medema JP, Vermeulen L (2013) Poor-prognosis colon cancer is defined by a molecularly distinct subtype and develops from serrated precursor lesions. Nat Med 19(5):614–618. https://doi.org/10.1038/nm.3174
4. Marisa L, de Reynies A, Duval A, Selves J, Gaub MP, Vescovo L, Etienne-Grimaldi MC, Schiappa R, Guenot D, Ayadi M, Kirzin S, Chazal M, Flejou JF, Benchimol D, Berger A, Lagarde A, Pencreach E, Piard F, Elias D, Parc Y, Olschwang S, Milano G, Laurent-Puig P, Boige V (2013) Gene expression classification of colon cancer into molecular subtypes: characterization, validation, and prognostic value. PLoS Med 10(5):e1001453. https://doi.org/10.1371/journal.pmed.1001453
5. Roepman P, Schlicker A, Tabernero J, Majewski I, Tian S, Moreno V, Snel MH, Chresta CM, Rosenberg R, Nitsche U, Macarulla T, Capella G, Salazar R, Orphanides G, Wessels LF, Bernards R, Simon IM (2014) Colorectal cancer intrinsic subtypes predict chemotherapy benefit, deficient mismatch repair and epithelial-to-mesenchymal transition. Int J Cancer 134(3):552–562. https://doi.org/10.1002/ijc.28387
6. Sadanandam A, Lyssiotis CA, Homicsko K, Collisson EA, Gibb WJ, Wullschleger S, Ostos LC, Lannon WA, Grotzinger C, Del Rio M, Lhermitte B, Olshen AB, Wiedenmann B, Cantley LC, Gray JW, Hanahan D (2013) A colorectal cancer classification system that associates cellular phenotype and responses to therapy. Nat Med 19(5):619–625. https://doi.org/10.1038/nm.3175
7. Schlicker A, Beran G, Chresta CM, McWalter G, Pritchard A, Weston S, Runswick S, Davenport S, Heathcote K, Castro DA, Orphanides G, French T, Wessels LF (2012) Subtypes of primary colorectal tumors correlate with response to targeted treatment in colorectal cell lines. BMC Med Genomics 5:66. https://doi.org/10.1186/1755-8794-5-66
8. Guinney J, Dienstmann R, Wang X, de Reynies A, Schlicker A, Soneson C, Marisa L, Roepman P, Nyamundanda G, Angelino P, Bot BM, Morris JS, Simon IM, Gerster S, Fessler E, De Sousa EMF, Missiaglia E, Ramay H, Barras D, Homicsko K, Maru D, Manyam GC, Broom B, Boige V, Perez-Villamil B, Laderas T, Salazar R, Gray JW, Hanahan D, Tabernero J, Bernards R, Friend SH, Laurent-Puig P, Medema JP, Sadanandam A, Wessels L, Delorenzi M, Kopetz S, Vermeulen L, Tejpar S (2015) The consensus molecular subtypes of colorectal cancer. Nat Med 21(11):1350–1356. https://doi.org/10.1038/nm.3967
9. Trinh A, Trumpi K, De Sousa EMF, Wang X, de Jong JH, Fessler E, Kuppen PJ, Reimers MS, Swets M, Koopman M, Nagtegaal ID, Jansen M, Hooijer GK, Offerhaus GJ,

Kranenburg O, Punt CJ, Medema JP, Markowetz F, Vermeulen L (2017) Practical and robust identification of molecular subtypes in colorectal cancer by immunohistochemistry. Clin Cancer Res 23(2):387–398. https://doi.org/10.1158/1078-0432.CCR-16-0680

10. Halling KC, Roche PC (2001) Immunohistochemical Analysis for hMLH1 and hMSH2 Expression in Colorectal Cancer. Methods Mol Med 50:81–86. https://doi.org/10.1385/1-59259-084-5:81

11. Parc YR, Halling KC (2001) Microsatellite instability testing. Methods Mol Med 50:69–79. https://doi.org/10.1385/1-59259-084-5:69

Check for updates

Chapter 12

Stool DNA Integrity Method for Colorectal Cancer Detection

Claudia Rengucci, Giulia De Maio, Maura Menghi, and Daniele Calistri

Abstract

Fluorescence long DNA (FL-DNA) is a non-invasive and simple-to-perform stool DNA test. This assay consists of a qualitative and quantitative real-time PCR (RT PCR) analysis. FL-DNA has great potential in colorectal cancer (CRC) lesions detection used alone or in combination with the standard CRC screening tool: immunochemical fecal occult blood test (iFOBT).

Key words FL-DNA, CRC, Stool DNA, Colonocytes, Screening

1 Introduction

Colorectal cancer (CRC) is a multistage process by which healthy colonic epithelium slowly develops into polyps or adenomas and over time progress into carcinomas [1]. Despite the high disease incidence, mortality is lower [2] thanks to the improvement of screening programs. The investigations used can be categorized into three broad groups: stool tests, endoscopic examinations and imaging tests [3, 4]. Due to the different technical limits, none of these methods is optimal. Recently, different stool DNA tests have been proposed alone or in combination with current routine diagnostic tests [5, 6].

Stool DNA tests are based on the continuously exfoliation of colonocytes into the fecal stream [7] whose DNA can be used to characterize the colonic epithelium [8]. Typically, healthy mucosa sheds apoptotic colonocytes, whereas diseased mucosa exfoliates nonapoptotic colonocytes. Fragments of 200 bp or more in length characterize nonapoptotic DNA. This DNA is called long DNA (L-DNA) and is become an utilizable biomarker for CRC early diagnosis.

In our laboratory, we developed the fluorescence long DNA (FL-DNA) method, a quality and quantitative evaluation of L-DNA based on fluorescence amplification of different genomic DNA regions by real-time PCR (RT PCR) [9].

Jean-François Beaulieu (ed.), *Colorectal Cancer: Methods and Protocols*, Methods in Molecular Biology, vol. 1765,
https://doi.org/10.1007/978-1-4939-7765-9_12,

Firstly, the DNA quality is assessed through the amplification of a control plasmidic DNA, added to each sample. A specific oligo-mix (FL-DNA Control Mix), containing primers complementary to the 150 bp insert flanking regions, amplifies the control plasmidic DNA in inhibitors-free samples only [10].

Later the quantitative evaluation of DNA is done by the co-amplification of sequences from 139 to 344 bp in length with two Oligo-mixes: FL-DNA MixA, specific for fragments 2 and 3 of *APC*, and exon 8 of *p53* and FL-DNA MixB, specific for fragment 4 of *APC* and exons 5 and 7 of *p53*, respectively [11].

The DNA concentration is measured through a reference standard curve expressed as ng/reaction [12]. DNA extraction can be performed through a manual or semiautomatic method depending on laboratory equipment and availability.

FL-DNA is a user-friendly, non-invasive and not expensive stool DNA test that could be performed in addition to the immunochemical-based fecal occult blood test (iFOBT) currently used in CRC screening programs. This combined approach showed a better prediction of CRC and/or high risk adenoma lesions [13].

2 Materials

2.1 Feces pre-treatment

The two feces pre-treatment protocols can be performed for both DNA extraction methods.

2.1.1 Feces pre-treatment within 2 hours from sample arrival

1. Stool Reagent 1(Diatech Pharmacogenetics).
2. Stool Reagent 2 (Diatech Pharmacogenetics).
3. Ethanol 100%.

2.1.2 Feces pre-treatment within 7 days from sample arrival

1. Stool Stabilizer [(0.5 mol/L Tris-HCL, 0.15 mol/L EDTA, 10 mmol/L NaCl (pH 9.0)].
2. Stool Reagent 2 (Diatech Pharmacogenetics).
3. Ethanol 100%.

2.2 DNA Extraction

2.2.1 Manual Method

1. Pre-lysis treatment: Helix Tissue Buffer (Diatech Pharmacogenetics), Helix Proteinase K (Diatech Pharmacogenetics).
2. Lysis treatment: Lysis Solution: 198 μL Helix Lysis Buffer and 22 μL di Helix Proteinase K (Diatech Pharmacogenetics), Binding Solution: 1279 μL di Helix Binding DNA and 21 μL di Helix DTT (Diatech Pharmacogenetics).
3. Separation: Binding Solution: 1279 μL di Helix Binding DNA and 21 μL di Helix DTT (Diatech Pharmacogenetics), Helix Wash 1 (Diatech Pharmacogenetics), Helix Wash 2 (Diatech Pharmacogenetics).
4. Elution: Helix Elution Buffer (Diatech Pharmacogenetics).

2.2.2 Automatic Method with Helix Extraction System®

1. Pre-lysis treatment: Helix Tissue Buffer (Diatech Pharmacogenetics), Helix Proteinase K (Diatech Pharmacogenetics).
2. Lysis, Separation and Elution treatment: Helix Lysis Buffer (Diatech Pharmacogenetics), Helix Proteinase K (Diatech Pharmacogenetics), Helix Binding DNA (Diatech Pharmacogenetics), Helix DTT (Diatech Pharmacogenetics), Helix Wash 1 (Diatech Pharmacogenetics), Helix Wash 2 (Diatech Pharmacogenetics), Helix Elution Buffer (Diatech Pharmacogenetics).

2.3 Real-Time PCR

1. MESA GREEN qPCR MasterMix Plus for SYBR® Assay No ROX (EUROGENTEC).
2. FL-DNA MixA or FL-DNA MixB (Diatech Pharmacogenetics).
3. FL-DNA Control Mix (Diatech Pharmacogenetics).
4. FL-DNA Control (Diatech Pharmacogenetics).
5. DNase–RNase-free Water.

3 Methods

Carry out all procedures at room temperature unless otherwise specified.

3.1 Feces pre-treatment

Stool samples can undergo two different treatments depending if they will be processed within 2 h from their arrival or they will be pretreated later (*see* **Note 1**).

3.1.1 Fresh feces pre-treatment within 2 hours from sample arrival

1. Dispense 900 μL of Stool Reagent 1 in a 2 mL tube an add 200 mg of fecal sample.
2. Vortex briefly and centrifuge at 5000 × *g* for 15 min at 4 °C.
3. Transfer the supernatant in a clean 2 mL tube. Add 930 μL of ethanol (100%) and 155 μL of Stool Reagent 2. Discard pellet.
4. Mix by inversion five times and centrifuge at 5000 × *g* for 15 min at 4 °C.
5. Remove supernatant paying attention to not remove any pellet, which may be not visible.
6. Proceed with DNA extraction or store pellet at −20 °C.

3.1.2 Frozen feces pre-treatment

1. If stool samples will be processed later they have to be stored at −80 °C in 30–50 mL of Stool Stabilizer, depending on the amount of material (*see* **Note 2**).
2. During the pretreatment, you can use directly the fecal sample starting from **step 2** of Subheading 3.1.1 protocol. This can be valid also for following extractions.

3.2 DNA Extraction

3.2.1 Manual Method

1. Set a thermomixer at 65 °C.
2. Add 500 μL Helix Tissue Buffer to the pellet. If pellet is not well suspended add further 100 μL Helix Tissue Buffer.
3. Vortex for 30 s until pellet is completely suspended.
4. Centrifuge at 13000 × *g* for 1 min.
5. Transfer 450 μL of supernatant in a new 2 mL tube and add 8 μL Helix Proteinase K.
6. Vortex and incubate for 30 min at 65 °C in agitation at 20 × *g*.
7. Vortex and spin samples.
8. Prepare for each sample 220 μL of Lysis Solution with 198 μL Helix Lysis Buffer and 22 μL Helix Proteinase K.
9. Prepare for each sample 1300 μL of Binding Solution with 1279 μL of Helix Binding DNA and 21 μL di Helix DTT.
10. Set a thermomixer at 70 °C and incubate Helix Elution Buffer until use.
11. Transfer 400 μL of prelysed sample in the Lysis Tube and add 220 μL Lysis Solution.
12. Vortex for 10–20 s and incubate 5 min at room temperature.
13. Incubate for 10 min at 70 °C in agitation at 20 × *g*.
14. Centrifuge briefly.
15. Add 800 μL Binding Solution.
16. Vortex for 10–20 s and incubates 5 min at room temperature.
17. Vortex for 10–20 s and centrifuge briefly.
18. Transfer 700 μL of lysed sample in the column inserted into the collection tube.
19. Centrifuge for 1 min at 13000 × *g*.
20. Empty the collection tube and transfer further 700 μL of lysed sample again into the same column.
21. Centrifuge for 1 min at 13000 × *g*.
22. Put the column in a clean collection tube and dispense 500 μL Binding solution.
23. Centrifuge for 1 min at 13000 × *g*.
24. Put the column in a clean collection tube and dispense 700 μL Helix Wash 1.
25. Centrifuge for 1 min at 13000 × *g*.
26. Put the column in a clean collection tube and dispense 600 μL Helix Wash 1.
27. Centrifuge for 1 min at 13000 × *g*.
28. Put the column in a clean collection tube and dispense 600 μL Helix Wash 2.

29. Centrifuge for 1 min at 13000 × *g*.
30. Put the column in a clean collection tube and centrifuge for 5 min at 13000 × *g*.
31. Transfer the column into the elution tube and add 60 μL warm Helix Elution Buffer.
32. Centrifuge for 1 min at 13000 × *g*.
33. Discard the column and proceed with the amplification or store the DNA at +2/+8 °C for max 2–3 days or at −35/−20 °C for a longer time.

3.2.2 Automatic Method with Helix Extraction System

1. Set a thermomixer at 65 °C.
2. Add 500 μL Helix Tissue Buffer to the pellet. If pellet is not well suspended add further 100 μL Helix Tissue Buffer.
3. Vortex 30 s or until pellet is completely suspended.
4. Centrifuge for 1 min at 13000 × *g*.
5. Transfer 450 μL of supernatant in a new 2 mL tube and add 8 μL Helix Proteinase K.
6. Vortex and incubate for 30 min at 65 °C in agitation at 20 g.
7. Vortex and spin.
8. Set a thermomixer at 70 °C and incubate Helix Elution Buffer until use.
9. Reagents volumes to be used (Helix Lysis Buffer + Helix Proteinase K, Helix Binding DNA + Helix DTT, Helix Wash 1, Helix Wash 2, and Helix Elution Buffer) are indicated by the instrument.
10. Transfer 400 μL of prelysed sample in a HES lysis plate and procede using Helix Extraction System® with protocol "*HELIX DNA strip vc400-ve60 v200807_stool*".
11. When elution is finished, proceed with the amplification or store DNA at +2/+8 °C for max 2–3 days or at −35/−20 °C for a longer time.

3.3 DNA Amplification

All samples should be amplified with **Control Amp-Mix** in order to evaluate the DNA quality (*see* **Note 3**).

3.3.1 Control Amp-Mix

1. Equilibrate the MG PreMix to room temperature and gently vortex it.
2. Prepare the Control Amp-Mix according to Table 1.
3. Carefully mix the Control Amp-Mix vortexing quickly, then centrifuge briefly.
4. Dispense 20 μL of Control Amp-Mix in each reaction tube, previously labeled.

Table 1
DNA amplification Control Amp-Mix

Control Amp-Mix	Volume for 1 sample (μL)
MG PreMix	12.5
FL-DNA Control Mix	1.0
FL-DNA Control	1.0
$MgCl_2$ 100	0.5
Water	5.0
Total volume	20.0

Table 2
DNA amplification Amp-Mix A and B

Amp-Mix A o B	Volume for 1 sample (μL)
MG PreMix	12.5
FL-DNA Mix A/FL-DNA Mix B	1.0
$MgCl_2$ 100	0.5
Water	6.0
Total volume	20.0

5. Add 5 μL of sample in each sample tube or 5 μL of water in the negative control tube.
6. Total reaction volume: 20 μL.

3.3.2 Amp-Mix A/Amp-Mix B

1. Prepare a suitable number of tubes considering that in each run it is necessary to include four standards (FL-DNA STD 5, 1, 0.3, 0.1 ng/rxn), clinical samples in duplicate and a negative control (water) for both Amp-Mix A and Amp-Mix B.
2. Prepare Amp-Mix A and Amp-Mix B according to Table 2.
3. Carefully mix both Amp-Mix vortexing quickly, then centrifuge briefly.
4. Dispense 20 μL of each Amp-Mix in the respective reaction tubes, previously identified.
5. Add 5 μL of sample (in duplicate) in each sample tube, 5 μL of water in the negative control tube or 5 μL of each standard in the four standard tubes.
6. Total reaction volume: 20 μL.

Table 3
The amplification thermal profile:

Hold	95 °C for 5 min
Cycling (35 cycles)	94 °C for 30 s/59 °C for 30 s/72 °C for 30 s (fluorescence acquisition in Green)/ 80 °C for 30 s (fluorescence acquisition in Green 2)
Melt	Temperature ramp from 72 to 95 °C with 1 °C increment every step. First step (premelt conditioning): 90 s; Next steps: 5 s each; fluorescence acquisition in Melt A channel on Green Melt; Optimize Gain before Melt in all reaction tubes to ensure that the highest raw fluorescence intensity is lower than 70.

3.3.3 Amplification

1. The amplification thermal profile has been optimized on Rotor-Gene Q and Rotor-Gene 6000 (Table 3).
2. Follow the instrument manual to set the following channels for fluorescence acquisition and amplification thermal profile:
3. "Green": source 470 nm—detector 510 nm—Gain 10.
4. "Green 2": source 470 nm—detector 510 nm—Gain 10.

3.4 DNA Quality Assessment

1. In Analysis, select Quantitation, Cycling A. Green. Activate Slope Correct and Dynamic Tube options and set Threshold at 0.15.
2. The negative control must have a Ct value between 15 and 20 ($15 \leq \text{WATER Ct} \leq 20$).
3. Calculate a ΔCt value for each sample according to the formula:

   $\Delta Ct = \text{Sample Ct} - \text{WATER Ct}$
4. Samples with a $\Delta Ct \leq 5$ can be considered inhibitors-free and can be amplified with Mix A and Mix B.
5. Samples with a $\Delta Ct > 5$ are not suitable to be amplified with Mix A and Mix B because of presence of inhibitors in the eluate. In this case a novel DNA extraction is recommended.

3.5 Quantitative Analysis

1. Set two different pages, one for Mix A and one for Mix B. Analyze data independently.
2. In Analysis select Quantitation and Cycling A, Green 2.
3. Identify as "Standard" FL-DNA STD 5, 1, 0.3, and 0.1 ng/rxn and as "Unknown" other samples.
4. Remove the "Auto-Find Threshold" option.
5. Activate Slope Correct and Dynamic Tube options and set Threshold at 0.15.
6. Click on Outlier Removal and select the lowest "NTC Threshold" value in order to maintain the WATER fluorescence curve

below threshold and to keep visible the fluorescence signal for FL-DNA STD 0.1 ng/rxn.

7. For an accurate quantitative analysis, **Efficiency** must be ≥0.75, R^2 must be ≥0.98.
8. All samples with a FL-DNA value ≥0.1 ng/rxn must be confirmed through the Melt Curve analysis in order to exclude any nonspecific amplification products.
9. In Analysis select Melt then Melt A and Green Melt. Exclude any Digital Filter.
10. Samples should show one or more peaks at temperature >80 °C only.
11. For each sample sum the average concentration of Mix A and the average concentration of Mix B, then multiply by 100 in order to have the final FL-DNA value.

3.6 Evaluation of FL-DNA Results Compared to iFOBT

FL-DNA results can also be used in combination with iFOBT tests to predict the presence of a tumor and/or high-risk adenomas (*see* **Note 4**). To combine these two analyses, we adopted the Fagan Nomogram approach. According to the diagnostic relevance of fecal hemoglobin and FL-DNA as independent variables, it is possible to test whether or not, and to what extent, the FL-DNA assay could improve iFOBT diagnostic accuracy.

1. iFOBT values can be divided into three main subgroups: negative, low positive and high positive. In a previous study these classes were: <100 ng/mL, 100–432 ng/mL, and >432 ng/mL [9].
2. FL-DNA results can be divided into three classes according to different values (*see* **Note 5**): low level, medium level and high level. Referring to a previous paper these classes can be: 0–9, 10–30, and ≥30 ng/reaction [9].
3. To estimate post-testprobability, i.e., the probability of disease in a subject after the diagnostic test results are known, it is necessary to estimate the pretest probability and to determine the likelihood ratio (*see* **Note 6**).

4 Notes

1. A bad initial fecal sample collection might compromise result validity. Fecal samples collected before the preparation for the colonoscopy should be transported at 4 °C to the biomolecular laboratory where they will be processed in max 7 days.
2. To preserve the DNA quality all the material must be covered.
3. Presence of PCR inhibitors, if not well evaluated, might cause not efficient results.

4. There are no data on large records that permit to evaluate kit FL-DNA effects on the mortality decrease in the population. Nowadays, colonoscopy is still considered as the reference standard method necessary to reduce CRC incidence and mortality.
5. Results reliability depends also from the procedures performed in preliminary steps: biological samples collection, samples preservation, and DNA extraction.
6. The pretest probability is the chance of having the disease before testing and this is usually related to the disease prevalence. The likelihood ratio is the ratio of the probability of the specific test result in people who do have the disease to the probability in people who do not. The posttest probability is consequently calculated by multiplying the likelihood ratio of the diagnostic test by the pretest probability.

FL-DNA [ng]	Hb $<$ 100 [ng/mL]	100 $\leq$ Hb $<$ 432 [ng/mL]	Hb $\geq$ 432 [ng/mL]
0–9	0.4%	4.1%	16.8%
10–30	1.2%	11.3%	37.4%
$\geq$30	24.2%	76.4%	93.8%

According to data obtain in Rengucci et al.'s study [9], in the negative-iFOBT subgroup, the pre-test probability of there being a tumor was around 13%, but FL-DNA did not add any useful information. Furthermore, in the low positive iFOBT subgroup, with its 12% overall probability of having cancer, the breakdown analysis as a function of the higher FL-DNA subgroup brings the probability of having a tumor to 76%. Specifically, in the high iFOBT subgroup, with its 38% overall probability of having cancer, breakdown analysis as a function of the high FL-DNA subgroup highlighted the probability of having colorectal cancer as 93%. The combination between colorectal cancer and high-risk adenomas increased the posttest probability values of having a disease in association with the higher FL-DNA values at 76%, 85%, and 94% for all the three main iFOBT subgroups, respectively.

Acknowledgment

This work was supported by Diatech Pharmacogenetics, Jesi (AN)—Italy.

References

1. Fearon ER, Vogelstein B (1990) A genetic model for colorectal tumorigenesis. Cell 61 (5):759–767
2. Ferlay J, Soerjomataram I, Ervik M, Dikshit R, Eser S, Mathers C, Rebelo M, Parkin DM, Forman D, Bray, F. GLOBOCAN 2012 v1.0, Cancer incidence and mortality worldwide: IARC CancerBase No. 11 [Internet]. Lyon, France: International Agency for Research on Cancer; 2013. Available from: http://globocan.iarc.fr. Accessed 10 Nov 2016.
3. Levin B, Lieberman DA, McFarland B et al (2008) Screening and surveillance for the early detection of colorectal cancer and adenomatous polyps, 2008: a joint guideline from the American Cancer Society, the US Multi-Society Task Force on Colorectal Cancer, and the American College of Radiology. Gastroenterology 134:1570–1595. https://doi.org/10.1053/j.gastro.2008.02.002
4. Quintero E, Castells A, Bujanda L et al (2012) Colonoscopy versus fecal immunochemical testing in colorectal-cancer screening. N Engl J Med 366:697–706. https://doi.org/10.1056/NEJMoa1108895
5. Bosch LJ, Carvalho B, Fijneman RJ et al (2011) Molecular tests for colorectal cancer screening. Clin Colorectal Cancer 10:8–23. https://doi.org/10.3816/CCC.2011.n.002
6. Ahlquist DA (2010) Molecular detection of colorectal neoplasia. Gastroenterology 138:2127–2139. https://doi.org/10.1053/j.gastro.2010.01.055
7. Ahlquist DA, Harrington JJ, Burgart LJ et al (2000) Morphometric analysis of the "mucocellular layer" overlying colorectal cancer and normal mucosa: relevance to exfoliation and stool screening. Hum Pathol 31:51–57
8. De Maio G, Rengucci C, Zoli W et al (2014) Circulating and stool nucleic acid analysis for colorectal cancer diagnosis. World J Gastroenterol 20:957–967. https://doi.org/10.3748/wjg.v20.i4.957
9. Rengucci C, De Maio G, Menghi M et al (2014) Improved stool DNA integrity method for early colorectal cancer diagnosis. Cancer Epidemiol Biomarkers Prev 23:2553–2560. https://doi.org/10.1158/1055-9965.EPI-14-0379
10. Calistri D, Rengucci C, Bocchini R et al (2003) Fecal multiple molecular tests to detect colorectal cancer in stool. Clin Gastroenterol Hepatol 1:377–383. https://doi.org/10.1053/S1542-3565(03)00186-1
11. Calistri D, Rengucci C, Lattuneddu A et al (2004) Detection of colorectal cancer by a quantitative fluorescence determination of DNA amplification in stool. Neoplasia 6:536–540. https://doi.org/10.1593/neo.04190
12. Calistri D, Rengucci C, Molinari C et al (2009) Quantitative fluorescence determination of long-fragment DNA in stool as a marker for the early detection of colorectal cancer. Cell Oncol 31:11–17. https://doi.org/10.3233/CLO-2009-0443
13. Calistri D, Rengucci C, Casadei Gardini A et al (2010) Fecal DNA for noninvasive diagnosis of colorectal cancer in immunochemical fecal occult blood test-positive individuals. Cancer Epidemiol Biomarkers Prev 19:2647–2654. https://doi.org/10.1158/1055-9965.EPI-10-0291

Check for updates

Chapter 13

RT-qPCR for Fecal Mature MicroRNA Quantification and Validation

Farid E. Ahmed, Nancy C. Ahmed, Mostafa M. Gouda, Paul W. Vos, and Chris Bonnerup

Abstract

By routinely and systematically being able to perform quantitative stem-loop reverse transcriptase (RT) followed by TaqMan® minor-groove binding (MGB) probe, real-time quantitative PCR analysis on exfoliated enriched colonocytes in stool, using human (*Homo sapiens*, hsa) micro(mi)RNAs to monitor changes of their expression at various stages of colorectal (CRC) progression, this method allows for the reliable and quantitative diagnostic screening of colon cancer (CC). Although the expression of some miRNA genes tested in tissue shows less variability in normal or cancerous patients than in stool, the noninvasive stool by itself is well suited for CC screening. An miRNA approach using stool promises to offer more sensitivity and specificity than currently used genomic, methylomic, or proteomic methods for CC screening.

To present an application of employing miRNAs as diagnostic markers for CC screening, we carried out global microarray expression studies on stool colonocytes isolated by paramagnetic beads, using Affymetrix GeneChip miRNA 3.0 Array, to select a panel of miRNAs for subsequent focused semiquantitative PCR analysis studies. We then conducted a stem-loop RT-TaqMan® MGB probes, followed by a modified real-time qPCR expression study on 20 selected miRNAs for subsequent validation of the extracted immunocaptured total small RNA isolated from stool colonocytes. Results showed 12 miRNAs (miR-7, miR-17, miR-20a, miR-21, miR-92a, miR-96, miR-106a, miR-134, miR-183, miR-196a, miR-199a-3p, and miR214) to have an increased expression in stool of CC patients, and that later TNM stages exhibited more increased expressions than adenomas, while 8 miRNAs (miR-9, miR-29b, miR-127-5p, miR-138, miR-143, miR-146a, miR-222, and miR-938) showed decreased expressions in stool of CC patients, which becomes more pronounced as the cancer progresses from early to late TNM stages (0–IV).

Key words Adenocarcinoma, Colon cancer, Colonocyte, Colorectal cancer, TaqMan

1 Introduction

CRC is the second and third most common malignancy in men and women, respectively, in developed and developing countries, including the USA and Europe [1, 2]. Mortality and morbidity from colon cancer represent a major health problem involving a malignant disease that is theoretically preventable through

Jean-François Beaulieu (ed.), *Colorectal Cancer: Methods and Protocols*, Methods in Molecular Biology, vol. 1765, https://doi.org/10.1007/978-1-4939-7765-9_13,

screening. Early detection would be greatly enhanced if accurate, practical, and cost-effective diagnostic biomarkers for this malignancy were available. Current screening methods (e.g., fecal occult blood test, FOBT) lack sensitivity [2, 3], are costly, with side effects and have low compliance, or may result in mortality (e.g., colonoscopy) [4]. An approach using miRNAs, which are relatively nondegradable when extracted from stool by commercially available kits and manipulated thereafter, would be preferable to a transcriptomic messenger (m)RNA-, mutation DNA-, epigenetic-, or a proteomic-based test [5].

Stool represents a challenging environment, as it contains many substances and certain inhibitors, which need to be removed for a successful PCR. Stool testing has several advantages over other screening methods, such as blood for example, as it is truly noninvasive and requires no unpleasant cathartic preparation, formal health care visits, or time away from work or routine activities. It reflects the full length of the colorectum and samples can be taken in a way that represents the right and left side of the colon. It is also believed that colonocytes are released continuously and abundantly into the fecal stream, contrary to blood that is released intermittently as in guaiac FOBT [6]; therefore, this natural enrichment phenomenon partially obviates the need to use a laboratory technique to enrich for tumorigenic colonocytes, as for example when blood is used for testing. Furthermore, because testing can be performed on mail-in-specimens, geographic access to stool screening is essentially unimpeded.

An optimal colon cancer screening test would be one that accurately detects advanced adenomas with a high chance of malignant progression [6]. Clinical management of adenomas entails removing them at the time of detection by colonoscopy. However, many eligible patients do not wish to undertake such an expensive and invasive test because of the need for bowel preparation, dietary restrictions, abdominal pain, and potential perforation of the colon [4]. Given the desirability of using a noninvasive test as an initial screen, molecular approaches [7] were developed. An miRNA approach in stool could meet the criteria for test acceptability as it is noninvasive, it requires ~1 g of stool, results are comparable to those for colon tissue, sampling on consecutive dates is not required, samples can be sent by mail in cold packs, the method can differentiate between normal tissue and colon adenomas/carcinomas, it has high sensitivity and specificity of detecting advanced polyps, and it can be automated [5], which makes it relatively inexpensive and more suited for early detection when compared to a test such as that for mutated DNA markers. Market availability of powerful high-throughput approaches for global miRNA characterization, such as microarrays and universally applicable quantification assays for miRNA expression such as qPCR, suggest that the validation pipeline that often encounters bottlenecks [6] is more efficient for an miRNA assay.

MiRNAs are small, noncoding sequences of 17–27 nucleotides long that regulate cell processes in ~30% of mammalian genes by imperfectly binding to the 3′ untranslated region (UTR) of target mRNAs, resulting in prevention of protein accumulation by either transcription repression, or by inducing mRNA degradation [8]. Many miRNA are thought to target hundreds of mRNAs. The market availability of powerful high-throughput approaches for global miRNA characterization, such as microarrays and simpler, universally applicable quantification assays for miRNA expression such as qPCR, suggests that the validation pipeline that often encounters bottlenecks [6] would be more efficient for an miRNA assay. MiRNAs operate in a complex regulatory network, and it is predicted that miRNAs together regulate thousands of human genes [8]. MiRNAs are transcribed as long primary precursor molecules (pri-miRNA) that are subsequently processed by the nuclear enzyme Drosha and other agents to the precursor intermediate miRNA (pre-miRNA), which in turn is processed in the cytoplasm by the protein Dicer to generate the mature single-stranded (ss) miRNA [9]. MiRNA functions have been shown to include development and apoptosis, cell cycle progression, so specific miRNAs are critical in oncogenesis. MiRNAs are biomarkers for classifying both solid [10] and liquid human tumors [11]. They play a role in cancer initiation and metastasis [12] and can function as either an oncogene or a tumor suppressor gene [13]. MiRNA genes are frequently located at fragile sites as well as minimal regions of loss of heterozygosity, minimal regions of amplification or common breakpoint regions, suggesting that miRNAs correctly classify human cancers of unknown primary origin, as well as poorly differentiated tumors [14], and promise to serve as biomarkers for cancer diagnosis, prognosis and response to therapy [11, 15].

It has been estimated that approximately 10^{10} normal adult colonic epithelial cells, each having a lifespan of 3–4 days, are shed daily from the lower two thirds of colon crypts, which makes colonocyte use to develop a CRC screening test an appealing, attainable goal [7]. As CRC miRNAs are identified in stool colonocytes by an approach, as presented herein, the validation of novel miRNA–mRNA target pairs within the pathways of interest could lead to discovery of cellular functions collectively targeted by differentially expressed miRNAs [16].

2 Materials

All solutions are prepared in sterile distilled water, using analytical grade reagents. Sodium azide is not added to reagents. For long-term storage, reagents are stored at −20 °C, and stool at −80 °C. Waste disposal regulations are strictly followed when disposing of waste material.

2.1 Stool Collection

1. Stool is collected in a jacket (Moore Medical, New Britain, CT, USA) to be placed on toilet seat.
2. A clean and sterile plastic spoon, or a solid brush is used to collect stool and place it in a small sterile plastic collection jar.
3. RNALater is used as RNA preservation solution.
4. A Stomacher® 400 EVO Laboratory Blender (Seward, UK).

2.2 Colonocyte Enrichment

For each sample:

1. 80 μL Invitrogen™/Dynabeads® (Carlsbad, CA, USA) immunoparamagnetic beads (DynaMag™-50), 600 nm in diameter, made of iron oxide particles and encapsulated with plastic polymer, exhibit superparamagnetism in the presence of an externally applied magnetic field) [17] were used.
2. 12 ng/mg magnetic beads of mouse IgG1 monoclonal anti-Ep-CAM antibody (Ab) Ber-Ep4 (Dako, Glostrup, Denmark).
3. Hank's solution (Thermo Fisher).
4. Fetal bovine serum (FBS).
5. 1 M Hepes buffer.
6. Nylon filter (pore size 512 μm).
7. Diff-Quick stain (Thermo Fisher).

2.3 Target Primers and TaqMan Probes

1. Stem-loop RT primers (Life Technologies/Thermo Fisher Scientific, Waltham, MA, USA) were obtained for each of the 20 selected miRNA genes [miRNAs [miRNA-7, miR-9, miR-16a, miRNA-17, miRNA-20a, miRNA-21, miR-29b, miRNA-92a, miR-106a, miRNA-127-5p, miRNA-134, miR-138, miRNA-143, miRNA-146a, miRNA-183, miRNA-196a, miRNA-199a-3p, miRNA-214, miRNA-222, and miR-938]].
2. TaqMan with minor grove binder (MGB) probes with non-fluorescence quencher at the 3′ end and the fluorescence dye FAM at the 5′ end (Life Technologies/Thermo Fisher Scientific) were also employed.

2.4 Extraction of Total RNA from Stool

1. Automatic or manual extraction of total RNA from stool was carried out using a guanidinium-based buffer and the RNeasy isolation Kit® (Qiagen, Valencia, CA, USA) [18].
2. NanoDrop-1000 (Thermo Fisher Scientific, Inc., Waltham, MA, USA).
3. Agilent 2100 Bioanalyzer (Agilent Technologies, Inc., Palo Alto, CA, USA) by the RNA 6000 Nano LabChip® [18, 19].

2.5 ss-cDNA Preparation

1. Sensiscript RT Kit® (Qiagen) for making a copy of ss-DNA.
2. TaqMan™ MicroRNA Reverse Transcription Kit, Universal Master Mix without UNG and TaqMan™ Assay.

3. A modified TaqMan®-based quantitative real-time PCR assay including miRNA-specific forward primer, reverse primer, and dye-labeled hydrolysis TaqMan® probes [20].

2.6 Semiquantitative Real-Time PCR

1. Real-time PCR equipment (we use Roche's PCR LightCycler's 480™, Mannheim, Germany) using 96 samples' plate.
2. Master mix: we use Universal Master Mix without UNG and TaqMan™ Assay (Life Technology).

2.7 Statistical Analysis

1. Lattice package in R (version 2.9.0, The R Foundation for Statistical Computing, http://cran.r-project.org), and S-plus software (Insightful Corporation, Seattle, WA).
2. Other packages such as GESS (Gene Expression Statistical System) published by NCSS (www.ncss.com).

3 Methods

All procedures are carried out at room temperature unless otherwise specified.

3.1 Acquisition of Stool Specimens

1. All Laboratory work is carried out and standardized under blind conditions and following guidelines for handling biohazardous material established by the Institution's Biological Safety Committee.
2. Stool samples (bowel movement. 20 g) are collected from consenting individuals before administering any laxative in a jacket, which can be placed in the toilet, then using a clean plastic spoon to collect samples from mucinous layers, which are rich in colonocytes, and from nonmucinous parts of stool, in order to have a representation of the entire colon (both right- and left-sided colon) [18, 19].
3. Participant then places 1 g of collected stool sample in a smaller clean urine container with 5 mL of the preservative RNA*Later*® that prevents fragmentation of the fragile mRNA and stored at −80 °C until RT-qPCR quantification is carried out randomly and blindly on all stored samples at once in order to prevent analytical bias [18, 19].

3.2 Colonocyte Enrichment

1. Approximately 1 g of thawed stool is homogenized in a Stomacher® 400 EVO Blender at 200 rpm for 3 min, with 40 mL of Hank's solution containing 10% FBS and 25 mM Hepes buffer (pH 7.35).
2. The homogenates is filtered through a nylon filter followed by addition of 80 μL of Dynal superparamagnetic polystyrene beads coated with the Ber-Ep4 anti-Ep-CAM antibody [21]

at a final concentration of 12 ng of Ab/mg magnetic beads (1 μg Ab/106 target cells).

3. The mixtures is incubated for 30 min on a shaking platform at room temperature.
4. A 100,000 colonocytes is enough to test all the 20 miRNA genes of interest (*see* **Note 1**)
5. To visualize colonocytes. a drop of the cell suspension is spread on a glass slide, dried and stained with Diff-Quick stain.
6. To estimate the number of colonocytes form which total small RNA will be extracted, use another drop of cell suspension placed in a hemocytometer, and count under the microscope.
7. The supernatant is removed and the pellet containing colonocytes is stored at −80 °C until small RNA extraction [21].

3.3 RNA Extraction and Ss-cDNA Preparation.

1. Extracting total small RNA from about 0.25 g of stored frozen stool (−80 °C) according to manufacture's specifications is carried out randomly and blindly at once in order to prevent analytical bias, using the guanidinium-based buffer provided with the RNeasy isolation Kit® [18].
2. Purity of total RNA is measured spectrophotometrically on NanoDrop-1000 at 2260 nm, 280 nm and 230 nm showing an OD $260_{nm}/280_{nm}$ ratio from 1.9 to 2.0, indicating that it is reasonably pure. OD 230_{nm} is also used for protein measurement [19].
3. The integrity of RNA is determined on an Agilent 2100 Bioanalyzer utilizing the RNA 6000 Nano LabChip® [18, 19] (*see* **Note 2**).
4. The Sensiscript RT Kit® is employed for making a copy of ss-DNA in a 7.5 μL RT reaction containing total RNA, 50 nm stem-loop RT primer, 1× RT buffer, 0.23 nm of each of dNTP, 3.33 U/μL multiscriptase reverse transcriptase, of which 2–3 μL is subsequently amplified by PCR [20].
5. The reaction, in a 96-well plate, is incubated in a 9700 thermocycler for 30 min at 16 °C, 30 min at 42 °C, 5 min at 85 °C to inactivate the Thermoscript RT, and formed ss-cDNA held at 4 °C.
6. A 2–3 μL of ss-cDNA is subsequently amplified by PCR (*see* **Note 3**). The use of nontemplate controls and RT-minus controls are also employed to confirm the correct performance of the RT reaction [20].

3.4 RT of Mature miRNAs

1. Total RNA is briefly exposed to RNAase-free DNAase I for 5 min.
2. RNA is then reverse-transcribed to a cDNA using a long gene-specific primer (i.e., the antisense PCR primer) at an elevated

temperature. A Sensiscript thermostable reverse transcriptase is employed at room temperature.

3. Briefly, a 7.5 μL RT reaction containing an antisense primer and a primer for the 18S rRNA internal control normalizer is heated to 80 °C for 5 min to denature the RNA, followed by 5-min incubation at 60 °C to anneal the primers. The reaction is cooled to room temperature, and the remaining reagents (5× buffer, dNTPs, DTT, RNAse inhibitor, Sensiscript) are added according to manufacturer's protocol. The reaction proceeds for 45 min at 60 °C, followed by a 5-min incubation at 85 °C to inactivate the Sensiscript [19, 20]. Commercial systems are also available (*see* **Note 4**).

3.5 qPCR of Mature miRNAs

This semiquantitative real-time qPCR assay (*see* **Note 5**) of mature miRNAs using TaqMan® MGB probes is specific for mature miRNAs (*see* **Note 6**) and discriminates among related miRNAs that differ by as little as one nucleotide, and is not affected by genomic DNA contamination [19, 20] (*see* **Notes 7** and **8**).

1. The 10 μL PCR reaction included 0.67 μL RT product (representing ~1 nm total RNA) (*see* **Note 9**), 1× TaqMan® probe, 1 μM of forward and 0.7 μm of reverse stem-loop RT primers (~50 nM each).
2. Reaction run conditions are as follows: 95 °C for 10 min, followed by 30 cycles of 95 °C for 15 s and 60 °C for 1 min. All reactions were run in triplicate [20].
3. Components for the assay are found in the TaqMan™ MicroRNA Reverse Reanscription Kit, Universal Master Mix without UNG and TaqMan™ Assay, from Applied Biosystems [20].
4. The melting temperature (T_m) of tailed forward primer at 5′ depends on the sequence composition of miRNA molecules (higher GC lead to higher T_m) [19] (*see* **Note 10**).
5. Because of inconsistent and inadequate selection of internal control for the normalization of miRNA expression in body fluid and excrement studies, a reference gene such as 18S ribosomal (r)RNA, can be used as a relative quantitative normalization standard because of the absence of pseudogenes and the weak variation in its expression [22], although other standards are also used (*see* **Note 11**).
6. The comparative cross point (CP) method, also called the E-method, for semiquantitative PCR analysis (*see* **Note 12**) is carried out using a Roche LightCycler (LC™), model 480 PCR instrument, utilizing the LC Relative Quantification Software™ [23, 24] (*see* **Note 13**).

7. The E-method [25] uses standard curves in which the relative target concentration is a function of the difference between crossing points (or cycle numbers) as calculated by the second derivative maximum, in which the Cycler's software algorithm (Roche v4.0 software for the LC™ model 480) identifies the first turning point of the fluorescent curve in the graph showing fluorescence *versus* cycle number [19, 20], which corresponds to the second derivative maximum calculation [26] (*see* **Note 14**).

3.6 Statistical Analysis

1. The miRNA expression data is first analyzed with parametric statistics such as Student t-test or analysis of variance (ANOVA) test, if the data distribution is random; or with nonparametric Kruskall–Wallis, Mann–Whitney, and Fisher exact tests, if the distribution is not random [27, 28]. If necessary, more complicated models such as multivariate analysis and logistic discrimination [29] can be employed.
2. For the corrected index, cross-validation is used to protect against overfitting [30].
3. The area under the receiver operating characteristic (ROC) curve, [in which sensitivity is plotted as a function of (1—specificity)], can be used to describe the trade-off between sensitivity and specificity [31].
4. Principal component analysis (PCA) method [32], which is a multivariate dimension reduction technique to simplify grouping of genes that show aberrant expression from those not showing expression, or a much reduced expression, can also be employed for data analysis.
5. If the miRNA gene panel (or a derived Predictive MicroRNA Index, PMI) [33], Table 1, is better than existing screening methods, all of the data generated can be used to assess the model so overfitting is not a concern. Figure 1 is a graphical representation of data presented in Table 1.

Table 1
Predictive MicroRNA Index (PMI)

Cancer cases	True positive (TP)	False negative (FN)
Normal subjects	False positive (FP)	True negative (TN)
$\%\text{Sensitivity} = \frac{TP}{TP+FN} \times 100$		
$\%\text{Specificity} = \frac{TN}{FP+TN} \times 100$		

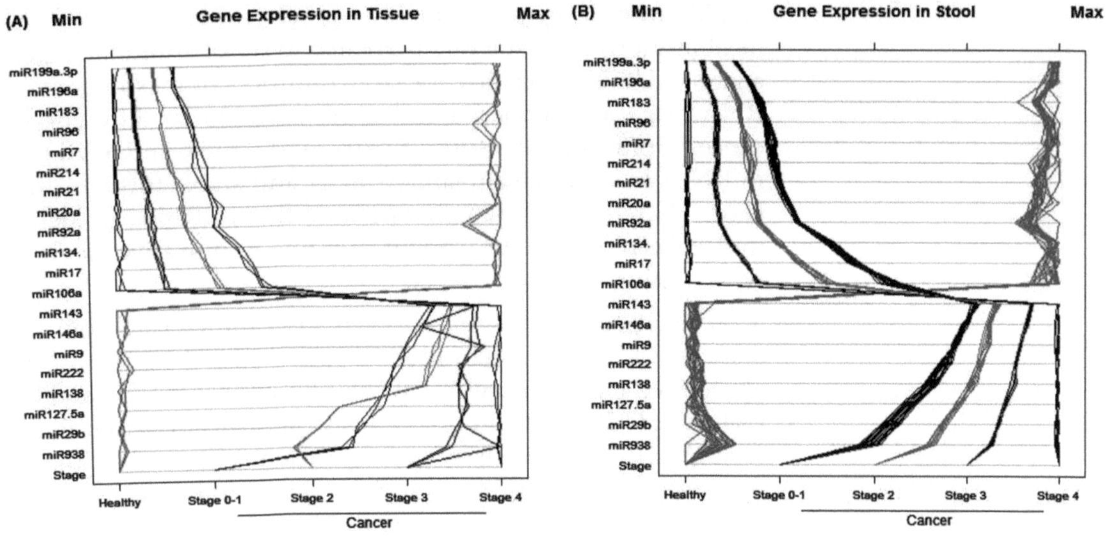

Fig. 1 TaqMan stem-loop primer. MicroRNA expression in tissue (**a**) and stool (**b**) samples taken from 12 healthy and 60 CC individuals, respectively. The stage of cancer is indicated by the bottom row of the panel. In stool, there were 20 normal healthy individuals (yellow lines), and 40 with colon cancer (TNM stages 0–4) represented by pink (stage 0–1), orange (stage 2), red (stage 3), and black (stage 4) lines, respectively. Instances of high expression appear on the right and those with low expression on the left. Expression by stem-loop RT-minor grove binding qPCR was measured by the comparative cross point (CP) or the E-method on a Roche LightCycler® 480 PCR instrument. Scales were chosen so the minimum values line up on the "Min" mark labeled at top left of the panel. The same is true for the maximum values, which line up under the mark labeled "Max" at top right of the panel. Data in tissue from three individuals are similar to those in stool, although they are higher in values for each stage of CC for comparison with stool samples. Adapted from [36]

4 Notes

1. Considering that each cell contains ~20 pg total RNA or 0.4 pg mRNA (equivalent to 0.36 pg ss-cDNA), only a few picograms of cDNA is needed per PCR reaction [18].
2. Isolation of colonocytes from stool, and comparing the Agilent electrophoretic (18S and 28S) patterns to those obtained from total RNA extracted from whole stool, and differential lysis of colonocytes by RT lysis buffer (Quagen), could be constructed as a validation that the electrophoretic pattern observed in stool (18S and (28S) is truly due to the presence of human colonocytes, and not due to stool contamination with *Escherichia coli* (16S and 23S) [34].
3. We believe that employing a two-step RT-PCR format permitting reverse transcription and amplification to be performed separately under optimal conditions, is particularly attractive for experiments that require the same RT product to be used for analysis of multiple transcripts [24, 35], as compared to a one-step format that allows both cDNA synthesis and PCR

amplification to be performed in a single tube, because of the flexibility provided for our particular type of multiparameter analysis. Unlike screening for large numbers of messenger (m) RNA, we use a modest number of miRNAs to differentiate cancer from normal tissue [7, 20], and unlike mRNA [18], miRNAs in stool remain largely intact and stable for detection [36]. Therefore, we are in the opinion that miRNAs are better molecules to use for developing a reliable noninvasive diagnostic screening for colon cancer.

4. Two main approaches are adopted in commercially available systems: (a) use of a stem-loop RT primer [19], or (b) use an alternative approach (miQPCR) developed by Castoldi and his colleagues [34], which uses T4 ligase activities to extend uniformly miRNAs' 3′ ends by addition of a linkage adapter that is used to anchor and prime cDNA synthesis, followed by qPCR to amplify specifically target amplicons.
   (a) The stem-loop RT primer approach was developed and commercialized by Applied Biosystems (currently Life Technologies/Thermo) for subsequent TaqMan probe-based qPCR. The 5′-end of the RT primer base-pair with a region several nucleotides from its own 3′-end to create a base-paired stem separated by an unpaired loop. All except the last few nucleotides at the 3′-end of the RT primer are universal, i.e., they contain the same sequence in all miRNA primers. The last few nucleotides that extend 3′ from the stem are complementary to the 3′-end of a target miRNA. Extension of the primer along an miRNA template creates a cDNA that can be amplified with an miRNA-specific forward primer and a universal reverse primer, the latter of which is complementary to the 5′-end of the stem-loop RT primer.
   (b) All other commercial miRNA qPCR methods, including Sigma's MystiCq® brand, use poly-A tailing to lengthen the miRNA, as described by Shi and Chiang [37]. Poly (A) Polymerase (PAP), a template-independent enzyme, catalyzes the transfer of adenosine residues from ATP to the 3′-end of any RNA. RT can then be performed using an oligo-dT primer. The oligo-dT primer includes an adapter sequence at its 5′-end, which enables subsequent qPCR with a forward primer that is complementary to a specific miRNA and a reverse primer that is complementary to the adapter sequence.

5. Real-time PCR analysis measures product kinetics by detecting them as they accumulate online at a dynamic range of target molecules at least five orders of magnitude as compared to a traditional PCR format, using Roche's PCR LightCycler's 480™ (LC). The method relies on spectral analysis to

distinguish among amplicons, allowing for high-throughput detection of either 96 or 384 samples. Employing a two-step format, permits reverse transcription and amplification to be performed separately under optimal conditions, and is used because of the flexibility that this method provides for multiparameter analysis [24].

6. Although miRNAs represent a relatively abundant class of transcripts, their expression level could vary among species and tissues [5, 10, 20, 35, 37]. A modified TaqMan-based quantitative real-time PCR assay has been used to quantify the RT product that includes miRNA-specific forward primer, reverse primer and a dye-labeled hydrolysis TaqMan® probes [20].

7. Better specificity and sensitivity of stem-loop primers compared to conventional linear ones occurs due to base stacking and spatial constraint on the stem-loop structure, which improves the thermal stability and extends the effective footprint of RT primer/RNA duplex that may be required for effective RT from relatively shorter traditional RT primers, and also prevents it from binding double strand (ds) genomic DNA molecules, and therefore prevent amplification of any potential genomic DNA contaminants present in the preparation [19].

8. Some noncoding RNAs that are longer than 100 nucleotides, can be detected and quantified by traditional RT-qPCR with the same techniques that are used for mRNA analysis. In contrast, short noncoding RNAs, such as micro and piwi RNAs, are essentially the length of a single PCR primer. As a consequence, a technique that modifies these short RNAs is needed for RT [5, 7, 18–20, 35, 37].

9. This study emphasized on a commonly accepted dogma of real-time PCR analysis, in which optimal data are achieved when each RT reaction is normalized to contain an equal amount of a starting total RNA [7, 17, 19, 22, 24].

10. The TaqMan minor-groove binding (MGB) probes are employed to increase the Tm of small probes, which also have a 5′ FAM and a 3′ MG [19, 20].

11. Four additional standards (RNU6B, RNU43, U6 and SNORD-96A) and three stably expressed human miRNA (let-7a, miR-16, miR 103, and an miRNA from the worm *C. elegans*) [22, 36] can also be used to ascertain unbiased normalization and elimination of spurious data. Alternate normalization methods using Global means or Quantile normalization, which could eliminate the need for endogenous controls are unrealistic as they can only be achieved by using very large datasets [38].

12. Absolute quantification of miRNA is unnecessary because constantly transcribed housekeeping genes effectively serve as

internal standards for accurate quantification of miRNA genes of interest; our own experience [7, 18, 19, 24] and others [15, 22, 35, 39] support that conclusion.

13. We used Roche's LightCycler (LC) 480™ for real-time PCR analysis of product as they accumulate (i.e., online) over a large dynamic range of target molecule (i.e., at least five orders of magnitude as compared to traditional end-point PCR) [35, 39], which allows for a higher sample throughput using 96 plates, precise product determination during the log/linear amplification phase, reduced labor and increased fluorescence.
14. The E method [25] was selected because it produces more accurate results than the $2^{-\Delta\Delta Ct}$ method [39], as it compensates for differences in target and reference gene amplification efficiency [$E = 10^{-1/\text{slope}}$] either within an experiment, or between experiments. Normalization against a housekeeping internal standard or in some cases against several standards is customarily employed in this method.

References

1. Ahmed FE (2003) Colon cancer, prevalence, screening, gene expression and mutation, and risk factors and assessment. J Environ Sci Health C 21:65–131
2. Jemal A, Siegel R, Ward E, Moss SM, Amar SS, Balfour TW, James PD, Mangham CA, Murray T, Xu J, Thun MJ (2007) Cancer statistics, 2007. CA Cancer J Clin 57:43–66
3. Smith A, Young GP, Cole SR, Bampton P (2006) Comparison of a brush-sampling fecal immunochemical test for hemoglobin with a sensitive guaiac-based fecal occult blood test in detection of colorectal neoplasia. Cancer 107:2152–2159
4. Gatto NM, Frucht H, Sundararajan V, Jacobson JS, Grann VR, Neugut AI (2002) Risk of perforation after colonoscopy and sigmoidoscopy: a population based study. J Natl Cancer Inst 95:230–236
5. Ahmed FE (2007) The role of microRNA in carcinogenesis and biomarker selection: a methodological perspective. Expert Rev Mol Diagn 7:569–603
6. Davies RJ, Freeman A, Morris LS, Bingham S, Dilworth S, Scott I, Laskey RA, Miller R, Coleman N (2002) Analysis of minichromosome maintenance proteins as a novel method for detection of colorectal cancer in stool. Lancet 359:1917–1919
7. Ahmed FE, Vos P (2004) Molecular markers for human colon cancer in stool and blood identified by RT-PCR. Anticancer Res 24:4127–4134
8. Lewis BP, Burge CB, Bartel DP (2005) Conserved seed paring, often flanked by adenosines, indicates that thousands of human genes are microRNA targets. Cell 120:15–20
9. Ruby JG, Jan CH, Bartel D (2007) Intronic microRNA precursors that bypass Drosha processing. Nature 448:83–86
10. Cummins JM, Velculescu VE (2006) Implication of microRNA profiling for cancer diagnosis. Oncogene 15:6220–6227
11. Calin GA, Ferracin M, Cimmino A, Dileva G, Shimiz M, Wojcik SE et al (2005) A microRNA signature associated with prognosis and progression in chronic lymphocytic leukemia. N Engl J Med 353:1793–1801
12. Calin GA, Croce CM (2006) MicroRNA signatures in human cancers. Nat Rev Cancer 6:857–866
13. Chang-Zheng C (2005) MicroRNAs as oncogenes and tumor supressors. N Engl J Med 353:1768–1771
14. Calin GA, Sevignai C, Dumitru CD, Hyslop T, Noch E, Yendamuri S et al (2004) Human microRNA genes are frequently located at fragile sites and genomic regions involved in cancers. Proc Natl Acad Sci U S A 101:2999–3004
15. Schepler T, Reinert JT, Oslenfeld MS, Christensen LL, Silahtaroglu AN, Dyrskjøt L et al (2008) Diagnostic and prognostic microRNAs

in Stage II colon cancer. Cancer Res 68:6416–6424

16. Lanza G, Ferracin M, Gafa R, Veronese A, Spizzo R, Pichiorri F et al (2007) mRNA/microRNA gene expression profile in microsatellite unstable colorectal cancer. Mol Cancer 6:54, 2007
17. Koga Y, Yasunaga M, Katayose S, Moriya Y, Akasu T, Fujita S, Yamamoto S, Baba H, Matsumura Y (2008) Improved recovery of exfoliated colonocytes from feces using newly developed immunoparamagnetic beads. Gastroenterol Res Practice. https://doi.org/10.1155/2008/605273
18. Ahmed FE, Vos PW, IJames S, Flake G, Sinar DR, Naziri W, Marcuard SP (2007) Standardization for transcriptomic molecular markers to screen human colon cancer. Cancer. Genom Proteom 4:419–432
19. Ahmed FE, iJames S, Lysle DL, Dobbs LJ Jr, Johnke RM, Flake G et al (2004) Improved methods for extracting RNA from exfoliated human colonocytes in stool and RT-PCR analysis. Dig Dis Sci 49:1889–1898
20. Chen C, Ridzon DA, Broomer AJ, Zhou Z, Lee DH, Nguyen JT et al (2005) Real-time quantification of microRNAs by stem-loop RT-PCR. Nucleic Acids Res 33:e179
21. Matsushita HM, Matsumura Y, Moriya Y, Akasu T, Fujita S, Yamamoto S et al (2005) A new method for isolating colonocytes from naturally evacuated feces and its clinical application to colorectal cancer diagnosis. Gastroenterology 129:1918–1927
22. Peltier HJ, Latham J (2008) Normalization of microRNA expression levels in quantitative RT-PCR assays identification of suitable reference RNA targets in normal and cancerous human solid tissues. RNA 14:844–852
23. LightCycler Software®, Version 3.5, Roche Molecular Biochemicals, Mannheim, Germany, 2001, p. 64–79.
24. Ahmed FE (2005) qRT-PCR: application to carcinogenesis. Cancer Genomics Proteomics 2:317–332
25. Tellman G (2006) The E-method: a highly accurate technique for gene-expression analysis. Nat Methods 3:1–2
26. Luu-The V, Paquet N, Calvo E, Cumps J (2005) Improved real-time RT-PCR method for high-throughput measurements using second derivative calculation and double correction. Biotechniques 38:287–293
27. Ripley BD. Classification. In: Encyclopedia of statistical sciences, Vol. 1. New York, NY: Wiley-Interscience Publication; 1997.
28. Moore DS, McCabe GP, Craig B (2009) Introduction to the practice of statistics, 6th edn. W.H. Freeman & Company, St. Louis, MO
29. Nagan CY, Yamamoto H, Seshimo I, Ezumi K, Terayama M, Hemmi H, Takemasa I, Ikeda M, Sekimoto M, Monden M (2007) A multivariate analysis of adhesion molecules expression in assessment of colorectal cancer. J Surg Oncol 95:652–662
30. Efron B, Tibshirani RJ (1993) An introduction to the bootstrap. Chapman and Hall, New York, NY
31. Hanley JA, McNeil BJ (1982) The meaning and use of the area under a receiver operating characteristic (ROC) curve. Radiology 143:29–36
32. Gabriel KR, Odoroff CL (1990) Biplots in biomedical research. Stat Med 9:469–485
33. DeMuth JP, Jackson CM, Weaver DA, Crawford EL, Durzinsky DS, Durham SJ, Zaher A, Phillips ER, Khuder SA, Willey JC (1998) The gene expression index cmyc x E2F-1/p21 is highly predictive of malignant phenotype in human bronchial epithelial cells. Am J Respir Cell Mol Biol 19:18–29
34. Benes V, Collier P, Kordes C, Stolte J, Rausch T, Muckentaler MU et al (2015) Identification of cytokine-induced mutation of microRNA expression and secretion as measured by a novel microRNA soecific qPCR assay. Sci Rep 5:11,590
35. Schmittgen TD, Lee EJ, Jiang J, Sarkar A, Yang L, Elton TS, Chen C (2008) Real-time PCR quantification of precursor and mature microRNA. Methods 44:31–38
36. Ahmed FE, Ahmed NC, Vos PW, Bonnerup C, Atkins JN, Casey M et al (2013) Diagnostic microRNA markers to screen for sporadic human colon cancer in stool: I. Proof of principle. Cancer. Genom Proteom 10:93–114
37. Shi R, Chiang VL (2005) Facile means for quantifying microRNA expression by real-time PCR. Biotechniques 29(4):519–524
38. Okugawa Y, Toiyama Y, Goel A (2014) An update on microRNA as colorectal cancer biomarkers: where are we and what's next? Expert Rev Mol Diagn 14(8):999–1021
39. Livak KJ, Schmittgen TD (2001) Analysis of relative gene expression data using real-time quantitative PCR and the $2^{-\Delta\Delta C_T}$ method. Methods 25:402–408
40. Wegman E (1990) Hyperdimensional data analysis using parallel coordinate. J Am Stat Assoc 85:644–675

Check for updates

Chapter 14

A Stool Multitarget mRNA Assay for the Detection of Colorectal Neoplasms

Elizabeth Herring, Shigeru Kanaoka, Eric Tremblay, and Jean-François Beaulieu

Abstract

Noninvasive screening methods for the detection of colorectal cancers (CRC) at curable stages rely on the identification of specific biomarkers. Our group has shown that mRNA stool assays represent a powerful and robust approach for the prediction of colorectal neoplasms. In this methodological chapter, we describe the procedures to isolate good quality stool RNA and the steps to evaluate the levels of specific host mRNA markers such as ITGA6, MYC, and GADD45B using TaqMan-based quantitative and droplet digital PCR approaches.

Key words Colorectal cancer, Diagnosis, mRNA, Stool, qPCR, ddPCR

1 Introduction

Although among the most deadly cancer types worldwide [1], colorectal cancer (CRC) is one that can be successfully treated when diagnosed before occurrence of metastases. Early and efficient detection is therefore a crucial factor for life saving [2–4]. Indeed, while the 5-year survival rate for localized CRC lesions is over 90%, it falls to near 10% for CRC that have spread to distant organs [5]. Colonoscopy is the gold standard for the detection of colorectal lesions with up to 95% sensitivity for CRC and 76% for adenomas. However, discomfort and unpleasant preparation procedures impact on compliance [6] and this invasive technique is not without risk and is expensive [7]. In the context where "the best screening test is one that gets performed" [8], the recent recommendations for CRC screening lists distinct strategies including noninvasive stool tests [9].

Fecal immunochemical testing (FIT) for occult blood has been implemented over the last few decades in several countries as a valid noninvasive screening procedure [9]. However, suboptimal lesion

Jean-François Beaulieu (ed.), *Colorectal Cancer: Methods and Protocols*, Methods in Molecular Biology, vol. 1765, https://doi.org/10.1007/978-1-4939-7765-9_14,

detection rates (66–80% sensitivity for CRC but less than 30% for advanced adenomas) and a significant proportion of false positives caused by benign conditions not related to cancer are limiting its utility [3, 10–12]. It is therefore imperative to explore alternate or complementary strategies with the potential to improve CRC screening performance, especially for the detection of cancers at their early stages. Based on the significant rate of tumor cell exfoliation into the colonic lumen, a parameter thought to be independent of blood release [13], a number of assays for the detection of fecal nucleic acid, proteins or other molecules have been experimented although none of them are yet explicitly recommended [9]. Significantly improving sensitivity of stool tests for both cancer and advanced adenoma detection over FIT alone, while keeping false positives at low levels, appears to be a reachable goal in the near future.

Herein, we present methodological advances on the detection of host mRNA in stools as a noninvasive testing assay for the detection of colorectal neoplasms. Although host mRNA only represents a minor part of total stool RNA and has been reported to be susceptible to degradation [3, 14, 15], our group has demonstrated that TaqMan quantitative PCR (qPCR) allows the detection of specific transcripts over represented in the stools of patients with cancers or advanced adenomas such as PTGS2 (COX-2), ITGA6, ITGA6A, MYC, and GADD45B [16, 17]. Droplet digital PCR (ddPCR) has also recently been used for the detection of ITGA6 and ITGA6A [18]. In this chapter, we describe the procedures to isolate stool RNA and evaluate the levels of specific host mRNA markers by qPCR and ddPCR.

2 Materials

2.1 General Equipment and Material List

2.1.1 Equipment

1. −20 °C laboratory freezer.
2. −80 °C laboratory freezer.
3. A laboratory balance.
4. 37 °C block heater or water bath.
5. A real-time qPCR machine.
6. A benchtop microcentrifuge with a rotor for eight-tube strips.
7. QX200 Droplet Generator (Bio-Rad) and accessories.
8. QX200 Reader (Bio-Rad).
9. PX1 PCR plate sealer and foil heat seals (Bio-Rad).
10. P2, P20, P200, and P1000 single channel pipettes.
11. An eight-channel adjustable volume pipette.
12. A polytron homogenizer.

13. A refrigerated microcentrifuge.
14. An absorption spectrophotometer with a 50 μL cuvette or a NanoDrop microvolume spectrophotometer.

2.1.2 Consumables

1. Thinwall, polypropylene tubes, 5 mL or more capacity.
2. Disposable P2, P20, P200, P1000 tips.
3. Disposable 5 mL pipettes.
4. 2 mL sterile screw top tubes.
5. 1.5 mL Eppendorf tubes.
6. 0.2 mL PCR tube strips and caps.
7. 96-well PCR plates and foil heat seal.

2.2 Molecular Biology Supplies

1. RiboZol.
2. Chloroform.
3. 70% ethanol: Add 30 mL of H_20 to 70 mL of 100% ethanol.
4. Reverse transcriptase.
5. Random hexamers.
6. TaqMan Gene Expression Assay.
7. RNase inhibitor.
8. Sterile RNase-free water.
9. TaqMan Gene Expression Reaction Mix.
10. ddPCR Supermix for Probes (Bio-Rad).
11. RNeasy Kit.
12. TaqMan Pre Amp Master Mix Kit.
13. Tris–EDTA (TE) buffer, molecular biology grade.

3 Methods

3.1 RNA Isolation

Isolate RNA using a modification of the Chomczynski and Sacchi method with both RiboZol (*see* **Note 1**) and the RNeasy kit as follows:

1. Add 3 mL of RiboZol to 5 mL tubes (*see* **Note 2**) containing 0.5 g of feces.
2. Homogenize the feces using a polytron.
3. Transfer the slurry to sterile 2.0 mL screw capped tubes (*see* **Note 3**) and microfuge at 12,000 × *g* for 5 min at 4 °C.
4. Transfer the supernatants to new sterile 2.0 mL tubes.
5. Add 0.3 mL of RiboZol and 0.3 mL of chloroform to each tube.

6. Shake the tubes vigorously for 30 s and then microfuge at 12,000 × *g* for 15 min at 4 °C.
7. Remove the aqueous phase from each tube (*see* **Note 4**) and transfer to fresh 2.0 mL tubes.
8. Add an equal volume of 70% ethanol to the tubes and vortex for 30 s.
9. Add the mixture to an RNeasy minispin column (*see* **Note 5**) and microfuge at 8000 × *g* for 15 s at room temperature.
10. Pipet 700 μL Buffer RW1 onto the column and microfuge for 15 s at 8000 × *g* to wash.
11. Transfer RNeasy column to a 2 mL collection tube.
12. Pipet 500 μL Buffer RPE onto the column and microfuge for 15 s at 8000 × *g* to wash.
13. Pipet 500 μL Buffer RPE onto the column and microfuge for 2 min at maximum speed to dry the RNeasy membrane.
14. Transfer the RNeasy column to a 1.5 mL tube and pipet 30 μL of RNase-free water directly onto the RNeasy membrane.
15. Microfuge for 1 min at 8000 × *g* to elute.
16. Measure the concentration of the RNA prep using an absorption spectrophotometer with a 50 μL cuvette or a NanoDrop microvolume spectrophotometer (*see* **Note 6**).

3.2 Reverse Transcription

1. Prepare samples on ice according to Table 1. Mix thoroughly and microfuge briefly to collect residual liquid from the walls of the tube (*see* **Note 7**).
2. Distribute the appropriate volume of master mix into individual reaction tubes.
3. Add template RNA to the individual tubes containing the master mix. Mix thoroughly and microfuge briefly.
4. Incubate for 60 min at 37 °C. Store cDNA at −20 °C.

3.3 Quantitative Polymerase Chain Reaction

1. Prepare a fresh master mix on ice according to Table 2 (*see* **Note 8**). Mix thoroughly and microfuge briefly to collect residual liquid from the walls of the tube.
2. Distribute the appropriate volume of master mix into individual reaction tubes of the 8 tube PCR strips.
3. Add 1 μL cDNA to each tube (*see* **Note 9**).
4. Cap the tubes with optical flat 8-cap strips (*see* **Note 10**).
5. Microfuge briefly in a benchtop microfuge fitted with a rotor for 8-tube strips to collect residual liquid from the walls of the tubes.

Table 1
Reverse transcription reaction components

Component	Volume/reaction	Final concentration
10× Buffer RT	6 μL	1×
dNTP Mix (5 mM each dNTP)	6 μL	0.5 mM each dNTP
Random hexamers (125 ng/μL)	6 μL	750 ng (per 60 μL reaction)
RNase inhibitor (10 units/μL)	3 μL	30 units (per 60 μL reaction)
Reverse transcriptase	3 μL	12 units (per 60 μL reaction)
RNase-free water	Variable	
Template RNA, added at **step 3**	Variable	0.375 μg
Total volume	60 μL	

Table 2
qPCR reaction components

Component	Volume/reaction (μL)	[Final]
Master Mix 2× TaqMan Gene Expression Reaction Mix	10	1×
20× TaqMan Gene Expression Assay	1	1×
RNase-free water	8	
cDNA from the reverse transcription reaction	1	Added at **step 3**

Table 3
Real-time PCR reaction parameters

	Hold	Hold	Cycle (45 cycles)
Temp	50 °C	95 °C	95 °C 60 °C
Time	2 min	10 min	15 s 1 min

6. Run the tubes in a real-time PCR instrument according to Table 3.
7. Analyze the results (*see* **Note 11**).

3.4 ddPCR Amplification

1. Prepare a fresh master mix on ice according to Table 4. Mix thoroughly and microfuge briefly to collect residual liquid from the walls of the tube.
2. Transfer 20 μL of the PCR reaction containing the sample nucleic acid, primers and probes (*see* **Note 12**) and the ddPCR Supermix to the middle row of a DG8 cartridge for a QX200 droplet generator.

Table 4
ddPCR reaction components

Component	Volume/reaction (μL)	[Final]
Master Mix 2× ddPCR Supermix for Probes (no dUTP)	10	1×
20× TaqMan Gene Expression Assay	1	1×
RNase-free water	8	
cDNA from the reverse transcription reaction	1	Added at **step 3**

3. Load 70 μL of droplet generator oil into the bottom wells of the DG8 cartridge.
4. Attach a gasket across the top of the DG8 cartridge and place it into the QX200 droplet generator (*see* **Note 13**).
5. After generating droplets, transfer the droplets from the top wells of the cartridge to a 96-well PCR plate by pipetting gently.
6. Heat seal the plate using Bio-Rad's PX1 PCR plate sealer and foil heat seal.
7. Place the PCR plate in a thermal cycler for PCR using an optimized protocol (*see* **Note 14**).
8. Following PCR amplification run the PCR plate in a QX200 droplet reader (*see* **Note 15**).
9. Use QuantaSoft software to analyze the data in each well (*see* **Note 16**).

3.5 Optional Preamplification Step

A multiplex preamplification of specific amplicons for analysis with TaqMan gene expression assays can be performed before PCRs.

1. Prepare a fresh master mix on ice according to Table 5. Mix thoroughly and microfuge briefly to collect residual liquid from the walls of the tube (*see* **Note 17**).
2. Distribute the appropriate volume of master mix into individual reaction tubes of the eight-tube PCR strips.
3. Add 5 μL cDNA to each tube.
4. Cap the tubes with optical flat eight-cap strips.
5. Microfuge briefly in a benchtop microfuge fitted with a rotor for eight-tube strips to collect residual liquid from the walls of the tubes.
6. Run the tubes in a real-time PCR instrument for 14 PCR cycles of 15 s at 95 °C, 4 min at 60 °C.
7. Dilute preamplification products 1:20 with TE Buffer, aliquot, and store at −80 °C.

Table 5
Preamplification reaction components

Component	Volume/reaction (μL)	[Final]
Master Mix 2× TaqMan PreAmp Master Mix	10	1×
20× TaqMan Gene Expression Assays pooled at final concentration of 0.2× in TE	1	1×
RNase-free water	4	
cDNA from the reverse transcription reaction	5	Added at **step 3**

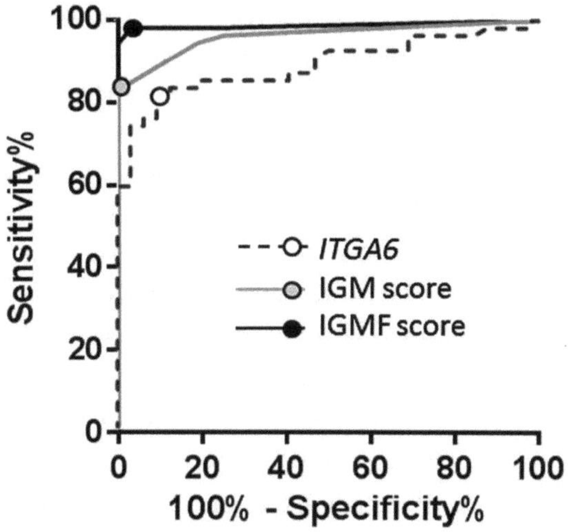

Fig. 1 ROC curves comparing detection of *ITGA6* transcript, a combination of three transcripts *ITGA6*, *GADD45B*, and *MYC* alone (IGM score) or with FIT (IGMF score) for the prediction of stage II and III colorectal cancers. For *ITGA6* alone, the area under the curve (AUC) was 0.890 while it is increased to 0.962 by the inclusion of two additional transcripts for the generation of the IGM score, and to 0.988 when the FIT results are included in the calculations (IGMF score). Accordingly, sensitivity and specificities were 89% and 91% for *ITGA6* alone, 83% and 100% for IGM score, and 98% and 97% for IGMF confirming the strength of the qPCR multitarget mRNA test in combination with FIT for the detection of colorectal cancers. Adapted from the data in [20]

3.6 Data Analysis

Data are analyzed using statistics package software such as Prism (GraphPad Software, La Jolla, USA). Comparisons of mRNA expression in stool samples from controls and patients with lesions are expressed as median with interquartile range and area under the receiver operating characteristic (ROC) curves are calculated. Sensitivities and specificities are expressed in % with a 95% confidence interval. Optimal cutoff values are calculated with Cutoff Finder [19]. Algorithms that combine distinct mRNA and/or FIT data can be used for the generation of specific scores (*see* **Note 18**; and Fig. 1 for an example).

4 Notes

1. Many companies provide a similar reagent under various names such as TriZol, QIAzol, and RiboZol. All are acid phenol/guanidine preparations and use the same protocol.
2. Any thinwall, polypropylene tube with a volume greater than 6 mL will do. The tube can be shortened with scissors to allow entry of the homogenizer probe if necessary.
3. Screw capped tubes are preferable to regular snap capped Eppendorf tubes as the chloroform added later in the procedure will be less likely to bleed through the screw cap.
4. RNA will be located exclusively in the upper aqueous phase. Carefully remove only about 80% of the clear upper aqueous phase avoiding contamination with protein, DNA, lipids, and carbohydrates that appear at the interface with the lower red phenol–chloroform phase.
5. RNeasy mini spin columns and all necessary solutions (RW1 and RPE) are provided with the RNeasy kit.
6. Dilute RNA preparation 1/10 to 1/100 depending on the yield. Measure optical density (OD) at 260 and 280 Hz to have an OD value between 0.1 and 1.
   (a) One A260 Unit of ssRNA = 40 μg/mL.
   (b) Concentration of ssRNA in sample: A260 × 40 μg/mL × dilution factor.
   (c) Pure RNA has an A260/A280 ≥ 2.0. A260/A280 of less than 2.0 means the preparation is contaminated with proteins and aromatic substances.
7. Recombinant reverse transcriptase (i.e. Superscript II, Omniscript, etc.) is genetically engineered for reduced RNase H activity, increased half-life and improved thermal stability offering higher cDNA yields, improved cDNA lengths, improved efficiency on GC-rich target RNAs and overall better performance than wild type enzymes.
8. TaqMan Gene Expression Assays consist of a pair of unlabeled PCR primers and a TaqMan probe with a FAM or VIC dye label on the 5′ end and a minor groove binder and nonfluorescent quencher on the 3′ end offering the highest specificity, greatest sensitivity and largest dynamic range of any gene expression technology.
9. Include negative and positive controls. A no-template control allows the detection of contamination of the PCR reagents. A positive control is necessary when amplifying a new target sequence to confirm that the primer-probe set works.
10. Tubes and caps are specific to each qPCR machine.

11. The results are presented as copy number. For qPCR, a standard reference curve is generated using serial fivefold dilutions of a cDNA stock solution of the target sequence quantified using a NanoDrop spectrophotometer.
12. The Bio-Rad droplet generator uses specially developed reagents and microfluidics to partition each sample into 20,000 nanoliter-sized droplets. Target DNA are distributed randomly into the droplets during the partitioning process.
13. The droplet generator takes about 2.5 min to process eight samples. Work quickly to have the tubes in the PCR machine within 1 h. To save time, a second cartridge can be prepared while the droplet generator is producing droplets with the first cartridge.
14. Optimizing the annealing temperature of the PCR assay is critical. Test a range of temperatures simultaneously using a thermal cycler with a thermal gradient feature. The optimal annealing temperature is the one that results in the largest fluorescence amplitude change between the positive and the negative droplets.
15. After PCR, the plate can be stored at 4 °C overnight. Do not store the plate for more than 3–4 days before running in the droplet reader. The droplet reader counts the PCR-positive and PCR-negative droplets to provide absolute quantification of target DNA. The reader measures fluorescence intensity of each droplet and detects the size and shape as the droplets pass the detector; droplets are excluded if they do not meet quality metrics.
16. The QuantaSoft software analyzes the data in each well; automatic thresholding determines concentrations and populates the data tables in the analysis mode of the software. The concentration reported is in copies/μL of the final 1× ddPCR reaction.
17. The preparation of the pooled 20× TaqMan Gene Expression Assays depends of the number of genes to be analyzed. In our lab, we have used pools of up to 20 commercially available TaqMan primer and probe mixtures for the preamplification step.
18. There are numerous ways to generate scores. One of the approaches used by our group [16] is based on the method previously described by Ng et al. [20] using the sum of the fold increase for each marker on a scale of 0–3 on the basis of three cutoff values (lower cutoff corresponding to a sensitivity of 80%, medium cutoff corresponding to a specificity of 90% and higher cutoff corresponding to a specificity of 99%).

Acknowledgments

The original studies were supported by Canadian Institutes of Health Research grants MOP 97836 and PPP 133373. JFB is the recipient of the Canada Chair in Intestinal Physiopathology and a member of the FRQS-funded Centre de Recherche of the Centre Hospitalier Universitaire de Sherbrooke.

The authors thank Bio-Rad Laboratories Canada and Dr. Katia Nadeau for the prolonged trial period with the ddPCR equipment and Dr. Sean C. Taylor for scientific advice.

References

1. Siegel RL, Miller KD, Jemal A (2016) Cancer statistics, 2016. CA Cancer J Clin 66(1):7–30. https://doi.org/10.3322/caac.21332
2. Maratt JK, Saini SD (2015) Colorectal cancer screening in the 21st century: where do we go from here? Am J Manag Care 21(7): e447–e449. doi:86282 [pii]
3. Robertson DJ, Imperiale TF (2015) Stool testing for colorectal cancer screening. Gastroenterology 149(5):1286–1293. https://doi.org/10.1053/j.gastro.2015.05.045. S0016-5085(15)00772-6 [pii]
4. Willyard C (2015) Screening: early alert. Nature 521(7551):S4–S5. https://doi.org/10.1038/521S4a. 521S4a [pii]
5. Manfredi S, Bouvier AM, Lepage C, Hatem C, Dancourt V, Faivre J (2006) Incidence and patterns of recurrence after resection for cure of colonic cancer in a well defined population. Br J Surg 93(9):1115–1122. https://doi.org/10.1002/bjs.5349
6. Schroy PC 3rd, Lal S, Glick JT, Robinson PA, Zamor P, Heeren TC (2007) Patient preferences for colorectal cancer screening: how does stool DNA testing fare? Am J Manag Care 13(7):393–400. doi:3337 [pii]
7. Lin JS, Piper MA, Perdue LA, Rutter CM, Webber EM, O'Connor E, Smith N, Whitlock EP (2016) Screening for colorectal cancer: updated evidence report and systematic review for the US Preventive Services Task Force. JAMA 315(23):2576–2594. https://doi.org/10.1001/jama.2016.3332
8. Ransohoff DF, Sox HC (2016) Clinical practice guidelines for colorectal cancer screening: new recommendations and new challenges. JAMA 315(23):2529–2531. https://doi.org/10.1001/jama.2016.7990
9. Force USPST, Bibbins-Domingo K, Grossman DC, Curry SJ, Davidson KW, Epling JW Jr, Garcia FA, Gillman MW, Harper DM, Kemper AR, Krist AH, Kurth AE, Landefeld CS, Mangione CM, Owens DK, Phillips WR, Phipps MG, Pignone MP, Siu AL (2016) Screening for colorectal cancer: US Preventive Services Task Force recommendation statement. JAMA 315(23):2564–2575. https://doi.org/10.1001/jama.2016.5989
10. Allison JE, Fraser CG, Halloran SP, Young GP (2014) Population screening for colorectal cancer means getting FIT: the past, present, and future of colorectal cancer screening using the fecal immunochemical test for hemoglobin (FIT). Gut Liver 8(2):117–130. https://doi.org/10.5009/gnl.2014.8.2.117
11. Hundt S, Haug U, Brenner H (2009) Comparative evaluation of immunochemical fecal occult blood tests for colorectal adenoma detection. Ann Intern Med 150(3):162–169
12. Lee JK, Liles EG, Bent S, Levin TR, Corley DA (2014) Accuracy of fecal immunochemical tests for colorectal cancer: systematic review and meta-analysis. Ann Intern Med 160(3):171. https://doi.org/10.7326/M13-1484. 1819122 [pii]
13. YJ Y, Majumdar AP, Nechvatal JM, Ram JL, Basson MD, Heilbrun LK, Kato I (2008) Exfoliated cells in stool: a source for reverse transcription-PCR-based analysis of biomarkers of gastrointestinal cancer. Cancer Epidemiol Biomarkers Prev 17(2):455–458. https://doi.org/10.1158/1055-9965.EPI-07-2515. 17/2/455 [pii]
14. Reck M, Tomasch J, Deng Z, Jarek M, Husemann P, Wagner-Dobler I, Consortium C (2015) Stool metatranscriptomics: a technical guideline for mRNA stabilisation and isolation. BMC Genomics 16:494. https://doi.org/10.1186/s12864-015-1694-y
15. Stauber J, Shaikh N, Ordiz MI, Tarr PI, Manary MJ (2016) Droplet digital PCR quantifies host inflammatory transcripts in feces reliably and reproducibly. Cell Immunol

303:43–49. https://doi.org/10.1016/j.cellimm.2016.03.007

16. Beaulieu JF, Herring E, Kanaoka S, Tremblay E (2016) Use of integrin alpha 6 transcripts in a stool mRNA assay for the detection of colorectal cancers at curable stages. Oncotarget 7 (12):14,684–14,692. https://doi.org/10.18632/oncotarget.7407
17. Hamaya Y, Yoshida K, Takai T, Ikuma M, Hishida A, Kanaoka S (2010) Factors that contribute to faecal cyclooxygenase-2 mRNA expression in subjects with colorectal cancer. Br J Cancer 102(5):916–921. https://doi.org/10.1038/sj.bjc.6605564. [pii]
18. Herring E, Kanaoka S, Tremblay E, Beaulieu JF (2017) Droplet digital PCR for quantification of ITGA6 in a stool mRNA assay for the detection of colorectal cancers. World J Gastroenterol 23(16):1–8. https://doi.org/10.3748/wjg.v23.i16.0000
19. Budczies J, Klauschen F, Sinn BV, Gyorffy B, Schmitt WD, Darb-Esfahani S, Denkert C (2012) Cutoff finder: a comprehensive and straightforward Web application enabling rapid biomarker cutoff optimization. PLoS One 7(12):e51862. https://doi.org/10.1371/journal.pone.0051862. PONE-D-12-12960 [pii]
20. Ng EW, Poon TC, Lam HS, Cheung HM, Ma TP, Chan KY, Wong RP, Leung KT, Lam MM, Li K, Ng PC (2013) Gut-associated biomarkers L-FABP, I-FABP, and TFF3 and LIT score for diagnosis of surgical necrotizing enterocolitis in preterm infants. Ann Surg 258 (6):1111–1118. https://doi.org/10.1097/SLA.0b013e318288ea96

Chapter 15

Colorectal Cancer Detection Using Targeted LC-MS Metabolic Profiling

Danijel Djukovic, Jiangjiang Zhang, and Daniel Raftery

Abstract

Colorectal cancer (CRC) is one of the most commonly diagnosed malignancies and causes of cancer death. While the mortality rates from CRC have steadily declined, 50,000 individuals in the USA (and many times this number worldwide) still succumb to this illness every year. Early detection of CRC is the most critical need for improving 5-year survival and cure rates. Currently available CRC diagnostic techniques often miss early stage disease such that only 40% of newly diagnosed CRC patients are treated for local disease, Therefore, development of new screening methods that are highly sensitive, specific, noninvasive and easily accessible are critically desired for the early diagnosis and significant reduction in death rate from CRC. In this chapter we describe a targeted LC-MS based metabolic profiling approach used for the discovery of CRC metabolite biomarker candidates, based on highly reproducible hydrophilic interaction liquid chromatography coupled to triple-quadrupole mass spectrometry (HILIC-LC-QQQ-MS). A partial least squares-discriminant analysis (PLS-DA) model was able to differentiate CRC patients from both healthy controls and polyp patients, as well as to distinguish CRC patients based on the cancer stage.

Key words Colorectal cancer (CRC), Polyps, Metabolomics, Targeted metabolic profiling, LC-MS, Metabolite biomarkers

1 Introduction

Colorectal cancer (CRC) is the third most commonly diagnosed malignancy and cause of death among both genders in the USA, with 135,430 annual diagnoses and 50,260 yearly casualties projected in 2017 [1]. The incidence and mortality rates have been in steady decline for the last 4 decades due to positive changes in lifestyle among the general population (e.g., reduction in smoking and red-meat consumption) as well as significant improvements in cancer diagnostics and medical treatments. Early detection of CRC is the most critical step in greatly improving 5-year survival and cure rates. When diagnosed in its early stages, 5-year survival rates are 90% for localized CRC (stages I and II) and 90% for regional CRC (stage III) [2]. However, at stage IV, 5-year survival rates are only

Jean-François Beaulieu (ed.), *Colorectal Cancer: Methods and Protocols*, Methods in Molecular Biology, vol. 1765, https://doi.org/10.1007/978-1-4939-7765-9_15,

14%. The three most effective diagnostic methods for CRC are family history screening, endoscopy (colonoscopy or sigmoidoscopy), and the fecal immunochemical test (FIT) [3]. Family history screening and FIT as noninvasive techniques are the most commonly used screening methods for CRC, but they have relatively low sensitivities and often miss the cancer in its early stages [4]. Endoscopy represents the gold standard for CRC diagnosis and is currently the most sensitive technique, but its major disadvantages include invasiveness, potential pain and discomfort, relatively high cost and accessibility. As a result, only 40% of newly diagnosed CRC patients are diagnosed and treated at localized stages (Stages I–III). The development of new screening methods that are highly sensitive, specific, noninvasive and easily accessible is highly desirable for the early diagnosis of CRC.

In the last decade, there have been many efforts made to develop new noninvasive tests such as stool DNA [5], microRNA [6] and gastrointestinal tract acid-446 (GTA-446) [7] for early CRC diagnosis. The stool DNA based method identifies four methylated genes and a mutant form of KRAS as CRC indicators with sensitivity and specificity of 0.85–0.90, respectively [5]. The microRNA study discovered two CRC-related biomarkers, microR-21 and microR-106b, that have higher expressions in the individuals with CRC vs. healthy controls [6]. The GTA-446 test is based on the discovery that this compound belonging to a recently identified family of circulating long-chain fatty acids is downregulated in the CRC-affected individuals compared to healthy controls [7].

A promising approach is provided by the field of metabolomics that focuses on the quantitative and qualitative studies of endogenous small molecules that are products of intracellular processes within a biological system. Generally, metabolite measurements in various biological samples including fluids, tissues, and cells are performed by either nuclear magnetic resonance (NMR) spectroscopy or mass spectrometry (MS) typically coupled to liquid chromatography (LC) or gas chromatography (GC). There is a great potential for metabolomics as a tool for biomarker discovery for cancer detection, therapeutic evaluation, and prognosis [8–10]. A number of recent LC-MS and GC-MS based metabolomics studies have focused on biomarker discovery for colorectal cancer (CRC) [11–17]. Many of these studies that use global, untargeted metabolite profiling approaches have reported outstanding performance; however, these results have yet to be validated in follow-on studies with additional patient samples.

The aim of this work is to describe the development and application of a targeted liquid chromatography-triple quadrupole mass spectrometry (LC-QQQ-MS) assay with broad coverage of the metabolome and high reproducibility. This assay was used in one of the more comprehensive metabolomics CRC biomarker discovery studies to date and was performed at the Northwest Metabolomics Research Center at the University of Washington, Seattle. Its findings were first reported by Zhu et al. [18, 19]. Our purpose here is to provide details of the methodology used to develop the assay, while more detailed information on the statistical analysis of the obtained data can be found in References [18, 19].

2 Materials

2.1 Clinical Samples

1. Serum samples were obtained from patients undergoing either colonoscopy for CRC screening or CRC surgery after overnight fasting and identical bowel preparation prior to their procedure. All serum samples were from newly diagnosed patients and were collected prior to any surgery or drug treatment (*see* **Note 1**).
2. In total, 234 subjects were recruited for this study, and they were grouped as CRC patients ($n = 66$), polyp patients ($n = 76$), or healthy controls ($n = 92$) based on the analysis of biopsied tissue. Patients were age and gender matched in each group (*see* **Note 2**).

2.2 Reagents

1. Methanol (MS grade), Acetonitrile (MS grade), ammonium acetate (MS grade), and acetic acid (LC-MS grade) were used.
2. Standard compounds are obtained from commercial sources corresponding to the list of measured metabolites (see http://depts.washington.edu/nwmrc/services/metabolite-list).
3. Stable isotope-labeled tyrosine and lactate (L-tyrosine-$^{13}C_2$ and sodium-L-lactate-$^{13}C_3$, Cambridge Isotope Labs, Tewksbury, MA) are used as internal standards. The purities of non-labeled standards should be >95–99% whereas the purities of the two ^{13}C-labeled compounds is typically >99% (*see* **Note 3**).

2.3 LC-MS/MS Instrumentation

1. The LC system is composed of two Agilent 1260 binary pumps, an Agilent 1260 autosampler, and Agilent 1290 column compartment containing a column-switching valve.
2. Chromatographic separations are performed in hydrophilic interaction chromatography (HILIC) mode on two Merck SeQuant ZIC-cHILIC columns (150 × 2.1 mm, 3.0 μm particle size) connected in parallel (*see* **Note 4**). This column arrangement allows one column to perform separation while the other column is reconditioned to be ready for the next injection.
3. MS ionization and data acquisition are performed using an AB Sciex QTrap 5500 mass spectrometer equipped with an electrospray ionization (ESI) source.

4. The instrument is controlled by ABI Analyst 1.5 software. Peak integration was performed using Sciex MultiQuant 2.1 software.

3 Methods

3.1 Sample Preparation

1. After thawing frozen samples at room temperature for 45 min, 50 μL place serum aliquot into a 2 mL Eppendorf vial.
2. Perform protein precipitation and metabolite extraction by adding 150 μL methanol to each serum sample; then vortex the mixture for 2 min, incubate at −20 °C for 20 min, and consequently centrifuge at 20,800 × *g* for 10 min. The supernatant is collected into a new 2 mL Eppendorf vial.
3. To the first vial containing the pellet, add another round of 300 μL methanol, and vortex the mixture for 10 min to allow thorough metabolite extraction. After centrifuging this mixture at 20,800 × *g* for 10 min, collect the supernatant and add to the same vial containing the previous supernatant.
4. Dry the combined supernatants from two rounds of extractions using a Vacufuge Plus evaporator (Eppendorf, Hauppauge, NY) (*see* **Note 5**).
5. Reconstitute the dried samples in 500 μL 5 mM ammonium acetate in 40% water/60% acetonitrile +0.2% acetic acid containing 5.13 μM L-tyrosine-$^{13}C_2$ and 22.54 μM sodium-L-lactate-$^{13}C_3$. The two isotope-labeled internal standards are added to each sample to monitor the LC-MS system performance.
6. Filter the samples through 0.45 μm PVDF filters (Phenomenex, Torrance, CA) prior to LC-MS analysis.
7. Extract a pooled mixture of serum from CRC patients, polyp patients, and healthy controls using the same procedure as above. This sample is used as the quality control (QC) sample and is injected every ten patient samples (*see* **Note 6**).

3.2 LC Conditions

1. Inject each sample twice, 10 μL for MS analysis using negative ionization mode and 2 μL for MS analysis using positive ionization mode.
2. The flow rate is set to 0.300 mL/min, the autosampler temperature is kept at 4 °C, the column compartment is set at 40 °C, and run time for both ionization modes is 20 min (40 min total time per sample) (*see* **Note 7**).
3. The mobile phase is composed of Solvents A (5 mM ammonium acetate in 90% H_2O/ 10% acetonitrile +0.2% acetic acid) and B (5 mM ammonium acetate in 90% acetonitrile/10% H_2O + 0.2% acetic acid). The gradient conditions for both separations are identical and are shown in Table 1.

Table 1
LC gradient conditions

Time segment, min.	Solvent A, %	Solvent B, %
0–2	25	75
2–5	From 25 to 70	From 75 to 30
5–9	70	30
9–11	From 70 to 25	From 30 to 75
11–20	25	75

3.3 MS Conditions

1. Targeted data acquisition is performed in multiple-reaction-monitoring (MRM) mode. In the described experiment, 99 and 59 MRM transitions were monitored in negative and positive mode, respectively (158 transitions in total, *see* http://depts.washington.edu/nwmrc/services/metabolite-list and Fig. 1).
2. The source and collision gas is N_2 (99.999% purity). The ion source conditions in negative/positive mode are typically as follows: curtain gas (CUR) = 25 psi, collision gas (CAD) = high (9 L/min), ion spray voltage (IS) = −3.8/3.8 KV, temperature (TEM) = 500 °C, ion source gas 1 (GS1) = 50 psi, and ion source gas 2 (GS2) = 40 psi.
3. The optimized MS conditions (precursor ion/product ion pairs, declustering potential, cell entrance potential, collision energy, and cell exit potential) for each metabolite are determined using standards by first direct injection and then by running them through the HILIC column (*see* Table 1).
4. Confirm the metabolite identities by spiking the pooled lab QC serum sample used for method development with mixtures of standard compounds (each mixture can contain five standard metabolites or possibly more) (*see* **Note 8**).
5. All the samples in this experiment were analyzed over a 12-day period and the retention times (RT) did not undergo any significant shift (each peak was within 6 s throughout 12 days of analysis). The extracted MRM peaks are integrated using Sciex MultiQuant 2.1 software.
6. The overall reproducibility of the assay is excellent. The interday (12 days of nonstop data acquisition) average coefficient of variation (CV) of metabolite peak areas under MRM curve is 11.0% while the intraday CVs are 4.1–6.7% (*see* Fig. 2). For the two metabolites that have corresponding stable isotope-labeled internal standards (lactate and tyrosine), the interday CV is under 4.0% for both.

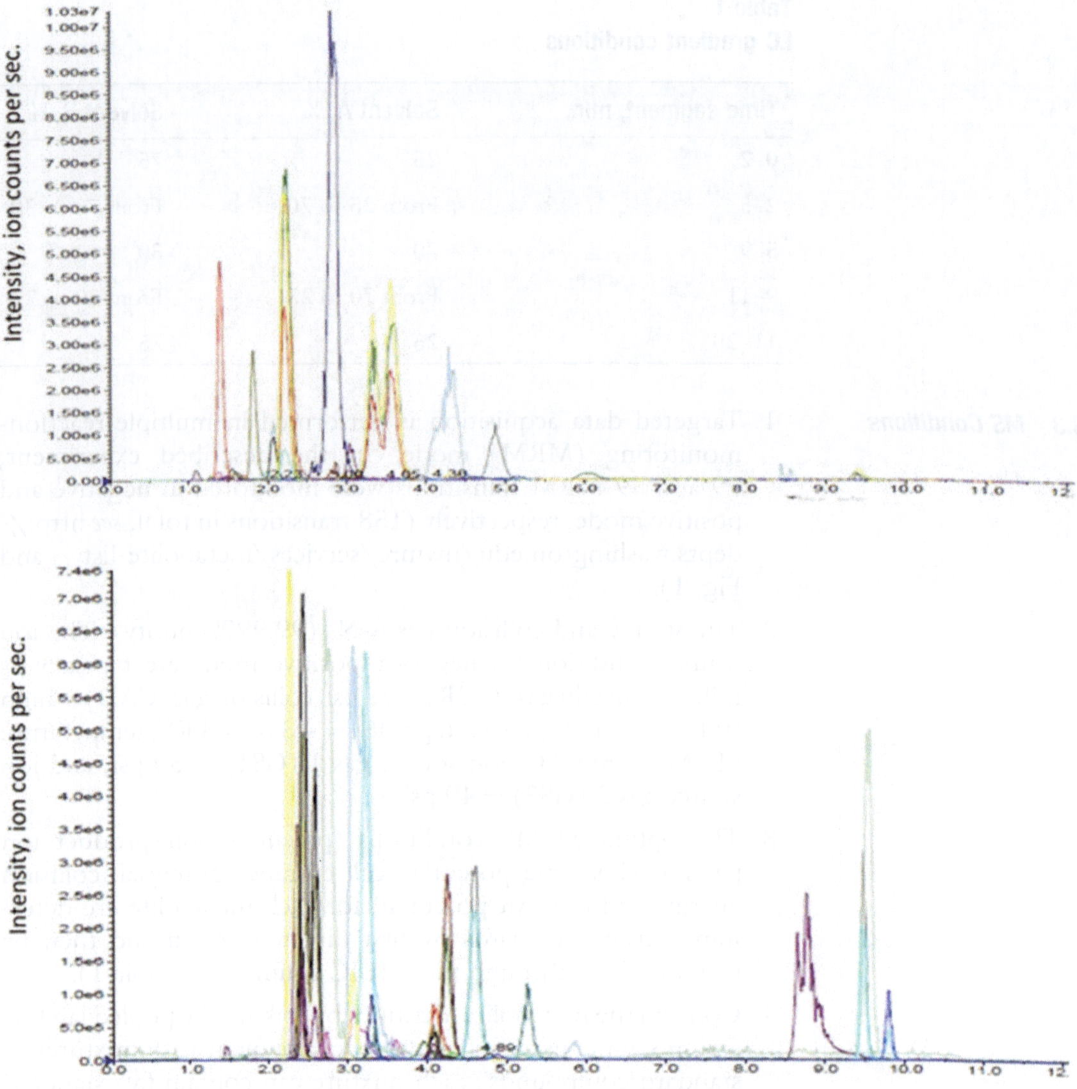

Fig. 1 Collected set of ion chromatograms for the targeted assay. Only first 12 min of the chromatogram is shown, as no peaks appear afterward

3.4 Data Analysis, Model Development, and Cross-Validation

1. Using the above described LC-MS assay, targeted screening of 154 metabolites and two stable isotope-labeled internal standards (156 MRM transitions) can be performed, covering more than 25 major metabolic pathways (e.g., TCA cycle, amino acid metabolism, and glycolysis). In total, 113 metabolites out of 158 targeted MRM transitions were measured in the serum samples (*see* **Notes 9** and **10**, and http://depts.washington.edu/nwmrc/services/metabolite-list).

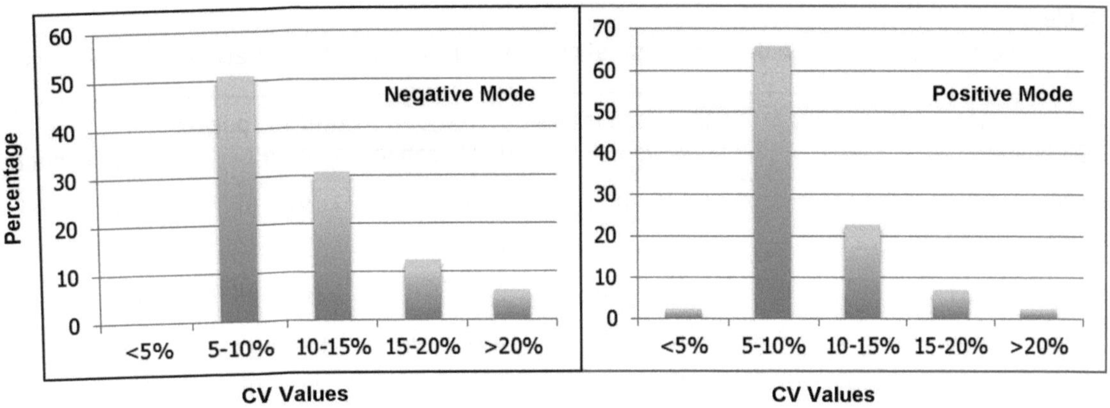

Fig. 2 Reproducibility of the targeted LC-MS assay as monitored using serum QC samples

2. After exporting from MultiQuant software, integrated spectral data are normalized using average values from the data from QC injections (1 QC injection per every ten study samples) on a metabolite by metabolite basis. In particular, metabolite levels are divided by the average value of the same metabolite measured in the QC samples. Typically, there are 4 QC samples per batch of 30 biological samples.
3. In this set of study samples, 42, 48, and 8 of measured metabolites showed statistical significance between CRC vs. healthy controls, CRC vs. polyps and healthy controls vs. polyps, respectively. Among these differential metabolites (some of which are shown in Table 2), 11 had $p < 0.001$ (with a fold change ranging from 0.75 to 2.73) when comparing the CRC patients to healthy controls, and 13 had $p < 0.001$ (with the fold change ranging from 0.77 to 3.22) when comparing the CRC patients to polyp patients.
4. Mann–Whitney U-tests, generation of receiver operator characteristics (ROC) curves, and calculation of sensitivity, specificity, and area under ROC curves (AUROC) can be conducted using JMP Pro10 (SAS Institute) or other readily available software packages.
5. In terms of multivariate statistical analysis, a number of options are available, and there are many software packages that can be utilized. We describe one approach to illustrate some of these analyses. Here, partial least squares-discriminant analysis (PLS-DA) and Monte Carlo Cross-Validation (MCCV, with in-house developed codes) were performed using Matlab software (installed with PLS toolbox. MCCV was applied with the data divided into the training (70%) and testing (30%) sets using 100 iterations. In each iteration, three specificities of the training set, 0.95, 0.85, and 0.75, were used to determine the thresholds of PLS-DA predicted Y values. The same

Table 2
List of metabolites that showed strong separation between CRC vs. Controls and CRC vs. Polyps

Metabolite	CRC vs. controls *p*-value	Fold change	CRC vs. polyps *p*-value	Fold change
Glyceraldehyde	1.52E−05	1.34	2.19E−07	1.41
N-Acetyl-glycine	7.70E−04	0.75		
Hippuric acid	8.46E−05	2.73	1.40E−05	3.22
Linolenic acid	3.32E−04	0.78	2.04E−04	0.77
Glycochenodeoxycholate	5.84E−05	1.42	9.22E−05	2.27
Glycocholate	4.25E−04	1.79	1.94E−04	3.01
Dimethylglycine			2.11E−04	0.78
Hydroxyproline/Aminolevulinate			9.09E−04	1.32
Glutamine			3.91E−04	0.92
Lysine	1.18E−04	0.88	5.00E−06	0.84
Glutamic acid	6.27E−04	1.22		
Methionine	1.16E−04	0.88	1.89E−06	0.85
Histidine	2.75E−06	0.81	2.57E−05	0.85
Arginine				
2′-deoxyuridine	8.10E−04	0.91	3.81E−05	0.89
Uridine			2.26E−05	0.84

thresholds were then applied to the test set to determine sensitivities and specificities. The sample classification could be classified as true class or as random permutation.

6. In order to identify CRC diagnostic serum biomarkers, multiple steps of metabolite selections, model building, and cross-validation are typically performed. Here, and at the beginning, individual metabolites that had $p < 0.05$ (Mann–Whitney U test) were selected as potential biomarker candidates and then AUROC, sensitivity, and specificity of each metabolite were determined in comparing CRC patients with healthy controls and CRC patients with polyp patients, respectively. No single metabolite proved to be both sensitive and specific (generally, AUROC >0.75) to separate CRC patients from either healthy controls or polyp patients. PLS-DA models with leave one out cross-validation were then applied to identify groups of biomarkers that could be used for diagnosing CRC patients. All metabolites that had $p < 0.05$ between groups (42 metabolites between CRC and control, and 48 metabolites between CRC and Polyp, respectively) were used for initial PLS-DA analysis.

Efforts were then made to simplify the model in consideration of more practical applications in clinical settings. PLS-DA variable importance in projection (VIP) plots were generated to evaluate the important metabolite biomarkers that contributed most to the separation of CRC patients from the other two groups in this study. When the VIP score threshold was set to 1, 13 metabolite biomarkers were selected for the separation between CRC patients and healthy control and 14 metabolite biomarkers were selected for the separation of CRC patients from polyp patients. Based on the VIP selection, a second PLS-DA model was built using only the metabolites that had VIP scores greater than 1. To evaluate the diagnostic power of the potential metabolic markers, ROC curves were generated, showing a good differentiation of CRC from healthy controls (AUROC = 0.90) and patients with polyps (0.93). Also in order to exam the robustness of our PLS-DA based CRC diagnostic models, Monte Carlo cross-validation (MCCV) was applied for the comparison of PLS-DA models using the true sample classifications to those with randomly permuted sample class information, and superior sensitivity from true sample classifications showed the robust diagnostic power of this metabolic profiling approach.

7. Clinical factors, such as gender, age, medication, and substance status have been proposed by other researchers as factors that could strengthen the metabolite biomarker models [18]. Here, four general clinical factors (age, gender, smoking, and alcohol status) were added to the model in an effort to improve its performance. Excellent AUROCs (0.93–0.95, respectively) for differentiating CRC patients from healthy controls or polyp patients.
8. The resulting PLS-DA model including the four clinical factors showed good performance for all CRC stages with all AUROCs $\geq$0.93, with the best performance for stage IV CRC (AUROC = 0.99).
9. Besides the diagnostic power of metabolite biomarkers for comparing CRC patients with healthy controls and polyp patients, the metabolite changes in CRC patients with different cancer stages can also be investigated. It was observed that glutamic acid, adenosine and aspartic acid were significantly altered across the cancer stages. A prediction model based on these three metabolites was developed, and it generated excellent clinical performance.

4 Notes

1. Patient recruitment and sample collection protocols were approved by the Purdue University and Indiana University School of Medicine Institutional Review Boards. Informed consent was provided by all subjects in the study according to the institutional guidelines.
2. Full demographic information can be found in Reference 18.
3. Additional internal standards can be added to the assay, including additional amino acids, organic acids and amines. In general, it is advisable to use ^{13}C or ^{15}N-labeled compounds, although some D-labeled compounds can also be used if the D are not labile. Also, the use of doubly (or more) labeled compounds detected as M + 2 or higher ions is advised so as to separate the detection of these compounds from metabolites with isotopic atoms that occur naturally (M + 1 species).
4. Excellent performance may also be obtained using Waters BEH Amide columns. In our experience, the Waters columns offer better reproducibility and significantly longer life span (2–3000 sample injections per column) than the ZIC-cHILIC columns. Users are also encouraged to try other, similar columns as technology evolves.
5. Drying times are typically 1.5–2 h but can be longer if the sample volumes are larger or the dryer is not working optimally. Alternatively, the extracted sample can be dried using a lyophilizer, or with nitrogen gas.
6. Typically, two pooled QC samples are used in the analysis. First, a "study QC" that consists of a mixture from a number of study samples from each group (10 or more from each group) is prepared and run once for every study sample. These QC samples provide the best match to the biological samples as they have essentially the same matrix and can be used both to verify good performance of the instrument during the run and for normalization of the study samples during data analysis. A second, "lab QC" is run at least once per sample batch to monitor the long time performance of the instrument. This QC is also a serum or plasma sample obtained commercially in a large lot, which is then aliquoted and frozen. This lab QC is prepared according to the standard protocol.
7. Typically, very few (none in this case) will have retention times above 12 min. However, the HILIC columns need additional time to regenerate. Thus 20 min was chosen as a compromise to allow reasonably high throughput (30 biological samples per day) and enough time for essentially complete regeneration so as not to degrade column performance.

8. Mixtures of standard compounds are made using compounds that have different masses and chromatograms to avoid ambiguity. Concentrations are used such that the roughly match those found in serum. Reference concentration values can be found in the Human Metabolome Database (www.hmdb.ca). Concentration values are compared to those obtained from the pooled lab QC sample to make sure they are in the proper range using MS analysis.
9. It is common for such assays to target more metabolites than are typically measured in a particular sample type. Here, this assay was developed to measure metabolites in both blood and cell/tissue samples, which sometimes have very different concentrations for the same metabolites. For example, it is often easier to measure nucleotides and coenzymes in cells than plasma/serum.
10. Some metabolites that could not be well chromatographically separated and had similar m/z values (<1 Da) were integrated as a single peak (e.g., malonic acid and 3-hydroxybutyric acid were reported as a single peak). Ultimately, choosing chromatographic conditions involves a trade-off among the metabolites that will be well detected and those that may overlap.

References

1. Siegel RL, Miller KD, Fedewa SA, Ahnen DJ, Meester RGS, Barzi A, Jemal A (2017) Colorectal cancer statistics, 2017. CA Cancer J Clin 67:177–193
2. Howlader N, Noone AM, Krapcho M (2016) SEER cancer statistics review, 1975-2013. National Cancer Institute, Bethesda, MD
3. Rex DK, Johnson DA, Anderson JC, Schoenfeld PS, Burke CA, Inadomi JM (2009) American College of Gastroenterology guidelines for colorectal cancer screening 2008. Am J Gastroenterol 104:739–750
4. Bond JH (2003) Colon polyps and cancer. Endoscopy 35:27–35
5. Ahlquist DA, Zou H, Domanico M, Mahoney DW, Yab TC, Taylor WR, Butz ML, Thibodeau SN, Rabeneck L, Paszat LF, Kinzler KW, Vogelstein B, Bjerregaard NC, Laurberg S, Sørensen HT, Berger BM, Lidgard GP (2012) Next-generation stool DNA test accurately detects colorectal cancer and large adenomas. Gastroenterology 142:248–256
6. Link A, Balaguer F, Shen Y, Nagasaka T, Lozano JJ, Boland CR, Goel A (2010) Fecal microRNAs as novel biomarkers for colon cancer screening. Cancer Epidemiol Biomark Prev 19:1766–1774
7. Ritchie SA, Tonita J, Alvi R, Lehotey D, Elshoni H, Myat S, McHattie J, Goodenowe DB (2013) Low-serum GTA-446 anti-inflammatory fatty acid levels as a new risk factor for colon cancer. Int J Cancer 132:355–362
8. Gu H, Nagana Gowda GA, Raftery D (2012) Metabolic profiling: are we en route to better diagnostic tests for cancer? Future Oncol 8:1207–1210
9. Nagana Gowda GA, Zhang S, Gu H, Asiago V, Shanaiah N, Raftery D (2008) Metabolomics-based methods for early disease diagnostics: a review. Expert Rev Mol Diagnost 8:617–633
10. Vander Heiden MG, Cantley LC, Thompson CB (2009) Understanding the Warburg Effect: the metabolic requirements of cell proliferation. Science 324:1029–1033
11. Qiu Y, Cai G, Su M, Chen T, Zheng X, Xu y NY, Zhao A, Xu LX, Cai S, Jia W (2009) Serum metabolite profiling of human colorectal cancer using GC-TOFMS and UPLC-QTOFMS. J Proteome Res 8:4844–4850
12. Tan B, Qiu Y, Zou X, Chen T, Xie G, Cheng Y, Dong T, Zhao L, Feng B, Hu X, Xu LX, Zhao A, Zhang M, Cai G, Cai S, Zhou Z, Xheng M, Zhang Y, Jia W (2013) Metabonomics identifies serum metabolite markers of

colorectal cancer. J Proteome Res 12:3000–3009
13. Cheng Y, Xie G, Chen T, Qiu Y, Zou X, Zheng M, Tan B, Feng B, Dong T, He P, Zhao L, Zhao A, Xu LX, Zhang Y, Jia W (2012) Distinct urinary metabolic profile of human colorectal cancer. J Proteome Res 11:1354–1363
14. Nishiumi S, Kobayashi T, Ikeda A, Yoshie T, Kibi M, Izumi Y, Okuno T, Hayashi N, Kawano S, Takenawa T, Azuma T (2012) A novel serum metabolomics-based diagnostic approach for colorectal cancer. PLoS One 7: e40459. https://doi.org/10.1371/journal.pone.0040459
15. Farshidfar F, Weljie AM, Kopciuk K, Buie WD, Anthony ML, Dixon E, Sutherland FR, Molckovsky A, Vogel HJ, Bathe OF (2012) Serum metabolic profile as a means to distinguish stage of colorectal cancer. Genome Med 4:42–54
16. Ritchie SA, Ahiahonu PWK, Jayasinghe D, Heath D, Liu J, Lu Y, Jin W, Kavianpour A, Yamazaki Y, Khan AM, Hossain M, Su-Myat KK, Wood PL, Krenitsky K, Takemasa I, Miyake M, Sekimoto M, Monden M, Matsubara H, Nomura F, Goodenowe DB (2010) Reduced levels of hydroxylated, polyunsaturated ultra long-chain fatty acids in the serum of colorectal cancer patients: implications for early screening and detection. BMC Med 8:13–32
17. Li F, Qin X, Chen H, Qiu L, Guo Y, Liu H, Chen G, Song G, Wang X, Li F, Guo S, Wang B, Li Z (2013) Lipid profiling for early diagnosis and progression of colorectal cancer using direct-infusion electrospray ionization Fourier transform ion cyclotron resonance mass spectrometry. Rapid Commun Mass Spectrom 27:24–34
18. Zhu J, Djukovic D, Deng L, Gu H, Himmati F, Chiorean EG, Raftery D (2014) Colorectal cancer detection using targeted serum metabolic profiling. J Proteome Res 13:4120–4130
19. Zhu J, Djukovic D, Deng L, Gu H, Himmati F, Chiorean EG, Zaid MA, Raftery D (2015) Targeted serum metabolite profiling for colorectal cancer progression monitoring. Anal Bioanal Chem 407:7857–7863

Check for updates

Chapter 16

Proteomic Profiling for Colorectal Cancer Biomarker Discovery

Paula Álvarez-Chaver, Loretta De Chiara, and Vicenta Soledad Martínez-Zorzano

Abstract

Nowadays, the ideal biomarker for colorectal cancer (CRC) has not been found. Two-dimensional electrophoresis (2-DE) and mass spectrometry (MS) are suitable techniques for searching new biomarkers. In this chapter, we describe methodology for biomarker discovery based on a proteomic approach. In addition, special attention is given to the sample preparation, including protein extraction, fractionation, and cleanup, as we consider this a critical step. Comparing the proteomic profile of tumor and mucosa, we identified the nucleoside diphosphate kinase A (NDKA) protein as a candidate biomarker for CRC. Finally, we validated NDKA with an ELISA kit using serum samples from individuals of a screening cohort. Our results suggest that serum NDKA is a potential biomarker for screening of CRC and premalignant advanced adenomas (AA).

Key words Colorectal cancer, Tissue, Serum, Biomarkers, Proteomics, Two-dimensional electrophoresis, Mass spectrometry, Western blot, ELISA immunoassay, Nucleoside diphosphate kinase A

1 Introduction

The search for new biomarkers is still a priority in colorectal cancer (CRC) research, because no biomarker has shown the desirable sensitivity and specificity for clinical use [1]. Proteomics includes powerful techniques aimed to find differences in protein expression between normal and disease states. We used two-dimensional electrophoresis (2-DE), a combination of isoelectrofocusing (IEF) with sodium dodecyl sulfate-polyacrylamide gel electrophoresis (SDS-PAGE), coupled to mass spectrometry (MS) identification, due to its capability of separating thousands of proteins in a single analysis (Fig. 1) [2, 3]. Regarding the sample, we choose tissue to be certain that differentially expressed proteins were altered in this pathology. Besides, we opted for a prefractionation of the sample prior to 2-DE in order to reduce its complexity and improve the search for a good biomarker. The protein nucleoside diphosphate

Jean-François Beaulieu (ed.), *Colorectal Cancer: Methods and Protocols*, Methods in Molecular Biology, vol. 1765, https://doi.org/10.1007/978-1-4939-7765-9_16,

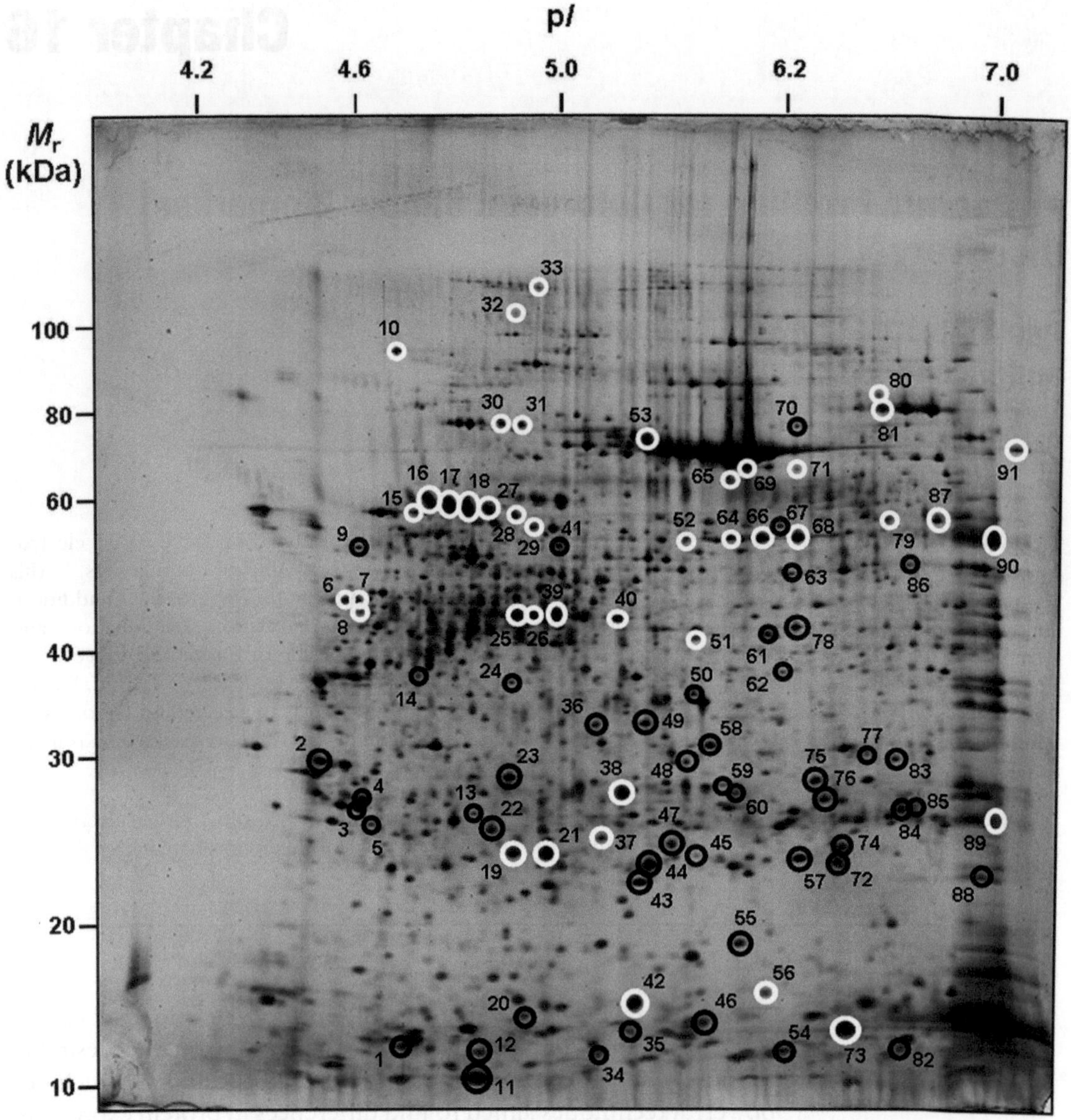

Fig. 1 Representative two-dimensional map of the hydrophilic protein fraction from a colorectal tumor. Spots overexpressed (black) and underexpressed (white) in colorectal tumors compared to mucosa are highlighted. *pI* isoelectric point, *Mr* experimental relative molecular mass. Reproduced from ref. [2] with permission from Elsevier

kinase A (NDKA) was found overexpressed in the hydrophilic fraction of CRC tumors, and was selected as an interesting candidate protein to be validated as a biomarker for this neoplasia. First, the increase of NDKA protein levels in tumor tissues was corroborated by Western blot (Fig. 2) [2]. Then, with the aim of evaluating the utility of NDKA for the discrimination of individuals with CRC or premalignant advanced adenomas (AA) from individuals with no

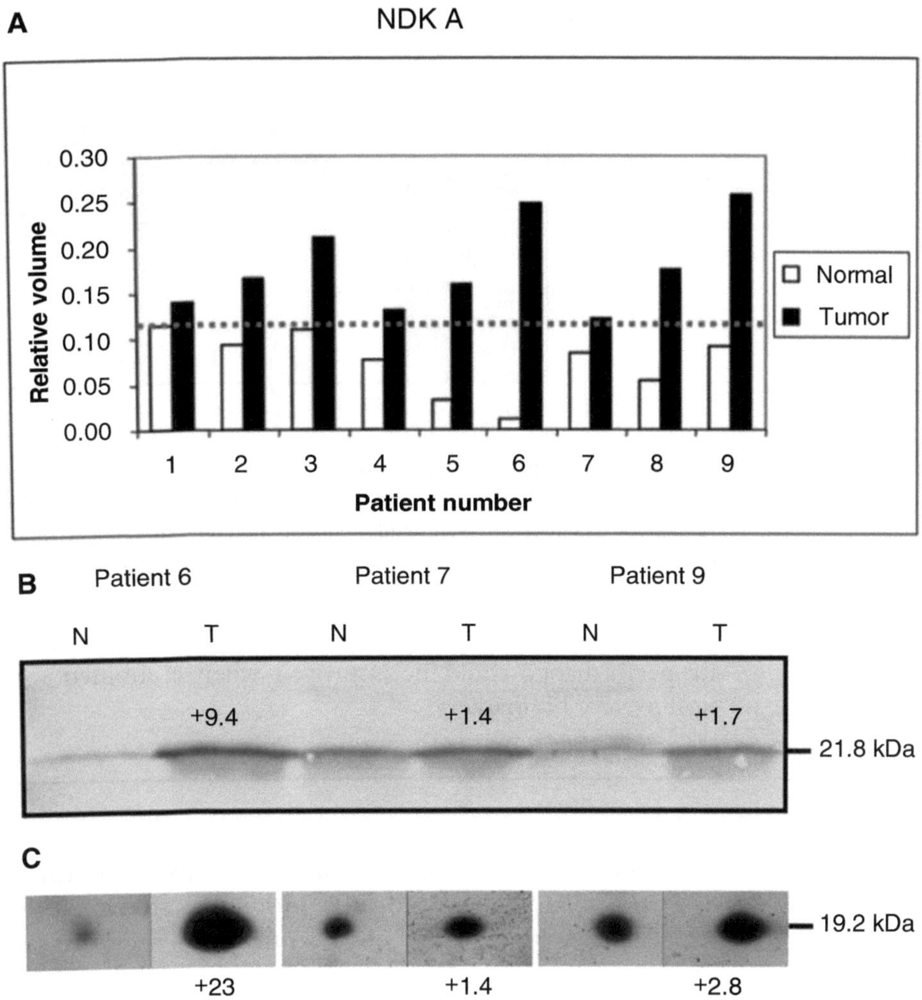

Fig. 2 NDKA expression in normal (healthy) and tumoral colorectal tissue. (**a**) and (**c**) show the expression of NDKA after 2D–PAGE and silver staining. The horizontal line in (**a**) shows the cutoff that could separate both groups. (**b**) is a Western blot after SDS-PAGE that shows the overexpression found in three of the same patients included in the 2D-PAGE analysis. *N* normal, *T* tumor. Reproduced from ref. [2] with permission from Elsevier

neoplasia, we measured NDKA serum concentration in a screening cohort using a commercial enzyme-linked immunosorbent sandwich assay (ELISA). Patients with CRC or AA showed elevated NDKA concentrations compared to individuals with no neoplasia (no colorectal findings, benign colorectal pathologies, and nonadvanced adenomas) (Fig. 3) [4].

Therefore, this chapter includes the protocols we used in a proteomic study focused on the search of new CRC biomarkers using tissue samples, concluding that this approach is a good strategy [5]. Upon validation, our results suggest that serum NDKA is a

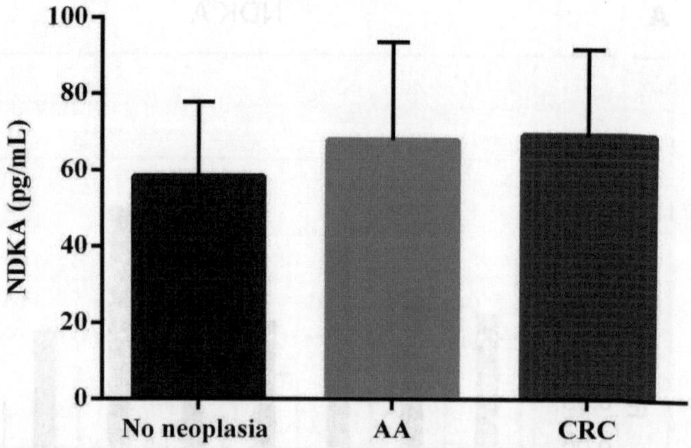

Fig. 3 Boxplot representation of serum NDKA levels in the screening cohort. Boxes represent mean values and whiskers indicate the standard deviation. *No neoplasia* includes no colorectal findings, benign pathologies, nonadvanced adenomas, *AA* advanced adenomas, *CRC* colorectal cancer

potential biomarker for the screening of CRC and AA. Its diagnostic performance could be improved when combined with other noninvasive biomarkers.

2 Materials

2.1 Samples

1. Paired samples of healthy colorectal mucosa and tumor tissue from CRC patients for the proteomic study (*see* **Note 1**). Tissues were stored at −80 °C until used.
2. Blood samples for the validation step were obtained using adequate tubes for serum collection, following the instructions of the tube manufacturer, as time for clotting, centrifugation time and speed (*see* **Note 2**).

2.2 Protein Extraction and Prefractionation

Store all reagents at room temperature unless otherwise indicated.

1. ReadyPrep™ Protein Extraction Kit (Membrane I) (Bio-Rad) that includes the following reagents:
   (a) Membrane protein extraction buffer 1 (M1): use directly. Store at 4 °C after opening (*see* **Note 3**).
   (b) Membrane protein extraction buffer 2 (M2): contains Triton X-114. Use directly. Store at 4 °C after opening (*see* **Note 3**).
2. Protease inhibitors: Complete™ Mini tablets (Roche). Store at 4 °C.
3. 1.5 mL microcentrifuge tubes.
4. Microcentrifuge capable of spinning at 12–16,000 × *g* at 4 °C.

5. Vortex mixer.
6. Sonicator and micro-tip to sonicate samples in small volumes.
7. Heat block/bath set at 37 °C.

2.3 Protein Precipitation and Cleanup

Store all reagents at room temperature unless otherwise indicated.

1. ReadyPrep™ 2-D Cleanup Kit (Bio-Rad) that includes the following reagents (*see* **Note 4**):
   (a) Precipitation agent 1. Care should be exercised when handling it because it is corrosive.
   (b) Precipitation agent 2.
   (c) Wash reagent 1.
   (d) Wash reagent 2. Store at −20 °C for at least 1 h prior to use. For convenience, store it in a − 20 °C freezer. Be careful in handling it because it is flammable and is an irritant (it contains acetone and trichloroacetic acid).
   (e) Wash two additive.
2. Protein solubilization buffer (PSB) diluent included in the ReadyPrep™ Protein Extraction Kit. Store at 4 °C after opening (*see* **Note 3**).
3. PSB powder included in the ReadyPrep™ Protein Extraction Kit. To make 2 mL of PSB add 1.1 mL of PSB diluent per gram of PSB powder.
4. 1.5 mL microcentrifuge tubes.
5. Microcentrifuge capable of spinning at 12–16,000 × *g* at 4 °C.
6. Vortex mixer.
7. Ultrapure water.

2.4 Protein Quantification

1. RC DC™ protein assay kit (Bio-Rad) that contains the DC Reagent S, DC Reagent A, RC Reagent I, RC Reagent II, DC Reagent B and Bovine Serum Albumin (BSA) as the standard.
2. Bradford protein assay (Bio-Rad) that contains the Bradford reactive and BSA as the standard.
3. 0.1 N HCl.
4. Ultrapure water.
5. 1.5 mL microcentrifuge tubes.
6. 10 mL glass tubes.
7. Microcentrifuge capable of spinning at 12–16,000 × *g*.
8. Vortex mixer.
9. Cuvettes for spectrophotometer.
10. Spectrophotometer to measure absorbance at 595–750 nm.

2.5 SDS–Polyacrylamide Gel

1. Resolving gel buffer: 1.5 M Tris–HCl, pH 8.8. Weigh 36.3 g of Tris and dissolve in 100 mL of Milli-Q (MQ) H_2O. Adjust pH with HCl and then complete up to 200 mL with MQ H_2O. Store at 4 °C (*see* **Note 5**).
2. Stacking gel buffer: 0.5 M Tris–HCl, pH 6.8. Weigh 12.2 g of Tris and dissolve in 100 mL of MQ H_2O. Adjust pH with HCl and then complete up to 200 mL with MQ H_2O. Store at 4 °C (*see* **Note 5**).
3. 30% acrylamide–bis solution, 37.5:1 (Bio-Rad) (2.6% cross-linker acrylamide: N, N′-methylene-bis-acrylamide). Store at 4 °C (*see* **Note 6**).
4. Sodium dodecyl sulfate (SDS): 10% solution in MQ H_2O. Weigh 10 g of SDS and dissolve in 100 mL of MQ H_2O (*see* **Note 7**).
5. Ammonium persulfate (APS): 10% solution in MQ H_2O. Weigh 0.05 g of APS in 500 μL of MQ H_2O (*see* **Note 8**).
6. N, N, N′, N′-tetramethyl-ethylendiamine (TEMED). Store at 4 °C.
7. Sucrose (*see* **Note 9**).
8. Mini-PROTEAN® Tetra Cell spacer plates of 0.75 mm thickness, short plates, and combs (Bio-Rad).
9. Mini-PROTEAN® Tetra Cell casting frame and casting stand (Bio-Rad).
10. PROTEAN II xi cell-casting stand with glass plate sandwich in alignment slot (Bio-Rad).
11. Gradient former to construct reproducible polyacrylamide gradient gels (model 485, Bio-Rad).
12. Ultrapure water.
13. Magnetic stirrer and stirring bars.
14. Laboratory hydraulic lift.
15. Precision scale.

2.6 SDS–Polyacrylamide Gel Electrophoresis (SDS-PAGE)

1. SDS reducing buffer 2×: 0.1 M Tris–HCl pH 6.8, 4% SDS, 0.2% bromophenol blue, 20% glycerol (87%), 10% β-mercaptoethanol. To prepare 2 mL mix 0.4 mL of 0.5 M Tris–HCl pH 6.8, 0.8 mL of 10% SDS, 0.2 mL of 2% bromophenol blue, 0.46 mL of 87% glycerol, and 0.2 mL of 100% β-mercaptoethanol (*see* **Note 10**).
2. Electrode buffer 5× pH 8.3: 25 mM Tris, 192 mM glycine, 0.1% SDS (*see* **Note 11**).
3. Bromophenol blue: 2% solution in MQ H_2O.
4. Prestained SDS-PAGE standards-low Range.
5. Mini-PROTEAN® Tetra Cell electrophoresis module and a power supply (Bio-Rad).

6. PROTEAN II xi cell electrophoresis module and a power supply (Bio-Rad).
7. Low melting point agarose.
8. Circulating cooler bath.

2.7 Isoelectro-focusing (IEF)

1. Rehydration buffer: 7 M urea, 2 M thiourea, 4% CHAPS (w/v).
2. Reducing agent dithiothreitol (DTT). Store at 4 °C.
3. Iodoacetamide (IAA).
4. Carrier ampholytes Bio-Lyte 3/10 (Bio-Rad). Store at 4 °C.
5. Bromophenol blue: 2% solution in MQ H_2O.
6. ReadyStrip™ IPG linear strips, 17 cm, pH 4–7 (Bio-Rad).
7. Protean IEF Cell focusing tray (Bio-Rad).
8. PROTEAN® IEF Cell (Bio-Rad).
9. Protean IEF Cell equilibration tray (Bio-Rad).
10. SDS-PAGE equilibration buffer: 6 M urea, 50 mM Tris pH 8.8, 2% SDS (w/v), 30% glycerol (v/v) (*see* **Note 12**).
11. Mineral oil.
12. Forceps.
13. Electrode wicks, precut, 4 mm × 20 mm.
14. Precision scale.
15. Rocker stirrer.

2.8 Silver Staining Procedure, Image Acquisition and Analysis

Prepare all solutions using ultrapure water and analytical grade reagents.

1. Plastic container of at least 25 mm × 25 mm × 5 mm.
2. Rocker stirrer.
3. Precision scale.
4. Fixating solution: 40% ethanol and 10% acetic acid. Final volume 500 mL.
5. Sensibilizing solution: 34 g of sodium acetate, 1.5 g of sodium thiosulfate and 150 mL of ethanol. Final volume 500 mL.
6. Silver nitrate solution: 0.5 g in a final volume of 500 mL.
7. Revealing solution: 22.5 g of sodium carbonate and 187.5 μL of formaldehyde 37% in a final volume of 750 mL.
8. Stop solution: 7.3 g of ethylenendiaminetetraacetic acid disodium salt dehydrate ($EDTA\text{-}Na_2\ 2H_2O$) in a final volume of 500 mL.
9. Calibrated densitometer (GS-800, Bio-Rad).
10. PDQuest 7.3.1 software package (Bio-Rad) to perform 2D image analysis.

2.9 Mass Spectrometry Protein Identification

Prepare all solutions using ultrapure water and analytical grade reagents. Store all reagents at room temperature unless otherwise indicated.

1. 30 mM potassium ferricyanide. Store at 4 °C and protected from light (cover the bottle with aluminum foil).
2. 100 mM sodium thiosulfate.
3. 25 and 50 mM ammonium bicarbonate. Store at 4 °C.
4. 100% acetonitrile (ACN).
5. 100% ethanol.
6. 10% formic acid (v/v).
7. 10 mM dithiothreitol (DTT), prepared in 50 mM ammonium bicarbonate. Store at 4 °C.
8. 55 mM iodoacetamide (IAA), prepared in 50 mM ammonium bicarbonate. Store at 4 °C.
9. Sequencing grade modified trypsin (Promega). Store at −20 °C.
10. Sterile scalpel.
11. Flow hood.
12. Eppendorf LoBind® tubes 0.5 mL.
13. Vortex mixer.
14. Speed-vac at 45 °C.
15. Eppendorf® thermomixer or a stove.
16. Ultrasonic bath.
17. Microcentrifuge capable of spinning at 12–16,000 × *g*.
18. Tubes for liquid chromatographic nano-electrospray tandem mass spectrometry (LC-nESI-MS/MS).
19. Mass spectrometer Q-TOF Global (Micromass-Waters).

2.10 Western Blotting, Immunodetection, Image Acquisition and Analysis

1. PVDF membranes 0.45 μm (Immobilon-P, Millipore).
2. Western blot transfer buffer containing Tris–glycine (25 mM Tris and 192 mM glycine, pH 8.3), 10% methanol (v/v), and 1.3 mM SDS (*see* **Note 13**).
3. 100% methanol.
4. Mini Trans-Blot® (Bio-Rad) and a power supply. The tank is part of Bio-Rad's modular Mini-PROTEAN® Tetra system. The unique different feature is the electrode module.
5. Blue cooling unit freeze at −20 °C.
6. Filter papers and fiber pads the same size as 1D gel and PVDF membrane (7 × 8 cm).
7. Magnetic stirrer and stirring bars.

8. 10× phosphate buffer solution (PBS) pH 7.4: 1.37 M NaCl, 27 mM KCl, 0.1 M Na_2HPO_4, and 20 mM KH_2PO_4 (*see* **Note 14**).
9. Tween 20.
10. Blocking solution: 5% (w/v) nonfat milk in 1× PBS pH 7.4.
11. Primary antibody: mouse anti-human NDKA MCA1865 antibody (AbD Serotec). We use a 1/2000 dilution (*see* **Note 15**).
12. Secondary antibody: goat anti-mouse IgG (H + L) conjugated with alkaline phosphatase (Bio-Rad). We use a 1/2000 dilution (*see* **Note 15**).
13. Chromogenic substrate nitroblue tetrazolium/5-bromo-4-chloro-3-indolyl phosphate (NBT/BCIP, Roche Diagnostics).
14. Calibrated densitometer (GS-800, Bio-Rad).
15. Quantity One 4.4.1 software package (Bio-Rad) to carry out 1D image analysis.

2.11 ELISA Immunoassay

Reagent volumes are calculated for the use of the complete 96-well assay plate (*see* **Note 16**).

1. Human Nucleoside Diphosphate Kinase A (NME1) ELISA kit (Cusabio) that includes an assay plate with 96-coated microwells and all the necessary reagents:
   (a) Solutions provided by the kit that do not require preparation: sample diluent, biotin-antibody diluent, HRP-avidin diluent, TMB substrate, and stop solution.
   (b) Standard NDKA solution: add 1 mL of sample diluent to the standard vial (*see* **Note 17**).
   (c) Biotin-antibody solution 1×: add 120 μL of biotin-antibody concentrate (100×) to 11.88 mL of biotin-antibody diluent. Gently mix (*see* **Note 18**).
   (d) Horseradish Peroxidase (HRP)-avidin solution 1×: add 120 μL of HRP-avidin concentrate (100×) to 11.88 mL of HRP-avidin diluent. Gently mix.
   (e) 1× wash buffer: add 8 mL of wash buffer concentrate (25×) to 192 mL of ultrapure water and mix (*see* **Note 19**).
   (f) Adhesive strip for 96-well plate.
2. Single channel pipettes (100, 200, 1000 μL) and multichannel pipette (8-channel, 200 μL).
3. Reagent reservoir polystyrene trays of 50 mL for each solution to use with multichannel pipette.
4. ELISA plate washer (microplate washer).
5. Plate incubator set at 37 °C.

6. Microplate reader measuring absorbance at 450, 570, and 630 nm.
7. Computer software for performing a four parameter logistic (4-PL) curve fit.
8. Paper towels.

3 Methods

3.1 Protein Extraction and Prefractionation by Phase-Partitioning

The ReadyPrep™ Protein Extraction Kit is used to obtain two fractions enriched in hydrophilic and hydrophobic proteins, based on the methods developed by Bordier [6] and Santoni et al. [7]. Protein extracts obtained after prefractionation were stored at −20 °C until analysis.

1. For improved cell lysis, sonicate tissue samples at 4 °C in membrane protein extraction buffer M1 (0.5 mL per 50 mg of tissue in a microcentrifuge tube). Add a cocktail of protease inhibitors to prevent proteolysis during extraction. Use an ultrasonic tip for small volumes. Sonicate the sample on ice with 30 s sonication and 1 min rest for each cycle, for a total of 3 cycles (*see* **Note 20**).
2. Add 0.5 mL of chilled protein extraction buffer M2 and vortex 4 times during 60 s, maintaining the tube on ice for 30–60 s between each vortexing step. Finally, incubate the tube on ice for 10 min.
3. Incubate the tube at 37 °C for 30 min, mixing the sample 3–4 times during incubation.
4. Centrifuge the tube at 14,000 × *g* for 5 min at room temperature to produce a top aqueous phase containing hydrophilic (HPL) proteins and a bottom detergent phase enriched in hydrophobic (HPB) proteins (*see* **Note 21**).
5. Remove and transfer the top aqueous phase to a clean tube and repeat **steps 2–4** with the bottom detergent phase to purify the HPB fraction. Again, remove the top aqueous phase and pool with the previously collected. Collect the bottom phase and transfer to a new tube (*see* **Note 22**).

3.2 Protein Quantification Before Cleanup: RC DC Protein Assay

Use the 1.5 mL microfuge tube assay protocol and make all incubations at room temperature (*see* **Note 23**).

1. Add 5 μL of DC Reagent S to each 250 μL of DC Reagent A (this mixture is called Reagent A') (*see* **Note 24**).
2. Prepare five dilutions of BSA from 0.27 to 1.36 μg/μL in a final volume of 25 μL (*see* **Note 25**).

3. Pipette 25 μL of samples into clean, dry microfuge tubes (*see* **Note 26**).
4. Add 125 μL of RC Reagent I into each tube, vortex and incubate for 1 min.
5. Add 125 μL of RC Reagent II into each tube, vortex and centrifuge at 15,000 × *g* for 5 min.
6. Discard the supernatant (*see* **Note 27**).
7. Add 127 μL Reagent A' to each tube, vortex and incubate for 5 min. Vortex again.
8. Add 1 mL of DC Reagent B to each tube, vortex and incubate for 15 min.
9. Read absorbance at 750 nm (*see* **Note 28**).

3.3 Protein Cleanup

The ReadyPrep™ 2D Cleanup Kit is used to precipitate proteins and remove extraction agents that could interfere with isoelectrofocusing (IEF) (i.e., ionic detergents, salts, nucleic acids, and lipids). Maintain sample tubes on ice unless otherwise indicated.

1. Transfer 1–500 μg of protein in a final volume of 100 μL into a 1.5 mL microcentrifuge tube (*see* **Note 29**).
2. Add 300 μL of precipitating agent 1 to the protein sample, vortex and incubate on ice for 15 min (*see* **Note 30**).
3. Add 300 μL of precipitating agent 2 to the mixture of protein sample and precipitating agent 1, vortex and incubate on ice for 15 min (*see* **Note 30**).
4. Centrifuge the tubes at maximum speed (>12,000 × *g*) for 5 min (*see* **Note 31**).
5. Remove and discard the supernatant with care, without touching the pellet.
6. Centrifuge for 15–30 s to collect any residual liquid at the bottom of the tube.
7. Add 40 μL of wash reagent 1 to the pellet, vortex and centrifuge at maximum speed (>12,000 × *g*) for 5 min (*see* **Note 32**).
8. Remove and discard the wash solution.
9. Add 25 μL of ultrapure water to the pellet and vortex (*see* **Note 33**).
10. Add 1 mL of wash reagent 2 and 5 μL of wash 2 additive. Vortex for 1 min (*see* **Note 34**).
11. Incubate the tube at −20 °C for 30 min. Vortex the tube for 30 s every 10 min during the incubation period.
12. Centrifuge the tubes at maximum speed (>12,000 × *g*) for 5 min. Carefully remove and discard the supernatant.

13. Briefly centrifuge the tube, remove and discard any remaining wash reagent (*see* **Note 35**).
14. Resuspend the pellet in the appropriate volume of PSB (*see* **Note 36**).
15. Vortex the tube and incubate at room temperature for 5 min. Vortex the tube again to fully resuspend the pellet.
16. Centrifuge the tubes at maximum speed (>12,000 × *g*) for 5 min at room temperature to clarify the protein sample (*see* **Note 37**).

3.4 Protein Quantification After Cleanup: Bradford Assay

1. Prepare four dilutions of BSA, from 0.27 to 1.36 μg/μL in 10 mL glass tubes (*see* **Note 38**).
2. Pipette 10 μL of samples into 10 mL glass tubes.
3. Add 10 μL of HCl 0.1 N into each tube (*see* **Note 39**).
4. Add 80 μL of H_2O into each tube.
5. Add 3.5 mL of Bradford reactive diluted 1/4 into each tube, vortex and incubate for 20 min at room temperature.
6. Read absorbance at 595 nm (*see* **Note 40**).

3.5 SDS Discontinuous Polyacrylamide Gel 1D Electrophoresis

1. Assemble the Mini-PROTEAN Tetra Cell casting stand and frame. Place a comb in the assembled gel cassette and make a mark in the glass plate to know up to where it will be filled with the resolving gel solution (1 cm below the comb).
2. Prepare a 12% resolving gel mixing 3.4 mL of ultrapure water, 2.5 mL of resolving gel buffer, 100 μL of SDS 10%, and 4 mL of acrylamide–bis mixture in a 50 or 100 mL beaker. After a few minutes in agitation, add 80 μL of a fresh 10% solution of ammonium persulfate (APS) and 7.5 μL of TEMED.
3. Add the resolving gel between the Mini-PROTEAN spacer and the short plates up to the mark made before (*see* **Note 41**).
4. Immediately overlay the solution smoothly with ultrapure water (*see* **Note 42**).
5. Allow the gel to polymerize for 45 min–1 h and then remove the water by introducing absorbent filter paper between the glass plates.
6. Prepare a 4% stacking gel mixing 6.1 mL of ultrapure water, 2.5 mL of resolving gel buffer, 100 μL of SDS 10%, and 1.3 mL of acrylamide–bis mixture in a 50 or 100 mL beaker. After a few minutes in agitation, add 80 μL of a fresh 10% solution of APS and 7.5 μL of TEMED.
7. Add the stacking gel between the Mini-PROTEAN spacer and the short plates up to the top edge of the short plate. Immediately insert a 10-well comb between the glass plates and allow the stacking gel to polymerize for 30–45 min.

8. Remove the comb carefully to avoid breaking the wells and fill them with electrode buffer 1× to preserve them until samples are loaded (*see* **Note 43**).
9. Mix protein samples with SDS reducing buffer 2× in a 1:1 ratio, vortex and heat at 100 °C for 5 min (*see* **Note 44**).
10. Assemble the electrophoresis module with short plates of each gel facing inward to create a functioning assembly. Fill the upper chamber of the assembly with electrode buffer 1× up to the edge of the outer gel plate, and add the remaining buffer in the tank (lower chamber) to the indicated level (2-gels line marking in the front of the tank).
11. Centrifuge the tubes to bring down the condensate and slowly load samples into wells to allow them to settle evenly on the bottom of the well (*see* **Note 45**).
12. Place the lid on the tank aligning the color-coded plugs and jacks, connect the electrical leads to the power supply and apply power to begin electrophoresis. First, we apply 90 V for 15 min so that the samples enter in the stacking gel and lineup. Then, we increase the voltage up to 150 V until the bromophenol blue dye in the samples reaches the bottom of the resolving gel.
13. When electrophoresis is finished, turn off the power supply, disconnect the electrical leads, remove the tank lid, lift the electrode assembly and discard the running buffer. Then, remove the gel cassette and separate the two glass plates using a spatula. Carefully, remove the stacking gel and transfer the resolving gel to a container with ultrapure water to remove traces of SDS-PAGE running buffer.
14. Continue following the Western blot protocol in Subheading 3.10.

3.6 Isoelectrofocusing (IEF)

The sample is prepared in 350 μL containing rehydration buffer, 0.3% DTT and 0.5% Byo-Lyte 3/10 ampholytes. In this volume, we load 60 μg of HPL protein fraction to rehydrate a 17 cm IPG linear strip, pH 4–7.

1. Weigh 0.001 g of DTT in an eppendorf tube, add 1.75 μL of Byo-Lyte 3/10 ampholytes, add protein sample and complete with rehydration buffer up to 350 μL. We also add traces of bromophenol blue to color the sample and visually follow the process of electrophoresis (*see* **Note 46**).
2. Vortex, centrifuge the tube to bring down the entire sample and pipette the sample along the tray channel of the cell focusing tray for active rehydration (*see* **Note 47**).
3. Open the IPG strip package and carefully remove the protective cover from the IPG strip using forceps. Discard the cover (*see* **Note 48**).

4. Gently place the IPG strip onto the sample, with the gel facing down and the correct orientation. Ensure that the gel is in contact with the electrodes (*see* **Note 49**).
5. Wait 15 min and then overlay the IPG strip with 1.5 mL of mineral oil to prevent evaporation during the rehydration process.
6. Cover the IEF cell-focusing tray with the lid and place it in the PROTEAN IEF cell. Rehydrate at 50 V and 20 °C for 12 h (*see* **Note 50**).
7. Program focusing protocol as follow: conditioning step at 250 V for 15 min, voltage lineal ramping from 250 to 10,000 V for 3 h and finally, the focusing step up to 60,000 Vh (in theory 10,000 V for 6 h). All steps at 20 °C. Press START to initiate the run (*see* **Note 51**).
8. When IEF has finished, remove the IPG strip from the tray and hold it vertically with forceps on a filter paper to let the mineral oil drain. Then transfer the strip with the gel facing up to a clean and dry equilibration tray (*see* **Note 52**).
9. Incubate the strip with 2.5 mL of SDS-PAGE equilibration buffer containing 1% DTT, for 10 min in agitation (use a rocker stirrer). Put the strip in another tray channel with new 2.5 mL of SDS-PAGE equilibration buffer containing 1% DTT and repeat incubation. Then, make two other incubations with 2.5 mL of SDS-PAGE equilibration buffer containing 2.5% IAA, for 10 min each.
10. Remove the IPG strip from the tray and hold it vertically with forceps on a filter paper to let the equilibration buffer drain, and continue with **step 9** of the next section (*see* **Notes 53** and **58**).

3.7 SDS 9–16% Gradient Polyacrylamide 2D Gel Electrophoresis

1. Assemble the PROTEAN II xi cell-casting stand with glass plate sandwich in alignment slot. Mark the short glass plate 0.5 cm under the short plate and 0.7 cm from each spacer, where the IPG strip will be placed (*see* **Note 54**).
2. Prepare a 9% light solution mixing 8.4 mL of acrylamide–bis mixture (30% total; 2.6% bis), 6.72 mL of resolving gel buffer (Tris–HCl 1.5 M, pH 8.8), 280 μL of SDS 10%, and 12.6 mL of ultrapure water. After a few minutes in agitation, transfer the solution to the reservoir chamber of the gradient former labeled "light" (*see* **Note 55**).
3. Prepare a 16% heavy solution. First, weigh 4.2 g of sucrose and dissolve it in a mixture of 15 mL of acrylamide–bis mixture (30% total; 2.6% bis), 6.72 mL of resolving gel buffer (Tris–HCl 1.5 M, pH 8.8), 280 μL of SDS 10%, and 3.7 mL of ultrapure water. When the sucrose is completely dissolved,

transfer the solution to the mixing chamber of the gradient former, labeled “heavy.”

4. Place a stirring bar in each chamber. Put the gradient former on a magnetic stirrer placed elevated, next to the PROTEAN II xi cell-casting stand with glass plate sandwich in alignment slot. Connect the tubing in the output and put a microtip at the end of the tubing, inserting it between glass plates of the sandwich gel (*see* **Note 56**).
5. Add 420 μL of a fresh 10% solution of ammonium persulfate (APS) and 28 μL of TEMED to each solution in agitation.
6. First open the stopcock and then the valve that connects both chambers. First, the 16% heavy solution will flow through the tubing and microtip to the gel sandwich, flowing to the bottom. Then, the heavy solution will gradually mix with the light solution, reducing the percentage of the solution that flows to the gel sandwich. At the end, the 9% light solution will flow into the gel sandwich. Fill the gel sandwich to the mark previously made on the glass plate and immediately close the stopcock, remove the tubing and overlay the solution smoothly with ultrapure water (*see* **Note 57**).
7. Flush the system of the gradient former with ultrapure water to prevent polymerization of residual acrylamide within system.
8. Allow the gel to polymerize for 45 min–1 h and then remove the water by introducing absorbent filter paper between the glass plates (*see* **Note 58**).
9. Prepare a low melting point agarose solution (*see* **Note 59**).
10. Add 500 μL of low melting point agarose solution on the top of the gel, between both glass plates. Then place the IPG strip centered on the gel between the marks previously made on the glass, pushing the strip down with forceps to immerse it in agarose, so that it is in contact with the gel. Then, cover the strip with the remaining agarose solution to seal the 17 cm IPG strip on top of the polymerized gel.
11. Assemble the electrophoresis module, pour some electrode buffer 1× into the upper buffer compartment, and check for buffer leaks prior to run. If the buffer appears to be leaking, remove the gel sandwich assembly and reattach (*see* **Note 60**).
12. If there are no leaks, fill the upper buffer compartment with electrode buffer 1×. Add the remaining electrode buffer in the tank. Connect the tubing from a circulating cooler to the cooling core of PROTEAN II xi cell, using water as the coolant to maintain temperature at 15 °C during electrophoresis.
13. Place the lid on the tank aligning the color-coded plugs and jacks, connect the electrical leads to the power supply and apply power to begin electrophoresis. First, apply 20 mA/gel, 100 V

for 15 min, so that the samples run from the strip to the resolving gel and line up. Then, increase the voltage up to 400 V, 40 mA/gel, until the bromophenol blue dye in the samples has reached the bottom of the resolving gel.

14. When electrophoresis is finished, turn off the power supply, disconnect the electrical leads, remove the tank lid, lift the electrode assembly and discard the running buffer. Then, remove the gel cassette, separate the two glass plates using a spatula and transfer the resolving gel to a plastic container with ultrapure water to remove traces of SDS-PAGE running buffer.
15. Discard washing water and continue following the silver-staining protocol (next section).

3.8 Silver Staining, Image Acquisition and Analysis

Incubate the gel at room temperature with agitation, unless otherwise indicated. We use a silver staining protocol compatible with MS analysis, modified from [8, 9].

1. Incubate gel in fixating solution, overnight.
2. Discard fixating solution and wash the gel with ultrapure water for 5 min.
3. Discard water and add sensibilizing solution. Incubate for 1 h without agitation.
4. Discard sensibilizing solution and wash the gel with ultrapure water for 10 min. Repeat the wash step five times.
5. Add silver nitrate solution and incubate without agitation for 30 min (*see* **Note 61**). Discard solution in a specific waste container.
6. Wash the gel with ultrapure water for 20 s three times and discard.
7. Add revealing solution and incubate for 15–20 min (*see* **Note 62**). Discard solution in a specific waste container.
8. Add stop solution and incubate for 10 min. Discard.
9. Store the gel in ultrapure water until image acquisition.
10. Acquire the 2D gel image with a calibrated densitometer (Fig. 1).
11. Compare protein patterns of normal and colorectal cancer tissue using a specific software for 2D protein analysis, such as PDQuest 7.3.1 (Bio-Rad) (*see* **Note 63**).

3.9 Mass Spectrometry Protein Identification

Carry out all digestion protein steps in a flow hood at room temperature, unless otherwise indicated. Wear gloves to prevent protein contamination of samples, primarily from skin keratins that could mask protein identification by MS. Be careful not to carry the small piece of gel when pipetting solutions.

1. Carefully place the gel on a sterile glass plate and excise the protein spots of interest using a sterile scalpel, placing each one in an Eppendorf LowBind® tube with 50 μL of ultrapure water (*see* **Note 64**).
2. Discard water and add 200 μL of a 1:1 mixture of 30 mM potassium ferricyanide and 100 mM sodium thiosulfate (dye-removing solution). Incubate for 5 min at room temperature (*see* **Note 65**).
3. Discard dye-removing solution and add 200 μL of ultrapure water. Incubate for 15 min.
4. Discard water and add 100 μL of 25 mM ammonium bicarbonate. Incubate for 20 min and discard.
5. Add 100 μL of a 1:1 mixture of 50 mM ammonium bicarbonate and 100% acetonitrile (ACN). Incubate for 20 min, discard and repeat.
6. Discard and add 100 μL of a new 1:1 mixture of 50 mM ammonium bicarbonate and 100% ethanol. Incubate for 20 min and discard.
7. Add 100 μL of 100% ethanol, incubate for 15 min and discard (*see* **Note 66**).
8. Air-dry ethanol residues for a few minutes, or use a vacuum desiccator or a speed-vac.
9. Add 200 μL of 10 mM DTT and incubate at 56 °C for 1 h.
10. Discard DTT solution and add 200 μL of 55 mM IAA. Incubate for 30 min.
11. Discard IAA solution and add 200 μL of 50 mM ammonium bicarbonate. Incubate for 15 min and repeat. Discard solution.
12. Add 100 μL of a 1:1 mixture of 50 mM ammonium bicarbonate and 100% ACN. Incubate for 30 min and discard.
13. Add 100 μL of 100% ACN, incubate for 10 min and discard (*see* **Note 66**).
14. Let the ACN residues evaporate for a few minutes. During these minutes, prepare the trypsin solution. Dilute a stock solution (0.2 μg/μL in 50 mM acetic acid) in 25 mM ammonium bicarbonate in a proportion of 0.2 μL of stock solution per 15 μL of 25 mM ammonium bicarbonate.
15. Add 15 μL of trypsin solution (~40 ng of trypsin) and incubate overnight at 37 °C in an Eppendorf® thermomixer or a stove (*see* **Note 67**).
16. Extract tryptic peptides from the gel matrix in three steps. First, add 20 μL of 10% (v/v) formic acid and incubate for 30 min. Recover the solution and transfer it to a new Eppendorf LoBind® tube. Then, add 10 μL of 100% ACN to the gel

spot and incubate for 15 min at 37 °C. Recover the solution and transfer it to the previous Eppendorf LoBind® tube where peptides extracted with formic acid were added. Finally, repeat the second step, adding again 10 μL of 100% ACN and incubating for 15 min at 37 °C. Recover the solution in the previously used Eppendorf LoBind® tube.

17. Dry the peptide solution in a speed-vac at 45 °C for 45–60 min. Store at −20 °C until MS analysis.
18. For MS analysis, redissolved peptides in 10 μL 0.1% formic acid/50% ACN, sonicate tubes in an ultrasonic bath for 10 min, centrifuge at 12–16,000 × *g* for 15 min and finally, transfer solution to tubes for liquid chromatographic nano-electrospray tandem mass spectrometry (LC-nESI-MS/MS).
19. Proceed to perform the liquid chromatographic nano-electrospray tandem mass spectrometry (LC-nESI-MS/MS) in a mass spectrometer Q-TOF Global.

3.10 Western Blotting and Immunodetection

After completion of SDS-PAGE, 1D gels were subjected to protein transfer by the western blot method in tank or wet [10].

1. Discard water and add 100 mL of western blot transfer buffer to the gel. Incubate for 20 min with gentle agitation.
2. Cut a piece of PVDF membrane of the same size as the 1D gel (7 × 8 cm). Place the membrane in a sterile and clean plastic container and activate with 100 mL 100% methanol (v/v) for 30 s, discard and then wash with 100 mL ultrapure water for 2 min. Finally equilibrate with 100 mL transfer buffer for 20 min.
3. Soak two sheets of filter paper and two fiber pads in transfer buffer.
4. Prepare the gel sandwich following these steps: (a) place one prewetted fiber pad on the gray side of the cassette; (b) place a sheet of filter paper on the fiber pad; (c) place the equilibrated gel on the filter paper; (d) place the prewetted membrane on the gel. Complete the sandwich by placing the other sheet of filter paper on the membrane and the other fiber pad.
5. Close and lock the cassette firmly, being careful not to move the gel and filter paper sandwich. Place the cassette in the electrode module (*see* **Note 68**).
6. Place the electrode module and the frozen blue cooling unit in the tank and fill it with transfer buffer up to the mark on the tank.
7. Place the tank on a magnetic stirrer and put a stirring bar in the tank to help maintain an even buffer temperature and ion distribution in the tank.

8. Put the lid, plug the cables into the power supply and run the blot at 100 V (limit of 1.6 A) for 1 h.
9. Upon completion of the transfer, disassemble the blotting sandwich and remove the membrane for immunodetection (*see* **Note 69**).
10. Block membrane with 100 mL of 5% (w/v) nonfat milk in 1× PBS pH 7.4 at room temperature for 2 h, in agitation.
11. Discard the solution and add 50 mL of 1/2000 mouse anti-human NDKA MCA1865 (AbD Serotec) primary antibody. Incubate overnight at 4 °C, in agitation.
12. Discard primary antibody solution and wash the membrane with 100 mL of 1× PBS pH 7.4 at room temperature for 5 min, in agitation. Repeat three times.
13. Discard and add 50 mL of 1/2000 goat anti-mouse IgG (H + L) secondary antibody conjugated with alkaline phosphatase. Incubate for 90 min at room temperature, in agitation.
14. Discard secondary antibody, wash twice with 100 mL of 1× PBS pH 7.4 for 5 min each, then with 100 mL of 0.05% (v/v) Tween-20 in 1× PBS pH 7.4 for 5 min, and finally wash twice with 100 mL of 1× PBS pH 7.4 for 30 s. Discard.
15. Add the chromogenic substrate nitroblue tetrazolium/5-bromo-4-chloro-3-indolyl phosphate (NBT/BCIP, Roche Diagnostics) and incubate at room temperature in darkness, without agitation (*see* **Note 70**).
16. Stop the development reaction discarding NBT/BCIP solution and washing with ultrapure water for 10 min in agitation.
17. Place the membrane on a clean filter paper with the signal side facing up to dry.
18. Acquire the image with a calibrated densitometer and use a specific software package to carry out 1D image analysis, such as the Quantity One 4.4.1.

3.11 ELISA Immunoassay

All reagents, solutions, samples, and assay plate should be at room temperature before use.

1. According to the planned assay layout, add 100 μL of each standard tube (St0, St1, St2, St3, St4, St5, St6, and St7) to the corresponding wells, duplicated.
2. Add 100 μL of each serum sample, in duplicate, in the corresponding wells. Cover plate with adhesive strip and incubate for 2 h at 37 °C, protected from the light (*see* **Note 71**).
3. Aspirate liquid from wells using an ELISA plate washer (*see* **Note 72**). Do not wash the plate.

4. Add 100 μL of biotin-antibody 1× solution to each well with a multichannel pipette. Cover the plate with a new adhesive strip and incubate at 37 °C for 1 h, protected from the light.
5. Aspirate liquid from wells using an ELISA plate washer (*see* **Note 72**). Wash the plate with 200 μL of 1× wash buffer per well with an ELISA plate washer (*see* **Note 73**). Allow the wash buffer to sit in the wells for 2 min. Aspirate liquid. Repeat the wash step two more times.
6. After the final wash, invert plate and tap onto paper towel to eliminate remaining liquid.
7. Add 100 μL of 1× HRP-avidin solution to each well with a multichannel pipette. Cover the plate with a new adhesive strip and incubate for 1 h at 37 °C, protected from the light.
8. Wash the plate as described previously, five times.
9. Add 90 μL of TMB substrate to each well with a multichannel pipette and incubate at 37 °C, protected from light (*see* **Note 74**).
10. Add 50 μL of stop solution to each well with a multichannel pipette. Measure OD with Microplate reader at 450 and 570 nm.
11. Subtract the OD values obtained at 570 nm from the readings at 450 nm, for each well (*see* **Note 75**).
12. Average the corrected OD according to duplicates for each standard (St0–St7) and samples. Subtract the averaged S0 (blank) to standards St1–St7 and samples.
13. Calculated serum NDKA concentration (pg/mL) in samples using a four-parameter logistic (4-PL) curve-fit (*see* **Note 76**).

4 Notes

1. When searching for noninvasive biomarkers, serum may seem the desirable sample. However, our experience has indicated that the use of serum complicates the attribution of a differentially expressed protein to a tissue-specific disease. Hence, we find that the best approach is to use tissue for the proteomic study, and then validate candidate biomarkers in serum samples. Healthy colorectal mucosa was obtained from the distal edge of the resection, at least 10 cm from the tumor.
2. Serum obtained after centrifugation should be immediately removed from the tube. If serum is not used fresh, make aliquots and store samples at −20 °C if used within 1 month, or at −80 °C for longer storage to avoid protein degradation and denaturalization. When freeze samples are used, allow to completely thaw. Hemolyzed serum samples are not

recommended for this ELISA immunoassay, as well as repeated freeze–thaw cycles.

3. Use aseptic microtips when handling buffers M1, M2 and PSB diluent to prevent contamination. The kit is based on the separation of membrane proteins by temperature-dependent phase partitioning using Triton X-114 detergent [6, 7].
4. The ReadyPrep™ Protein Extraction Kit (Membrane I) (Bio-Rad) provides sufficient reagents to perform 50 extractions of 50 mg of tissue, but provides only one ReadyPrep 2-D cleanup kit that it is not enough to clean all fractions obtained. Cleanup is a critical step in the preparation of samples to remove extraction agents that could interfere with the IEF (i.e., ionic detergents, salts, nucleic acids, and lipids).
5. We use 1 N HCl to lower the pH slowly. At the beginning, we usually use concentrated HCl (10 N), adding slowly drop by drop until approaching the required pH, and then use the less concentrated HCl to adjust the pH. Store the resolving gel buffer for only 2 weeks because no sodium azide is added, and therefore, fungi can easily grow. We only use stacking gel buffer for 1D gel electrophoresis to concentrate or stack proteins between the two buffer gels and obtain high-resolution separations. In 2-DE we find a good resolution for a broader separation range with gradient resolving gels of 9–16% acrylamide–bis.
6. In the case liquid reagent is not available, prepare 30% acrylamide–bis-acrylamide as follows: weigh 29.2 g of acrylamide and 0.8 g of bis-acrylamide to prepare 100 mL of solution. It is mandatory to wear a mask and weigh acrylamide in a chemical fume hood because it is a very dangerous carcinogenic neurotoxin. Also, use safety glasses, gloves, lab coat, close-toed shoes, and other protective equipment appropriate for the task. Mixing and transferring to a bottle should also be done inside the fume hood. Store acrylamide–bis solution at 4 °C in a bottle covered with aluminum foil and prepare fresh each month.
7. Particular caution must be taken when weighing SDS because it causes skin irritation and respiratory sensitization by inhalation. Therefore, use a mask and weigh the powder in a chemical fume hood.
8. APS solution should be made fresh daily and store at 4 °C or on ice. We prefer preparing a new solution each time before use.
9. We use sucrose to prepare a dense solution for 9–16% gradient polyacrylamide gels.
10. When mixing SDS reducing buffer 2× with the sample in a 1:1 ratio, the final concentration of the buffer is 1×. We prepare

aliquots of 200 μL of SDS reducing buffer 2× and store them at −20 °C.

11. Stir the mixture slowly so that it does not form much foam because of the SDS. Store at 4 °C and dilute to 1× with ultrapure water for electrophoresis. For 1D electrophoresis, we prepare 1 L of electrode buffer 1× (150 mL of electrode buffer 5× and 750 mL of water). This volume is enough to run up to two gels in a Mini-PROTEAN tetra tank. For 2D electrophoresis, we prepare 1.5 L of electrode buffer 1×.
12. We use two SDS-PAGE equilibration buffers, one with 1% DTT (v/v) and the other with 2.5% IAA (v/v), to reduce and to alkylate sulfhydryl groups of cysteines in proteins, respectively. We prepare 10 mL of fresh SDS-PAGE equilibration buffer and use half to dissolve 0.05 g of DTT and the other half to dissolve 0.125 g of IAA. We add 100 μL of bromophenol blue 2% to the last one to color the IPG strip.
13. We prepare transfer buffer with SDS detergent to increase transfer efficiency. However, SDS may precipitate at temperatures below 10 °C, so the buffer temperature has to be higher.
14. We prepare 10× PBS as a stock solution and store at room temperature. Dilute to 1× for western blotting and store at 4 °C.
15. We prepare primary and secondary antibody dilutions in the blocking solution.
16. Before starting, plan the assay layout to determine the total number of wells needed. Each column contains eight wells (12 columns × 8 wells) that can be used separately. Unused wells should be kept inside the ziploc at 4 °C. Calculate the appropriate volumes for each solution according to the number of wells planned to use. Always include the seven standards detailed (*see* **Note 17**). Duplicates for all standards and samples are recommended.
17. The NDKA standard should be prepared at the moment for each assay. Before using, give a brief spin and then proceed to add the sample diluent. Very gently mix for complete reconstitution (do not vortex). Wait for 15 min before starting to use the standard solution. Prepare each standard dilution in a separate 1.5 mL tube (labeled as St0, St1, St2, St3, St4, St5, St6, and St7). Pipette 250 μL of sample diluent to each tube (St0–St6). Tube St7 corresponds to the undiluted, reconstituted standard (1200 pg/mL). For preparing the serial twofold dilutions, gently mix the tube before pipetting the next standard dilution. Pipette 250 μL of reconstituted standard in tube St6, place 250 μL of St6 in St5 tube, and so on, up to tube St1 that is the lowest concentration. Tube St0 corresponds to the zero standard (0 pg/mL). Concentration in tubes is as follows: St7 = 1200 pg/mL; St6 = 600 pg/mL; St5 = 300 pg/mL;

St4 = 150 pg/mL; St3 = 75 pg/mL; St2 = 37.5 pg/mL; St1 = 18.75 pg/mL.

18. The biotin-antibody solution 1× sometimes has a turbid appearance. Warm the solution at room temperature and carefully mix until solution is uniform.
19. The wash buffer concentrate (25×) sometimes forms crystals. Before using, make sure crystals have completely dissolved. Let it warm at room temperature and gently mix.
20. The sample-to-buffer volume ratio may be adjusted depending on the sample used. Insufficient volume of protein extraction buffer M1 may result in poor cell lysis, low hydrophilic protein yield and contamination of the membrane protein fraction with cytoplasmic proteins. We use a stepped titanium micro-tip of 5/32″ (3.9 mm) diameter and apply ultrasonic vibrations to sample in a continuous mode. The power output should not exceed 150 watts since working at a greater power could damage or even break the micro-tip. It is very important to chill the tube on ice for 1 min between each sonication to prevent heating of the sample.
21. Carefully remove the tubes from the centrifuge to prevent the phases from mixing.
22. It is important to traverse the interface to correctly recover the lower phase. If protein fractions are not used immediately, make aliquots and freeze at −20 °C. It is also convenient to separate a 5–10 μL aliquot for protein quantification. The pellet obtained at the end of this procedure is an additional source of membrane proteins that can be stored at −20 °C for analysis.
23. This assay allows accurate protein quantification in the presence of detergents, reducing agents and other substances that typically interfere with other protein assays. It is mandatory to quantify samples in order to verify that the amount of protein does not exceed the maximum recommended for the cleaning method to be effective.
24. Prepare fresh Reagent A' for each assay because it precipitates easily. Each standard or sample assayed requires 127 μL of this reagent.
25. Prepare the standard curve for each assay using the BSA standard included in the kit (1.36 μg/μL). We use 5, 10, 15, 20, and 25 μL of BSA, completing with ultrapure water to a final volume of 25 μL. Concentration corresponds to 0.27, 0.54, 0.82, 1.01, and 1.36 μg/μL.
26. We measure two different volumes of samples in duplicate (5–10 μL), completing with ultrapure water up to 25 μL.

27. Discard the supernatant by inverting the tubes and allow the liquid to drain completely from the tubes.
28. Absorbance can be measured at 650–750 nm.
29. Usually we get approximately 200 μL of each protein fraction, so we use two tubes, cleaning 100 μL at a time. When the amount of protein in the sample was higher than 5 μg/μL, we made a dilution before cleaning.
30. Do not touch the sample with the pipette tip when adding the precipitating solution. Proteins may precipitate on the tip causing sample loss.
31. Remove the tube as soon as centrifugation has finished so that the pellet does not disperse. We always place the tubes in the same orientation in the centrifuge so that the protein pellet remains on the same side of the tube after each spin, reducing protein loss.
32. It is important to vortex vigorously to ensure entire pellet is thoroughly washed. Position the tube in the centrifuge as before.
33. Protein pellets will not dissolve in ultrapure water.
34. Protein pellets will not dissolve in wash reagent 2. Wash reagent 2 should be prechilled at −20 °C for at least 1 h before use. We prefer to store it in the freezer at least the day before use. If wash reagent 2 is not completely chilled, quantitative recovery may be affected.
35. After centrifugation, the pellet will appear white. We air-dry the pellet for no more than 5 min at room temperature because an overdried pellet will be difficult to resuspend. After drying, the pellet is translucent.
36. PSB is included in the ReadyPrep™ 2D Cleanup Kit and contains 7 M urea, 2 M thiourea, and 4% CHAPS (w/v). We resuspend HPB and HPL protein pellets in 50–100 μL of PSB, respectively, because we usually get twice the amount of HPL protein than HPB protein.
37. We quantify protein samples immediately after cleanup in order to make as many aliquots as possible since once the sample is thawed it is not recommended to refreeze it.
38. Prepare the standard curve for each assay using BSA standard provided by the kit (1.36 μg/μL). We use 2, 4, 8, and 10 μL of BSA in a final volume of 10 μL, that correspond to 0.27, 0.54, 1.08, and 1.36 μg/μL. Use PSB provided with 2D Clean-up kit to complete up to the final volume of 10 μL. We measure 10 μL of samples in duplicate (only one volume because of the limitation of the sample after cleaning).

39. Bradford protein assay is a simple colorimetric assay for measuring total protein concentration and is based on the color change of Coomassie brilliant blue G-250 dye in response to various concentrations of protein. We used a modification of the method because many detergents and basic protein buffers interfere with the assay. We chose medium acidification by adding 10 μL of 0.1 N HCl to each reaction tube.
40. Absorbance can be measured at 465–595 nm.
41. Add the solution smoothly to prevent it from mixing with the air.
42. This overlay prevents inhibition of acrylamide polymerization in contact with atmospheric oxygen and helps to level the resolving gel.
43. We mark with permanent marker the bottom of each well to facilitate the loading of samples. Another option is to use Bio-Rad's patented sample loading guide, placing it between the two gels in the electrode assembly to locate the sample wells.
44. As we use SDS reducing buffer 2×, we mix equal volumes of sample and buffer. We prepare samples in a final volume of 20 μL (10 μL of sample and 10 μL of SDS reducing buffer 2×) because we need to load as much protein as possible. Besides, we find 20 μL is the maximum sample volume per well, using spacer plates of 0.75 mm, to avoid cross-contamination between adjacent wells. For Western blotting, we make 1D gels loading 50 μg of protein per well.
45. Since the gel is going to be used for western blotting, load prestained protein standard at least in one well. They allow the visualization of the electrophoresis, and after blotting, we can determine the mass values of the protein bands in our samples.
46. The optimal rehydration volume and protein load depends on the sample, the length of the IPG strip and the stain protocol used. For silver staining, the recommended range of protein load for a 17 cm IPG strip is 50–80 μg. We have good results loading 60 μg of HPL protein fraction for analytical gels. For preparative gels, i.e., those for MS analysis, we load 120 μg of protein.
47. The loaded sample should extend in a line along the whole length of the channel, taking care not to introduce any bubbles.
48. Always wear gloves when handling IPG strips to prevent protein contaminations, primarily from skin keratin.
49. IPG strips are marked with a "+" and the pH range at the end, that must be on the positive pole. This mark should be legible if IPG strip is placed correctly with the gel side down. Take care

not to get sample onto the plastic backing of the IPG strip because the gel will not absorb that amount of sample. If this happens, lift the strip up and down from one end until the air bubbles move to the end and out.

50. After 6 h we stop the active rehydration, wet two paper wicks with water, lift the ends of the IPG strip with forceps and carefully insert a paper wick between the IPG strip and each electrode. This is important to avoid electrode damage during IEF because of the presence of salts in the sample. Total salt concentration in the sample should not exceed 10 mM. Then, we program the PROTEAN IEF cell again with the remaining 6 h of active rehydration and focusing protocol. We use the default cell temperature of 20 °C, with a maximum current of 50 μA/IPG strip.

51. We believe it is better to select total volt-hours as total time, since the time required for ramping will depend on the sample composition, and the current is maintained at 50 μA/IPG strip (PROTEAN IEF default setting). Thus, for example, if salt concentration in the sample is high, the resistance will be higher and therefore the proteins will take longer to focus. We add a final holding step that maintains the voltage at 500 V until the user stops the run. This prevents protein drift. The total time required for IEF, including active rehydration, is 21 h and 15 min.

52. IPG strips can be stored at −20 °C after IEF, washing them before storage with ultrapure water. Nevertheless, we always proceed directly to the equilibration step and the SDS-PAGE.

53. During the equilibration step, we prepare the low melting point agarose solution to seal the strip to the gel of the second dimension, and SDS-PAGE 1× electrode buffer.

54. Always use the alignment slot to properly orient the gel sandwich. Failure to use this slot for alignment can result in casting leaks pouring the resolving gel, or electrode buffer leaks during the run.

55. Before adding the solution, make sure the stopcock of the mixing chamber and the valve that connects both chambers are closed. Otherwise, the light solution will spill and pass from the mixing chamber (labeled "light") to the reservoir chamber (labeled "heavy").

56. Place the gradient former above the top of the gel sandwich to pour the gel solution. We use a hydraulic laboratory lift.

57. We find a better resolution of the protein spots in our samples with 9–16% gradients gels compared to continuous gels.

58. To adjust 2D–PAGE protocol times, we prepare the 9–16% SDS gradient polyacrylamide 2D gels on the evening of the day

before, and leave them polymerizing overnight (**steps 1–8** in Subheading 3.7).

59. We recommend preparing this solution fresh each day. We weigh 0.015 g of low melting point agarose and dissolve it in 3 mL of electrode buffer 1× in agitation, at 40–50 °C. This quantity is enough to cover a 17 cm IPG strip. Wait until the solution is tempered to avoid damaging the strip, but without cooling it too much, otherwise it will be solid.
60. This is especially important because the electrophoresis lasts for 5–6 h. If a slow leak is occurring, electrophoresis can stop.
61. Add the silver nitrate solution in one corner of the plastic container, never on the gel, as it could cause background staining.
62. Add the revealing solution in one corner of the plastic container, never on the gel, as it could cause background staining. For our samples, we find that the optimum development time is between 15 and 20 min. Stop the development when the background begins to increase without detecting more spots, when strong spots begin to burn.
63. We use the software PDQuest 7.3.1 (Bio-Rad), normalizing the intensity of each spot in a gel as a proportion of the total protein intensity detected for the entire gel (relative volume).
64. Cut the spots around the area with silver dye without carrying excess acrylamide gel since this interferes in the MS analysis. We find it is better to puncture the spots with the tip of the scalpel to facilitate the entry of trypsin in the gel for the enzymatic digestion of proteins. We use Eppendorf LoBind® tubes because they improve the recovery rate of peptides compared to standard tubes.
65. Prepare the mixture fresh each day.
66. In this step, the spot will shrink because the solution dehydrates the piece of gel. Therefore, be careful not to discard the spot together with the solution, losing the sample.
67. Sequencing grade modified trypsin (Promega) is supplied lyophilized and has to be stored at −20 °C. To maintain maximum enzyme activity, dispense it into single-use aliquots after reconstituting and store at −20 °C for up to 1 month.
68. The Mini Trans-Blot® module accommodates two cassettes for electrophoretic transfer. Although we do not transfer proteins of two gels at the same time, we place both cassettes in the electrode module, one of them only with prewetted pads and filter papers (without gel and membrane).
69. For immunodetection, place the membrane with the side that was in contact with the gel facing up. This facilitates the

binding of antibodies and the chromogenic substrate. We stain the gel with coomassie blue in order to test the efficiency of the transfer.

70. We use one tablet of NBT/BCIP dissolved in 10 mL of water. The 5-bromo-4-chloro-3-indolyl phosphate (BCIP) is the substrate of the alkaline phosphatase enzyme conjugated with the secondary antibody, and is bounded to the chromogenic substrate nitroblue tetrazolium (NBT). During incubation, check the signal every few minutes to determine when to stop the development reaction.

71. During incubation periods, temperature should be carefully controlled. Therefore, a plate incubator set at 37 °C is highly recommended. The assay plate should also be protected from light during incubations.

72. If an ELISA plate washer (microplate washer) is not available, microwells can be completely emptied manually. To do so, firmly invert the plate flicking the content over the sink or an appropriate container filled with disinfectant. Cautiously shake the plate several times to ensure wells are completely emptied. Immediately, place the plate inverted on paper towel to allow elimination of residues.

73. Washes can be performed manually if an ELISA plate washer is not available. Several methods have been described, including dipping, wash bottles with single or multiple nozzles and multichannel pipette [11]. Among these, the latter is the most recommended to avoid cross-contamination between wells. Use a multichannel pipette to dispense 200 μL of wash buffer 1× to each well strip. Allow 2 min to sit and then completely eliminate liquid from wells as described before (*see* **Note 72**). The wash steps are critical in an ELISA for its good performance since unbounded reagents are eliminated at this stage.

74. It is highly recommended to follow the color development on the plate for each assay. Measure optical density (OD) at 630 nm every 5 min, monitoring the development of a dark blue color in the highest standard (St7). The reaction should be stopped when St7 has reached an OD of 0.9. The establishment of a fixed period to stop the reaction is not convenient since the development of color varies with temperature and laboratory conditions.

75. The use of the 450 nm reading without correction can lead to higher NDKA concentration values. Therefore, the reading at 570 nm is recommended to avoid less accurate results.

76. A 4-PL curve-fit is highly recommended for accurate results. Many software capable of generating this fit are freely available online, and provide step-by-step instructions to calculate concentrations. According to our experience, serum samples do

not require a dilution for testing. However, samples with a concentration higher than St7 (1200 pg/mL) require a dilution to obtain an accurate concentration value. Use several samples at different dilutions to decide the optimal dilution for your samples. On the other hand, in the case of samples with NDKA serum concentration below the lowest standard (St1: 18.75 pg/mL), it is more accurate to report concentration as <18.75 pg/mL.

References

1. Duffy MJ, Lamerz R, Haglund C et al (2014) Tumor markers in colorectal cancer, gastric cancer and gastrointestinal stromal cancers: European group on tumor markers 2014 guidelines update. Int J Cancer 134:2513–2522
2. Alvarez-Chaver P, Rodríguez-Piñeiro AM, Rodríguez-Berrocal FJ et al (2011) Selection of putative colorectal cancer markers by applying PCA on the soluble proteome of tumors: NDK A as a promising candidate. J Proteome 74:874–886
3. Görg A, Weiss W, Dunn MJ (2004) Current two-dimensional electrophoresis technology for proteomics. Proteomics 4:3665–3685
4. Otero-Estévez O, De Chiara L, Barcia-Castro L et al (2016) Evaluation of serum nucleoside diphosphate kinase A for the detection of colorectal cancer. Sci Rep 6:26703. https://doi.org/10.1038/srep26703
5. Alvarez-Chaver P, Otero-Estévez O, Páez de la Cadena M et al (2014) Proteomics for discovery of candidate colorectal cancer biomarkers. World J Gastroenterol 20:3804–3824
6. Bordier C (1981) Phase separation of integral membrane proteins in Triton X-114 solution. J Biol Chem 256:1604–1607
7. Santoni V, Kieffer S, Desclaux D et al (2000) Membrane proteomics: Use of additive main effects with multiplicative interaction model to classify plasma membrane proteins according to their solubility and electrophoretic properties. Electrophoresis 21:3329–3344
8. Heukeshoven J, Dernick R (1985) Simplified method for silver staining of proteins in polyacrylamide gels and the mechanism of silver staining. Electrophoresis 6:103–112
9. Shevchenko A, Wilm M, Vorm O et al (1996) Mass spectrometric sequencing of proteins silver-stained polyacrylamide gels. Anal Chem 68:850–858
10. Towbin H, Staehelin T, Gordon J (1979) Electrophoretic transfer of proteins from polyacrylamide gels to nitrocellulose sheets: procedure and some applications. Proc Natl Acad Sci U S A 76:4350–4354
11. Crowther JR (2009) The Elisa Guidebook. Series title: Methods in Molecular Biology, vol Vol. 515, 2nd edn. Humana Press, New York

Chapter 17

Tumor-Derived Microparticles to Monitor Colorectal Cancer Evolution

Diane Mege, Laurence Panicot-Dubois, and Christophe Dubois

Abstract

Colorectal cancer is the most common gastrointestinal cancer and the second-most common cause of cancer-related death worldwide. Microparticles are small vesicles known to be implicated in tumor growth, the development of metastases, and cancer-associated procoagulant activity. We have reported a specific hallmark of microparticles in colorectal and pancreatic cancers, the so-called "microparticulosome." We have also reported on variations in the microparticulosome in the case of the occurrence of a thromboembolic event. Here, we describe our flow cytometry-based methods for identifying and characterizing tumor-derived microparticles and thereby monitoring colorectal cancer evolution.

Key words Microparticle, Tumor-derived microvesicle, Colorectal cancer, Tissue factor, Fibrin

1 Introduction

Colorectal cancer (CRC) is the most common gastrointestinal cancer and the second-most common cause of cancer-related death worldwide. Like all solid tumors, CRC is associated with thromboembolic events, but at lower rates (5%) than pancreatic cancer (20%), for example [1]. The occurrence of cancer-associated thromboembolic events leads to a worse prognosis.

Microparticles (MPs) are small vesicles (0.1–1 μm diameter) that are produced and released by the exocytic blebbing of the activated and apoptotic cell membrane from most, if not all, types of cells. After cell activation or apoptosis induces an increase in the cytosolic calcium concentration, some cytoskeletal changes and a loss of phospholipid asymmetry in the membrane occurs. Five enzymes are involved in regulating the cell membrane phospholipid asymmetry and are implicated in MP generation: gelsolin, aminophospholipid translocase, floppase, scramblase and calpain. When the calcium concentration rises in the cytosol, gelsolin and calpain are activated and cleave cytoskeletal filaments. Simultaneously, scramblase is activated and translocase is inhibited. These two

Jean-François Beaulieu (ed.), *Colorectal Cancer: Methods and Protocols*, Methods in Molecular Biology, vol. 1765, https://doi.org/10.1007/978-1-4939-7765-9_17,

enzymes were implicated, along with floppase, in aminophospholipid (phosphatidylserine and phosphatidylethanolamine) transport from the outside layer of the cell membrane to the inside. During cell activation this balance is compromised, leading to the expression of aminophospholipids on the exterior membrane surface (the "flip-flop" mechanism). These cytoskeletal and membrane surface changes will allow for the budding of the membrane and thus the production of MPs [2].

MPs are known to be involved in tumor growth, the development of metastases and cancer-associated procoagulant activity, primarily through the expression of Tissue Factor (TF) and phosphatidylserine at their surface [3–5]. Using a mouse model of pancreatic cancer, we have reported that the expression of TF is inhibited by cancer cells and thus MPs are decreased during platelet-rich thrombus formation and blood coagulation cascade activation, and the growth of the tumor is then strongly diminished [6]. By using a mouse model of pancreatic cancer, we also observed that in the presence of an antiplatelet drug, the MPs did not accumulate at the site of thrombosis, and primary tumor growth and metastasis formation were reduced [7]. More recently, we have reported a specific hallmark of MPs in CRC and pancreatic cancer in comparison with benign colorectal and pancreatic diseases and healthy subjects, which is the so-called "microparticulosome." This microparticulosome was based on a combined characterization of the total circulating MPs, the subtypes (from platelets, endothelial cells, leukocytes, and erythrocytes), the procoagulant (bearing TF and/or fibrin), and the tumor-derived (bearing mucin 1, podoplanin, CEA, or CA19-9) MPs. We have observed that the microparticulosome changed with the evolution of the disease and tended to exhibit the signature that is observed for benign diseases or healthy subjects in the case of CRC remission (Table 1) [8]. We also reported variations in the microparticulosome during the occurrence of a thromboembolic event, particularly with the fibrin-bearing MPs [12]. We characterized and quantified the MPs using flow cytometry, which is more specific and reproducible than other available techniques, including immune-enzymatic ELISA tests, nanoparticle tracking analysis, electronic microscopy, spectroscopy, and chromatography. Here, we describe our methods for identifying and characterizing tumor-derived MPs to monitor CRC evolution.

2 Materials

2.1 Preparation of MPs from Human Blood (see Note 1)

1. Citrated tubes 9NC for blood sample (*see* **Note 2**).
2. Eppendorf centrifuge.
3. Haemolyse tubes with caps (Deltalab).

Table 1
Evolution of "microparticulosome" with remission of colorectal cancer (CRC) in 11 patients, adapted from Mege et al. [8]

	PREOPERATIVE CRC	REMISSION CRC	p value
Total MPs	100%	100%	0.1
Subpopulations			
PMP	63%	69%	0.4
EMP	0.03%	0.8%	0.003
EryMP	6%	2%	0.08
LeuMP	0.1%	0.2%	0.3
Procoagulant MPs			
TF positive	1%	0.4%	0.2
Fibrin positive	0.4%	1%	0.1
Tumor MPs			
MUC1 positive	0.09%	0%	0.1
PODO positive	0.5%	1%	0.1
CEA positive	0.2%	0%	0.002
CA19-9 positive	0%	0%	0.1

Percentages of MPs are given relative to total MPs, for each group. Statistically significant for p-value ≤ 0.05. Color code: from high (light grey) to intermediate (grey) and low (dark grey) levels of MPs
Total MPs Annexin V+ MPs, *PMPs* platelet-derived MPs (Annexin V+/CD41+), *EMPs* endothelial-derived MPs (Annexin V+/CD31+/CD41−), *EryMPs* erythrocyte-derived MPs (Annexin V+/CD235a+) (Annexin V+/CD11b+/CD235a−), *LeuMPs* leukocyte-derived MPs (Annexin V+/CD11b+/CD235a−), *TF positive* Annexin V+/TF+, *Fibrin positive* Annexin V+/Fib+, *MUC positive* AnnexinV+/MUC+, *CEA positive* AnnexinV+/CEA+, *CA 19-9 positive* Annexin +/CA19-9+

4. 3 mL Pasteur pipettes.
5. 1 mM prostacyclin (PGI2) stock solution in 50 mM Tris–HCl, pH 9.4. Store at −80 °C.
6. Tyrode (133 mM NaCl, 2.7 mM KCl, 11.9 mM $NaHCO_3$, 0.36 mM NaH_2PO_4-H_2O, 10 mM HEPES, 5 mM glucose, pH 7.4). Store at −20C.
7. 1.5 mL Eppendorf tubes reference and cryotubes.
8. Liquid nitrogen and azote tank.
9. −80 °C freezer.

2.2 Flow Cytometric Analysis of Platelet-Poor Plasma (PPP) Samples

Please remember that for each sample, another is required to control results (*see* **Note 3**).

1. Sample tubes for Flow Cytometer (Beckman Coulter).
2. Megamix-plus SSC beads (BioCytex).

Table 2
Antibodies and their isotypes (with volumes in μL) to characterize microparticles

Antigen	Antibody	Volume (μL)	Isotype	Volume (μL)	Fluorochrome
Annexin V	BioLegend®	10	BioLegend®	10	Pacific Blue
	Tau technologies®	10 (dil 1/100)	Tau technologies®	10 (dil 1/100)	FITC
Anti-CD41	Beckman Coulter®	2.5	Anti-CD41 (Beckman Coulter®)	2.5	PC7
Anti-CD31	Beckman Coulter®	10	Anti-IgG1 (Beckman Coulter®)	10	PE
Anti-CD11	Beckman Coulter®	2.5	Anti-IgG1 (Beckman Coulter®)	2.5	APC
Anti-CD235	Beckman Coulter®	2.5	Anti-IgG1 (Beckman Coulter®)	2.5	APC
Anti-TF	Abcam®	5 (dil 1/10)	Anti-IgG2 (homemade)	5 (dil 1/10)	488[a]
Anti-fibrin	Harvard[b]	5 (dil 1/10)	Anti-IgG2 (homemade)	5 (dil 1/10)	488[a]
Anti-mucin 1	Novocastra®	5 (dil 1/20)	Anti-IgG2 (Novocastra®)	5 (dil 1/5)	647
Anti-podoplanin	BioLegend®	10	Anti-IgG2 (BioLegend®)	2.5	PE
Anti-CEA	Abcam®	5	Anti-IgG1 (Beckman Coulter®)	10	PE
Anti-CA-19-9	Novocastra®	5 (dil 1/40)	Anti-IgG2 (Novocastra®)	5 (dil 1/5)	647

MPs Microparticles, *FITC* Fluoresceine isothiocyanate, *TF* Tissue Factor, *CEA* Carcinoembryonic antigen, *CA 19-9* Carbohydrate Antigen 19-9, *dil* dilution in phosphate-buffered saline or calcium buffer
[a]Homemade antibodies were labeled using an Alexa Fluor labeling kit
[b]Gift from Pr Furie, Harvard Medical School, Boston, USA, Hybridoma 59D8

3. Antibodies and their isotypes are summarized in the Table 2.
4. Phosphate-buffered saline without calcium and magnesium for dilution of the antibodies (and isotypes) (Gibco).
5. The annexin V and the calcium buffer 1× (Tau technology).
6. Paraformaldehyde (16%) stock solution (Pierce).
7. CytoCount beads (Dako).
8. Gallios flow cytometer setup as described.
9. Kaluza software.

3 Methods

3.1 Preparation of MPs from Human Blood

1. Collect venous blood samples in citrated tubes from the peripheral blood from fasted patients (*see* **Note 4**).
2. Store the blood samples in a vertical position at room temperature and prepared within 2 h following the drawing [9] (*see* **Note 5**).

3. Use the following standardized centrifugation protocol for the preparation of PPP samples (*see* **Note 6**):
   (a) Centrifuge the citrate blood (200 × *g* for 15 min).
   (b) Recover the upper yellow phase, which is the platelet-rich plasma (PRP), with a plastic Pasteur pipette in a new tube (see **Note** 7).
   (c) Add 4 μL PGI2 to PRP samples (see **Note 8**).
   (d) Centrifuge the PRP samples (1100 × *g* for 15 min) to obtain the PPP fractions.
   (e) Centrifuge the PPP samples (7000 × *g* for 3 min).
4. 700 μL PPP aliquots are snap-frozen (*see* **Note 9**) and stored at −80 °C until ready for the measurements.

3.2 Flow Cytometric Analysis of PPP Samples

1. The different types of MPs are characterized using a combination of annexin V and specific antibodies against the cells of origin, TF or fibrin, mucin 1, podoplanin, CEA, and CA19-9.
2. Each specific antibody is matched with an isotype control antibody (*see* **Note 3**), which are labeled with an appropriate fluorescent dye (as detailed in Table 2).
3. The MP labeling is based on a 30-min incubation of patient PPP (30 μL) with Annexin V and the appropriate antibodies (volumes in Table 2) in the dark (*see* **Note 10**).
4. Add a 300 μL volume of calcium buffer (*see* **Note 11**) and incubate for 3 min.
5. Add 100 μL of paraformaldehyde (16%) to fix each sample (*see* **Note 12**).
6. Add 30 μL of CytoCount beads (*see* **Note 13**).
7. Measure the samples and associated controls within an hour using flow cytometer such as the Gallios flow cytometer [10].
8. Set the flow cytometer and MP gating using the Megamix beads.
9. Analyze the sample with suitable software (we use the Kaluza software [11]); concentrations are expressed as the number of MPs/μL of PPP.

4 Notes

1. Although not considered herein, preanalytic parameters are important for the interpretation of results between series [8].
2. Venous blood samples have to be collected in tubes with anticoagulant, to avoid clot. We used citrated tubes, whereas others used EDTA or CDTA tubes.

3. One control is required for each sample, using isotype control antibody, in order to evaluate nonspecific binding by antibodies.
4. Patients who had consumed nothing for 6 h.
5. Blood samples have to be stored in a vertical position at room temperature and prepared within 2 h following the drawing, to avoid aggregation and clot as described by Lacroix et al. [9].
6. This standardized protocol based on three successive centrifugations allows obtaining nearly exclusively MPs.
7. To avoid mixing the lower phase (red) with the PRP, two millimeters of PRP were dispensed into the tube.
8. This is use to prevent platelet activation.
9. Liquid nitrogen freezing before conservation at −80 °C avoids creation of water crystals which could be considered as MPs and thus induce an overassessment of MPs levels.
10. The MP labeling needs to be performed without light to avoid fluorochrome excitation, which would cause the labeling to fade.
11. Calcium improves the binding of annexin V to phosphatidylserine.
12. Paraformaldehyde prevents activation of MPs and thus labeling failure.
13. The use of calibrated fluorescent beads covering the size range of MPs and weakly adjustments of flow cytometer parameters provide reproducible MPs counts.

References

1. Chew HK, Wun T, Harvey D et al (2006) Incidence of venous thromboembolism and its effect on survival among patients with common cancers. Arch Intern Med 166:458–464
2. Piccin A, Murphy WG, Smith OP (2007) Circulating microparticles: pathophysiology and clinical implications. Blood Rev 21:157–171
3. van Doormaal FF, Kleinjan A, Di Nisio M et al (2009) Cell-derived microvesicles and cancer. Neth J Med 67:266–273
4. Rak J (2010) Microparticles in cancer. Semin Thromb Hemost 36:888–906
5. D'Souza-Schorey C, Clancy JW (2012) Tumor-derived microvesicles: shedding light on novel microenvironment modulators and prospective cancer biomarkers. Genes Dev 26:1287–1299
6. Thomas GM, Panicot-Dubois L, Lacroix R et al (2009) Cancer cell-derived microparticles bearing P-selectin glycoprotein ligand 1 accelerate thrombus formation in vivo. J Exp Med 206:1913–1927
7. Mezouar S, Darbousset R, Dignat-George F et al (2015) Inhibition of platelet activation prevents the P-selectin and integrin-dependent accumulation of cancer cell microparticles and reduces tumor growth and metastasis in vivo. Int J Cancer 136:462–475
8. Mege D, Panicot-Dubois L, Ouaissi M et al (2016) The origin and concentration of circulating microparticles differ according to cancer type and evolution: A prospective single-center study. Int J Cancer 138:939–948
9. Lacroix R, Judicone C, Mooberry M et al (2013) Standardization of pre-analytical variables in plasma microparticle determination: results of the International Society on Thrombosis and Haemostasis SSC Collaborative workshop. J Thromb Haemost 11:1190–1193
10. Robert S, Lacroix R, Poncelet P et al (2012) High-sensitivity flow cytometry provides access

to standardized measurement of small-size microparticles—brief report. Arterioscler Thromb Vasc Biol 32:1054–1058

11. Lacroix R, Robert S, Poncelet P et al (2010) Standardization of platelet-derived microparticle enumeration by flow cytometry with calibrated beads: results of the International Society on Thrombosis and Haemostasis SSC Collaborative workshop. J Thromb Haemost 8:2571–2574
12. Mege D, Crescence L, Ouaissi M, Sielezneff I, Guieu R, Dignat-George F, Dubois C, Panicot-Dubois L (2017) Fibrin-bearing microparticles: marker of thrombo-embolic events in pancreatic and colorectal cancers. Oncotarget 8(57):97394–97406

Part III

Recent Advances in Colorectal Cancer Therapeutics

Check for updates

Chapter 18

Molecular Testing for the Treatment of Advanced Colorectal Cancer: An Overview

Patrick S. Lin and Thomas J. Semrad

Abstract

Concurrent with an expansion in the number of agents available for the treatment of advanced CRC, there has been an increase in our understanding of selection biomarkers to optimize the management of patients with this disease. For CRC patients being considered for anti-EGFR therapy, expanded RAS testing is the standard of care to determine the subset of patients who can benefit from cetuximab or panitumumab in conjunction with chemotherapy. A small fraction of patients have HER2 amplification where emerging data suggest treatment with drugs targeting this alteration. Although advanced CRC patients who harbor the BRAF V600E mutation have a poorer prognosis, they are eligible for combinatorial therapy targeting EGFR/BRAF or BRAF/MEK within the MAP kinase signaling pathway. Once primarily thought to be a negative prognostic marker, BRAF V600E mutation is now considered as a positive predictive factor with an opportunity for clinical intervention. A growing body of evidence also supports MSI testing as clinical benefits with immune checkpoint blockade by cancer immunotherapy have been demonstrated in MSI-high patients whose tumors exhibit high mutational burden. It has been established that UGT1A1*28 polymorphism is associated with irinotecan toxicity, but this test is rarely performed as the management strategy has not been identified. No established predictive biomarker for anti-VEGF therapy has yet to be discovered.

It is becoming increasingly apparent that our growing understanding of biomarkers is revolutionizing and improving our strategies in the treatment of advanced CRC. Traditional nonselective cytotoxic chemotherapy is gradually being augmented and even in some cases supplanted by selective targeted agents based on our increasing understanding of tumor signaling and mechanism at the molecular level. The prospect of personalized medicine in directing treatment approaches that are optimally beneficial for patients brings tremendous excitement to the growing field of cancer therapeutics. As discussed in this chapter, the concurrent development of molecular biomarkers with new treatment strategies holds great promise of precision medicine in improving outcomes for patients with advanced CRC.

Key words Colorectal cancer, RAS, BRAF, Microsatellite instability, Chemotherapy, Immunotherapy, Predictive biomarker, Prognostic biomarker

1 Introduction

The American Cancer Society estimates that there will be 135,430 new cases of colon or rectal cancer in the United States for 2017 [1]. Colorectal cancer (CRC) is the second leading cause of cancer-

Jean-François Beaulieu (ed.), *Colorectal Cancer: Methods and Protocols*, Methods in Molecular Biology, vol. 1765, https://doi.org/10.1007/978-1-4939-7765-9_18,

related deaths in men and third leading cause in women in the USA, with anticipated 50,260 deaths alone in 2017 [1]. The systemic treatment of advanced CRC has evolved over the last several decades, resulting in survival outcomes of 30 months or more in recent clinical trials [2, 3]. In population based studies, CRC death rates have declined by 34% among individuals aged 50 years and older in recent years, but there are striking sociodemographic differences in outcome and a rise in distal colon cancers among younger adults [4].

A complete review of the treatment of advanced CRC is beyond the scope of this chapter. Nonetheless, a broad overview is required to understand and guide the utilization of molecular biomarkers in advanced CRC. The spectrum of potential systemic therapies for patients with advanced CRC now includes cytotoxic chemotherapy as well as biologic agents targeting vascular endothelial growth factor (VEGF) and the epidermal growth factor receptor (EGFR). Cytotoxic chemotherapy agents with activity for the treatment of advanced CRC include 5-fluorouracil (5-FU), oxaliplatin, irinotecan, and trifluridine/tipiracil [5–8]. Approved anti-EGFR monoclonal antibodies are cetuximab (recombinant mouse/human) and panitumumab (human) [9, 10]. Anti-VEGF agents are differentiated based on target specificity and route of administration; they include bevacizumab, ziv-aflibercept, ramucirumab, and regorafenib [11–14]. Most recently, cancer immunotherapy has been intensely explored, with the programmed death 1 (PD-1) monoclonal antibodies having recently established a role in the management of a subset of patients with advanced CRC [15]. Additionally, the paradigm of biologic agents targeting growth factor receptor signaling has been extended to HER2 [16].

The expansion of this menu of active agents for the treatment of advanced CRC underlies improvements in survival for patients with this disease. Nonetheless, it has created challenges for the practicing oncologist to choose the optimal therapy and the appropriate treatment sequence for individual patients. Therefore, the development and use of molecular tests associated with survival regardless of therapy (prognostic biomarkers) and to identify patients more or less likely to benefit from a specific intervention (predictive biomarkers) has become increasingly critical for both drug development and for the selection of treatment for individual patients. In this chapter, we will focus on current and emerging molecular biomarkers that enable clinicians to refine treatment strategies in patients with advanced CRC (Table 1).

Table 1
Summary of candidate molecular markers for the treatment of advanced colorectal cancer

Marker	Prognostic/ Predictive	Associated therapy	Comment
UGT1A1*28 polymorphism	Predictive	Irinotecan	Associated with toxicity but management strategies not standardized
RAS mutation	Predictive	EGFR Antibodies	Strongly predictive for absent activity. Prognostic implications debated.
PI3K pathway alterations	Predictive	EGFR Antibodies	Predictive relevance not established, conflicting data
EGFR expression and amplification	Predictive	EGFR Antibodies	Abandoned, insufficient data
HER2 amplification	Predictive	HER2 therapy	Pending confirmation in larger studies
BRAF V600E	Prognostic and predictive	MAP kinase pathway combinations	Poor prognosis in advanced disease, selection marker for new treatment combinations
VEGF and circulating angiogenic factors	Predictive	Anti-VEGF agents	No established marker
Microsatellite Instability	Prognostic and predictive	Immune checkpoint inhibitors	Improved prognosis in early stage patients and strongly predictive of response to programmed death-1 targeted agents
Consensus Molecular Subtyping	Prognostic	Unknown	Ongoing studies testing predictive implications.

2 Testing for the Treatment of Advanced CRC

2.1 Molecular Tests for Cytotoxic Chemotherapy

2.1.1 UGT1A1

Irinotecan-based therapy in the form of FOLFIRI is a common choice of upfront chemotherapy in the treatment of advanced CRC [6]. The efficacy and toxicity associated with irinotecan-based therapy has garnered research interest in an enzyme called uridine diphosphate glucuronosyltransferase (UGT) 1A1 that is involved in irinotecan metabolism. Through glucuronidation, UGT1A1 inactivates SN-38, an irinotecan metabolite. Accordingly, the UGT1A1*28 polymorphism is associated with reduced protein expression and corresponding decreased glucuronidation, leading to bioavailable retention of SN-38. Initial studies demonstrated that drug toxicity was significantly increased in patients with one or two alleles of UGT1A1*28 [17]. Unfortunately, the management strategies for patients homozygous or heterozygous for this allele have not been standardized. In a study of 250 patients with advanced CRC treated with FOLFIRI, 8.8–45.6% of the cohort were homozygous and heterozygous respectively for UGT1A1*28 [18]. This polymorphism was associated with increased risk of hematologic toxicity in the first cycle of treatment but without statistically significant effect in subsequent cycles of therapy. UGT1A1 genotype has also been used to determine and guide maximal tolerable dose of irinotecan in a 3-week regimen [19]. Beside the established association of UGT1A1*28 polymorphisms with irinotecan-associated toxicity, it has also been hypothesized that the reduced rate of irinotecan metabolism may actually be a predictive biomarker for treatment response. Indeed, in the abovementioned study of advanced CRC patients treated with FOLFIRI, clinical response was increased in the UGT1A1*28 homozygous group [18]. However, this did not confer a statistically significant increase in survival. Currently, the optimal treatment with irinotecan based on UGT1A1 status remains incompletely defined [20]. The utility of UGT1A1*28 polymorphism in assessing irinotecan-associated toxicity and treatment response will likely require a better understanding of population pharmacogenomics of allelic frequencies and variations observed in different populations [21].

2.2 Molecular Tests for Targeting the EGFR Pathway

2.2.1 RAS

Activation of the EGFR (HER1; ERBB1) signaling pathway is observed in a variety of malignancies. Constitutive EGFR signaling results from receptor dimerization after binding to ligands such as EGF, amphiregulin, or epiregulin. Autophosphorylation results in an intracellular signal that is transduced through several enzymatic pathways. The dominant pathway involves the activation of the G-protein intermediate RAS, and subsequent signaling through BRAF, MEK, and ERK (the MAP kinase pathway). Mutations in the RAS family of proto-oncogenes (KRAS, NRAS, HRAS) result in constitutive activation of MAP kinase pathway signaling that is independent of activation of receptor tyrosine kinases such as EGFR. Since the EGFR antibodies cetuximab and panitumumab bind to the extracellular domain of EGFR to result in receptor internalization and block signaling, it has been hypothesized that mutations in RAS render the activity of EGFR antibodies irrelevant. Indeed, multiple studies have shown that cetuximab and panitumimab improve PFS and OS in metastatic CRC patients with wild-type KRAS but not those with mutated KRAS [22, 23]. These findings were subsequently confirmed in prospective-retrospective analyses of large clinical trials that randomized patients to treatment with or without EGFR antibodies. For instance, in the CRYSTAL trial that compared initial treatment with the combination of leucovorin, 5-FU, and irinotecan (FOLFIRI) to the same regimen with cetuximab, there was a significant interaction between KRAS mutation status and survival outcome [24]. Subsequent meta-analyses following systematic literature review have confirmed pooled survival advantage with anti-EGFR therapy for patients with wild-type KRAS over those harboring the KRAS mutation [25–29]. Therefore, KRAS mutation testing has been integrated into guideline-based management of advanced CRC [30, 31].

The most common RAS mutations in colon cancer occur in codons 12 and 13 of KRAS, and are present in 35–45% of cases. However, not all nonmutated KRAS in codons 12 and 13 benefit from anti-EGFR therapy [32]. Patients who have wild-type KRAS in codons 12 and 13 but mutated KRAS in codons 59, 61, 117, 146 or mutated NRAS do not respond to anti-EGFR treatment as compared to those without any RAS mutations. These results suggest that "expanded" RAS testing involving the above-mentioned codons (and corresponding exons) must be performed in determining the subset of patients who will benefit from anti-EGFR antibody. While no single study is statistically powered to evaluate the treatment by biomarker interaction for each of these additional mutations individually, cetuximab and panitumumab would be the appropriate treatment for advanced CRC patients who are wild type for all known RAS mutations [32, 31].

Although the use of anti-EGFR therapy is standard of care for patients with nonmutated KRAS CRC, there is no equivalent targeted therapy for patients with mutated KRAS. However, Tran et al. recently described a case whereby a patient with metastatic CRC was treated with CD8+ T cell infusion targeting mutant KRAS G12D and HLA-C*08:02 [33]. This antitumor immunotherapy led to regression of all lung metastases followed by progression in one lesion due to tumor immune evasion from eventual loss of HLA-C*08:02. The significance of this finding has been debated given the questionable prevalence of mutant KRAS G12D and HLA C*08:02 combination, but certainly raises the therapeutic potential of immunotherapy use in the future as we assess other KRAS mutations and HLA alleles [34]. Strategies that harness a T-cell response against mutated tumor antigens may be of clinical utility in advanced CRC patients harboring KRAS mutations. Furthermore, this has the opportunity to turn RAS from a negative selection biomarker for anti-EGFR therapy to a positive selection biomarker for novel immune therapies.

2.2.2 PI3K Pathway Alterations

Despite expanded RAS testing, many CRC patients do not exhibit response to anti-EGFR therapy. In addition to the RAS pathway, EGFR signaling is mediated through a distinct pathway that involves phosphoinositide-3-kinase (PI3K), AKT and PTEN. Accordingly, some studies have focused their efforts on these downstream effectors in this signaling pathway. Similar to the rationale for how RAS pathway mutations impact upstream EGFR-directed therapy, mutations in the PI3K pathway have been evaluated as a predictive marker for the efficacy of EGFR antibody therapy. Additionally, mutations in PIK3CA have been associated with response to aspirin therapy.

The PIK3CA gene encodes the α-catalytic domain of PI3K and is mutated in 10–20% of CRCs. The relevant mutations in PIK3CA occur in either exon 9 (the helical domain) or in exon 20 (the kinase domain). Initial studies came to conflicting conclusions regarding the potential utility of PIK3CA mutations to confer resistance to EGFR-targeted therapy [35, 36]. Of note, the presence of a mutation in PIK3CA does not exclude RAS mutations, complicating the interpretation of results that are not stratified by RAS. In a large study of 773 patients with evaluable specimens treated with EGFR antibody therapy, PIK3CA mutations overall were associated with a lower response rate in KRAS wild-type patients (17.7% vs. 37.7%; OR 0.35; 95% CI 0.13–0.83; $p = 0.015$) but not with reduced PFS or OS [37]. The effect may have been diluted by exon 9 mutations as response, PFS and OS were all statistically reduced in patients with exon 20 mutations compared to wild type patients. Nonetheless, only nine patients with exon 20 PIK3CA mutations but without RAS mutation were analyzed in the study. Moreover, a subsequent study on a subset of patients from the original cetuximab monotherapy phase III study did not find any effect of PIK3CA mutations as a predictive marker for benefit [38].

Several observational studies have demonstrated an association between aspirin use and reduced CRC mortality [39–41]. Subsequently, two cohort studies showed that post-treatment aspirin use confers improved survival for CRC patients who harbor the PIK3CA mutation [42, 43]. Unfortunately, these findings were not corroborated by a separate cohort study [44]. Accordingly, there is insufficient evidence at this time to recommend PIK3CA mutation analysis as a predictive marker either to select against anti-EGFR therapy or for posttreatment aspirin use.

2.2.3 EGFR (ERBB1) Expression and Amplification

Based on the mechanism of action, it was predicted that EGFR protein expression would be required for any activity of EGFR antibodies in metastatic CRC. Accordingly, only EGFR-expressing CRC was allowed on the initial clinical trials [45]. However, subsequent analyses did not demonstrate a correlation with EGFR expression and response [46]. Indeed, response to an EGFR antibody was observed in tumors that did not have immunohistochemically detectable expression of EGFR [47]. Therefore, expression of EGFR was abandoned as a predictive marker for the benefit of cetuximab or panitumumab in advanced CRC. Similarly, EGFR copy number has been described as a poor candidate for development as a predictive marker of the efficacy of EGFR antibody therapy [48], despite at least one small study suggesting a provocative interaction between copy number and outcome [49].

2.2.4 HER2 (ERBB2) Expression and Amplification

In contrast to the findings for EGFR monoclonal antibodies, the findings from a number of preclinical studies inferred the potential use of HER2 as a predictive marker in the management of advanced CRC. Mouse models of HER2-amplified, cetuximab-resistant xenografts were treated with different HER2-directed therapies [50, 51]. Single agent treatment with either anti-HER2 antibodies or HER2 tyrosine kinase inhibitors was ineffective in these preclinical models of advanced CRC. However, the combination of the two HER2-targeted therapies exhibited durable clinical response as measured by sustained decrease in tumor size. Extrapolating from the benefit of combined therapy with trastuzumab (antibody) and lapatinib (tyrosine kinase inhibitor) seen in the treatment of breast cancer [52], Sartore-Bianchi et al. showed in a multicenter, open-label, phase 2 trial that combined trastuzumab and lapatinib is highly active in the treatment of KRAS wild type, HER2-positive metastatic CRC [16]. Thirty percent of patients with advanced CRC with HER2 overexpression or amplification exhibited objective response and disease control. Furthermore, the extent of HER2 gene copy number appeared to be associated with response to treatment. CRC patients who harbored high HER2 gene copy number exhibited statistically higher rate of PFS than those with low-to-no HER2 amplification. Considering that regorafenib or trifluridine/tipiracil have response rates less than 5% [12, 8, 53], the above mentioned study with the combinatorial use of trastuzumab and lapatinib holds significant promise for patients in search of third or fourth-line therapies. More importantly, the study supports HER2 testing in KRAS wild-type CRC patients with a potentionally actionable target. Certainly, a phase III randomized study with head-to-head comparisons is required to confirm the benefit of HER2-directed therapies in treatment-refractory patients with advanced CRC.

2.3 Molecular Tests for Targeting the MAP Kinase Signaling Pathway

BRAF activating mutations occur in approximately 14% of patients with localized stage II and III CRC, and 8% of patients with advanced/metastatic disease [31]. Many studies over the years have evaluated the prognostic and predictive value of BRAF mutations in CRC patients. Several meta-analyses showed that advanced CRC patients who harbor the BRAF mutation have decreased PFS and OS as compared to those with wild-type BRAF [54, 55]. Poorer outcomes after recurrence were also seen in patients with stage II and II CRC harboring a BRAF mutation [56].

Although BRAF mutation is a poor prognostic factor, an increasing body of evidence suggests that BRAF mutation may be a predictive factor for treatment strategies. Given that patients with metastatic CRC with BRAF mutation have particularly poor outcomes, one study with molecular subgroup analysis suggests the use of FOLFIRINOX as first-line therapy followed by clinical trial [57]. Using analogous reasoning to that described for RAS mutations, the BRAF V600E mutation, immediately downstream of RAS, has been evaluated as a negative predictive marker for the efficacy of EGFR antibodies. Based on meta-analyses, there is insufficient evidence to support BRAF mutation testing as predictive marker for use of anti-EGFR therapy alone [58, 59]. However, early clinical trials suggest combinatorial use of EGFR, BRAF, MEK inhibitors with improved outcomes [60–62]. Triple therapy comprising panitumumab, dabrafenib, trametinib improves PFS and OS compared to panitumumab plus either dabrafenib or trametinib [63]. Kopetz et al. demonstrated that combined EGFR and BRAF V600E inhibition with irinotecan, cetuximab, vemurafenib markedly improved PFS over irinotecan and cetuximab alone (HR 0.42, 95% CI 0.26 to 0.66, $P < 0.001$) [64]. The use of triple therapy that included a BRAF V600E inhibitor exhibited statistically higher disease control rate over double therapy without it (67% vs. 22%, $P < 0.001$). With the abovementioned studies, it is becoming increasingly apparent that BRAF mutation analysis should be standard of care in upfront molecular testing as dual inhibition toward EGFR/BRAF or BRAF/MEK are promising strategies in the treatment of CRC harboring BRAF V600E mutation. That said, acquired resistance to combinatorial therapy has been reported requiring ongoing research into resistance mechanisms along the MAPK signaling pathway [65–67].

2.4 Molecular Tests for Selecting Anti-VEGF Therapy

The search for a molecular selection marker for the benefit of anti-VEGF strategies is a cautionary tale about the challenge of marker development in complex biologic environments. The initial biomarker development studies focused on tumor expression levels of VEGF as a potential predictor of responsiveness to bevacizumab. Neither VEGF expression by in situ hybridization nor expression by immunohistochemistry correlated with outcome in the pivotal AVF2107g study that established the role of bevacizumab in advanced CRC [68]. Similarly, VEGF, VEGFR1, or VEGFR2 expression by immunohistochemistry in either tumor cells or stroma did not correlate with outcome in the NO166966 study of XELOX and FOLFOX with or without bevacizumab [69]. Due to the lack of success of the tumor-based biomarker approach, investigators queried the levels of VEGF-A and other circulating factors associated with angiogenesis. No clear evidence for a predictive benefit of any circulating factor exists [70, 71]. The most provocative data was generated from a panel of plasma angiogenic factors collected from patients treated on a phase II study of FOLFIRI plus bevacizumab [72]. Similar to other studies, both baseline VEGF and VEGFR2 were not associated with outcome. However, elevations in certain alternative angiogenic factors including bFGF, PlGF, and HGF were observed in subsets of patients immediately before radiographic evidence of disease progression. Intratumoral expression of these pathways have been confirmed on progression on anti-VEGF therapy [73], but these data do not yet provide a mechanism to identify patients likely to respond to VEGF therapy nor allow for selection of alternative therapies.

2.5 Emerging Molecular Tests for Immunotherapy

Approximately 15% of CRCs have evidence of defective DNA mismatch repair (dMMR) manifested as microsatellite instability (MSI). While some of these tumors are a result of hereditary defects in DNA mismatch repair enzymes (Hereditary Non-Polyposis Colorectal Cancer HNPCC aka Lynch Syndrome), others arise from sporadic pathogenesis. Patients with deficient MMR CRC with loss of MLH1 should undergo BRAF V600E mutation analysis to assess the risk for Lynch syndrome [31]. In sporadic CRC, dMMR is most commonly caused by epigenetic silencing via CpG methylation of MLH1 promoter. In Lynch Syndrome, dMMR is secondary to a germline mutation of one of the four mismatch repairs genes, namely MLH1, MSH2, MSH6, PMS2, or equivalently in EPCAM which is immediately upstream of MSH2. Via an unknown mechanism, BRAF mutations are more commonly associated with epigenetic MMR gene silencing and rarely occur with germline-based dMMR. Accordingly, the presence of a BRAF mutation in a dMMR CRC strongly suggests a sporadic pathogenesis and less likely Lynch Syndrome [74]. Therefore, BRAF mutation testing in this setting has clinical implications as identification of patients with HNPCC necessitates further testing among family members for appropriate screening [31].

Current data suggest that defective DNA mismatch repair confers an improved prognosis in most stages of CRC, but there is also evidence that these tumors are relatively resistant to 5-FU monotherapy in the adjuvant setting [75]. The utility of MSI testing to direct treatment in advanced CRC was not well established until a landmark finding reported in 2015. Consistent with the idea that tumors with high mutational burden may be more responsive to immunotherapy, MSI-high CRC associated with dMMR exhibits clinical response to agents targeting PD-1/PD-L1 [76, 15]. Given that somatic mutations are more likely to occur in mismatch repair-deficient CRC than in mismatch repair-proficient cancers, and are more likely to be recognized by patient's own immune system as "mutation-associated neo-antigens", Le et al. hypothesized and showed that MSI-high CRC are responsive to immune checkpoint blockade of PD-1 receptor [15]. With pembrolizumab, the immune-mediated overall response rate and progression free survival were 40% and 78%, respectively for mismatch repair-deficient CRC, and 0% and 11% for mismatch repair-proficient CRC. In this study, high somatic mutation loads as established by whole exome-sequencing were associated with prolonged PFS following PD-1 blockade. Accordingly, mismatch repair status predicted clinical benefit of immune checkpoint blockade supporting MSI testing in the management of patients with advanced CRC.

Since this landmark finding, a number of preliminary studies are lending further support for MSI testing for metastatic CRC given clinical benefits from immune checkpoint blockade. At the 2017 Gastrointestinal Cancers Symposium, Hochster et al. showed in an open-label, multicenter phase Ib trial that patients with MSI-high metastatic CRC exhibited a 40% overall response rate per RECIST criteria with combination of atezolizumab and bevacizumab [77]. At the same meeting, Overman et al. provided an update of the phase II CheckMate-142 trial and demonstrated antitumor activity of nivolumab in patients with metastatic CRC, with overall response rate of 31.1% and median progression free survival of 9.6 months [78]. These studies affirm the growing body of evidence that MSI testing should become standard of care in advanced CRC as high tumor burden from high mutational load confers treatment sensitivity to immune checkpoint blockade. Accordingly, there is already some preliminary debate on whether 1st line therapy for MSI-high patients should involve chemotherapy or immunotherapy. Findings from randomized clinical trials will be required to further delineate the appropriate course of treatment in this molecularly defined subset.

Moreover, Bendell et al. showed combination of atezolizumab and cobimetinib resulted in a meaningful clinical response in KRAS mutated metastatic CRC [79]. MEK inhibition by cobimetinib may be able sensitize KRAS mutated tumors to atezolizumab by increasing MHC I expression on tumor cells and promoting CD8+ T cell accumulation. Accordingly, as MSI has rapidly become an established marker of potential sensitivity to immune checkpoint inhibitors, other molecular markers are being sought to define subgroups with sensitivity to immune-based combination therapy. The results of a phase III study of this combination (NCT02788279) compared to regorafenib in refractory KRAS mutated advanced CRC are eagerly awaited.

2.6 Gene Expression Profiling

Recognizing that single molecular events only partly define the molecular architecture of CRC, an international expert collaboration sought to define intrinsic molecular subtypes of CRC using gene expression profiling. Multiple prior attempts to stratify CRC showed little agreement with each other and did not result in a useful single consistent classification system [80–86]. The resulting consensus molecular subtyping (CMS) system includes four different subtypes of CRC [87, 88]. CMS1 (MSI Immune) involves a subgroup with high frequency of MSI, hypermutation, and evidence of strong immune activation. CMS2 (Canonical) is an epithelial subtype that involves prominent activation of signaling in WNT and MYC pathways. CMS3 (Metabolic) is an epithelial signature that contains some MSI, but less immune activation with frequent KRAS mutations and metabolic dysregulation. CMS4 (Mesenchymal) is a mesenchymal subtype that has increased expression of genes involved in the epithelial-to-mesenchymal transition (EMT) with prominent TGF-β activation. This subtype is consistent associated with worse prognosis. Of note, a significant fraction (13%) of tumors has mixed features and could not be classified.

This CMS classification system is perhaps the most robust gene classification system developed to date, and is the subject of significant ongoing research. The prognostic implications have been validated in several clinical trials [89–91]. However, the utility of the system will require the ability to define treatment effect. Early studies suggest the possibility of differential treatment effect of VEGF and EGFR inhibitors in CMS subgroups, although this data remains very limited [90, 91]. It should be recognized that this system was not trained to predict treatment efficacy; therefore, any potential prediction of therapeutic benefit reflects differential activity in disease subtypes which may or may not be able to be resolved to simpler biomarker-by-treatment effects.

References

1. Siegel RL, Miller KD, Jemal A (2017) Cancer Statistics, 2017. CA Cancer J Clin 67(1):7–30
2. Heinemann V, von Weikersthal LF, Decker T, Kiani A, Vehling-Kaiser U, Al-Batran SE, Heintges T, Lerchenmuller C, Kahl C, Seipelt G, Kullmann F, Stauch M, Scheithauer W, Hielscher J, Scholz M, Muller S, Link H, Niederle N, Rost A, Hoffkes HG, Moehler M, Lindig RU, Modest DP, Rossius L, Kirchner T, Jung A, Stintzing S (2014) FOLFIRI plus cetuximab versus FOLFIRI plus bevacizumab as first-line treatment for patients with metastatic colorectal cancer (FIRE-3): a randomised, open-label, phase 3 trial. Lancet Oncol 15(10):1065–1075
3. Venook AP, Niedzwiecki D, Lenz H-J, Innocenti F, Mahoney MR, O'Neil BH, Shaw JE, Polite BN, Hochster HS, Atkins JN, Goldberg RM, Mayer RJ, Schilsky RL, Bertagnolli MM, Blanke CD, Cancer, Leukemia Group B S, ECOG (2014) CALGB/SWOG 80405: phase III trial of irinotecan/5-FU/leucovorin (FOLFIRI) or oxaliplatin/5-FU/leucovorin (mFOLFOX6) with bevacizumab (BV) or cetuximab (CET) for patients (pts) with KRAS wild-type (wt) untreated metastatic adenocarcinoma of the colon or rectum (MCRC). ASCO Meeting Abstracts 32(15_suppl):LBA3
4. Siegel RL, Miller KD, Fedewa SA, Ahnen DJ, Meester RG, Barzi A, Jemal A (2017) Colorectal cancer statistics, 2017. CA Cancer J Clin 67 (3):177–193
5. Cunningham D, Glimelius B (1999) A phase III study of irinotecan (CPT-11) versus best supportive care in patients with metastatic colorectal cancer who have failed 5-fluorouracil therapy. V301 study group. Semin Oncol 26(1 Suppl 5):6–12
6. Douillard JY, Cunningham D, Roth AD, Navarro M, James RD, Karasek P, Jandik P, Iveson T, Carmichael J, Alakl M, Gruia G, Awad L, Rougier P (2000) Irinotecan combined with fluorouracil compared with fluorouracil alone as first-line treatment for metastatic colorectal cancer: a multicentre randomised trial. Lancet 355(9209):1041–1047
7. Hochster HS, Hart LL, Ramanathan RK, Childs BH, Hainsworth JD, Cohn AL, Wong L, Fehrenbacher L, Abubakr Y, Saif MW, Schwartzberg L, Hedrick E (2008) Safety and efficacy of oxaliplatin and fluoropyrimidine regimens with or without bevacizumab as first-line treatment of metastatic colorectal cancer: results of the TREE Study. J Clin Oncol 26 (21):3523–3529
8. Mayer RJ, Van Cutsem E, Falcone A, Yoshino T, Garcia-Carbonero R, Mizunuma N, Yamazaki K, Shimada Y, Tabernero J, Komatsu Y, Sobrero A, Boucher E, Peeters M, Tran B, Lenz HJ, Zaniboni A, Hochster H, Cleary JM, Prenen H, Benedetti F, Mizuguchi H, Makris L, Ito M, Ohtsu A, Group RS (2015) Randomized trial of TAS-102 for refractory metastatic colorectal cancer. N Engl J Med 372(20):1909–1919
9. Douillard JY, Siena S, Cassidy J, Tabernero J, Burkes R, Barugel M, Humblet Y, Bodoky G,

Cunningham D, Jassem J, Rivera F, Kocakova I, Ruff P, Blasinska-Morawiec M, Smakal M, Canon JL, Rother M, Oliner KS, Wolf M, Gansert J (2010) Randomized, phase III trial of panitumumab with infusional fluorouracil, leucovorin, and oxaliplatin (FOLFOX4) versus FOLFOX4 alone as first-line treatment in patients with previously untreated metastatic colorectal cancer: the PRIME study. J Clin Oncol 28(31):4697–4705

10. Jonker DJ, O'Callaghan CJ, Karapetis CS, Zalcberg JR, Tu D, Au HJ, Berry SR, Krahn M, Price T, Simes RJ, Tebbutt NC, van Hazel G, Wierzbicki R, Langer C, Moore MJ (2007) Cetuximab for the treatment of colorectal cancer. N Engl J Med 357 (20):2040–2048
11. Van Cutsem E, Tabernero J, Lakomy R, Prenen H, Prausova J, Macarulla T, Ruff P, van Hazel GA, Moiseyenko V, Ferry D, McKendrick J, Polikoff J, Tellier A, Castan R, Allegra C (2012) Addition of aflibercept to fluorouracil, leucovorin, and irinotecan improves survival in a phase III randomized trial in patients with metastatic colorectal cancer previously treated with an oxaliplatin-based regimen. J Clin Oncol 30(28):3499–3506
12. Grothey A, Van Cutsem E, Sobrero A, Siena S, Falcone A, Ychou M, Humblet Y, Bouche O, Mineur L, Barone C, Adenis A, Tabernero J, Yoshino T, Lenz HJ, Goldberg RM, Sargent DJ, Cihon F, Cupit L, Wagner A, Laurent D, Group CS (2013) Regorafenib monotherapy for previously treated metastatic colorectal cancer (CORRECT): an international, multicentre, randomised, placebo-controlled, phase 3 trial. Lancet 381(9863):303–312
13. Hurwitz H, Fehrenbacher L, Novotny W, Cartwright T, Hainsworth J, Heim W, Berlin J, Baron A, Griffing S, Holmgren E, Ferrara N, Fyfe G, Rogers B, Ross R, Kabbinavar F (2004) Bevacizumab plus irinotecan, fluorouracil, and leucovorin for metastatic colorectal cancer. N Engl J Med 350 (23):2335–2342
14. Tabernero J, Yoshino T, Cohn AL, Obermannova R, Bodoky G, Garcia-Carbonero R, Ciuleanu TE, Portnoy DC, Van Cutsem E, Grothey A, Prausova J, Garcia-Alfonso P, Yamazaki K, Clingan PR, Lonardi S, Kim TW, Simms L, Chang SC, Nasroulah F, Investigators RS (2015) Ramucirumab versus placebo in combination with second-line FOLFIRI in patients with metastatic colorectal carcinoma that progressed during or after first-line therapy with bevacizumab, oxaliplatin, and a fluoropyrimidine (RAISE): a randomised, double-blind, multicentre, phase 3 study. Lancet Oncol 16(5):499–508
15. Le DT, Uram JN, Wang H, Bartlett BR, Kemberling H, Eyring AD, Skora AD, Luber BS, Azad NS, Laheru D, Biedrzycki B, Donehower RC, Zaheer A, Fisher GA, Crocenzi TS, Lee JJ, Duffy SM, Goldberg RM, de la Chapelle A, Koshiji M, Bhaijee F, Huebner T, Hruban RH, Wood LD, Cuka N, Pardoll DM, Papadopoulos N, Kinzler KW, Zhou S, Cornish TC, Taube JM, Anders RA, Eshleman JR, Vogelstein B, Diaz LA Jr (2015) PD-1 blockade in tumors with mismatch-repair deficiency. N Engl J Med 372(26):2509–2520
16. Sartore-Bianchi A, Trusolino L, Martino C, Bencardino K, Lonardi S, Bergamo F, Zagonel V, Leone F, Depetris I, Martinelli E, Troiani T, Ciardiello F, Racca P, Bertotti A, Siravegna G, Torri V, Amatu A, Ghezzi S, Marrapese G, Palmeri L, Valtorta E, Cassingena A, Lauricella C, Vanzulli A, Regge D, Veronese S, Comoglio PM, Bardelli A, Marsoni S, Siena S (2016) Dual-targeted therapy with trastuzumab and lapatinib in treatment-refractory, KRAS codon 12/13 wild-type, HER2-positive metastatic colorectal cancer (HERACLES): a proof-of-concept, multicentre, open-label, phase 2 trial. Lancet Oncol 17(6):738–746
17. Iyer L, Das S, Janisch L, Wen M, Ramirez J, Karrison T, Fleming GF, Vokes EE, Schilsky RL, Ratain MJ (2002) UGT1A1*28 polymorphism as a determinant of irinotecan disposition and toxicity. Pharmacogenomics J 2 (1):43–47
18. Toffoli G, Cecchin E, Corona G, Russo A, Buonadonna A, D'Andrea M, Pasetto LM, Pessa S, Errante D, De Pangher V, Giusto M, Medici M, Gaion F, Sandri P, Galligioni E, Bonura S, Boccalon M, Biason P, Frustaci S (2006) The role of UGT1A1*28 polymorphism in the pharmacodynamics and pharmacokinetics of irinotecan in patients with metastatic colorectal cancer. J Clin Oncol 24 (19):3061–3068
19. Innocenti F, Schilsky RL, Ramirez J, Janisch L, Undevia S, House LK, Das S, Wu K, Turcich M, Marsh R, Karrison T, Maitland ML, Salgia R, Ratain MJ (2014) Dose-finding and pharmacokinetic study to optimize the dosing of irinotecan according to the UGT1A1 genotype of patients with cancer. J Clin Oncol 32(22):2328–2334
20. Fujita K, Sparreboom A (2010) Pharmacogenetics of irinotecan disposition and toxicity: a review. Curr Clin Pharmacol 5(3):209–217

21. Xu C, Tang X, Qu Y, Keyoumu S, Zhou N, Tang Y (2016) UGT1A1 gene polymorphism is associated with toxicity and clinical efficacy of irinotecan-based chemotherapy in patients with advanced colorectal cancer. Cancer Chemother Pharmacol 78(1):119–130
22. Karapetis CS, Khambata-Ford S, Jonker DJ, O'Callaghan CJ, Tu D, Tebbutt NC, Simes RJ, Chalchal H, Shapiro JD, Robitaille S, Price TJ, Shepherd L, Au HJ, Langer C, Moore MJ, Zalcberg JR (2008) K-ras mutations and benefit from cetuximab in advanced colorectal cancer. N Engl J Med 359 (17):1757–1765
23. Lievre A, Bachet JB, Le Corre D, Boige V, Landi B, Emile JF, Cote JF, Tomasic G, Penna C, Ducreux M, Rougier P, Penault-Llorca F, Laurent-Puig P (2006) KRAS mutation status is predictive of response to cetuximab therapy in colorectal cancer. Cancer Res 66(8):3992–3995
24. Van Cutsem E, Kohne CH, Lang I, Folprecht G, Nowacki MP, Cascinu S, Shchepotin I, Maurel J, Cunningham D, Tejpar S, Schlichting M, Zubel A, Celik I, Rougier P, Ciardiello F (2011) Cetuximab plus irinotecan, fluorouracil, and leucovorin as first-line treatment for metastatic colorectal cancer: updated analysis of overall survival according to tumor KRAS and BRAF mutation status. J Clin Oncol 29(15):2011–2019
25. Chen J, Ye Y, Sun H, Shi G (2013) Association between KRAS codon 13 mutations and clinical response to anti-EGFR treatment in patients with metastatic colorectal cancer: results from a meta-analysis. Cancer Chemother Pharmacol 71(1):265–272
26. Mao C, Yang ZY, Hu XF, Chen Q, Tang JL (2012) PIK3CA exon 20 mutations as a potential biomarker for resistance to anti-EGFR monoclonal antibodies in KRAS wild-type metastatic colorectal cancer: a systematic review and meta-analysis. Ann Oncol 23 (6):1518–1525
27. Petrelli F, Coinu A, Cabiddu M, Ghilardi M, Barni S (2013) KRAS as prognostic biomarker in metastatic colorectal cancer patients treated with bevacizumab: a pooled analysis of 12 published trials. Med Oncol 30(3):650
28. Ren J, Li G, Ge J, Li X, Zhao Y (2012) Is K-ras gene mutation a prognostic factor for colorectal cancer: a systematic review and meta-analysis. Dis Colon Rectum 55(8):913–923
29. Vale CL, Tierney JF, Fisher D, Adams RA, Kaplan R, Maughan TS, Parmar MK, Meade AM (2012) Does anti-EGFR therapy improve outcome in advanced colorectal cancer? A systematic review and meta-analysis. Cancer Treat Rev 38(6):618–625
30. Benson AB 3rd, Venook AP, Cederquist L, Chan E, Chen YJ, Cooper HS, Deming D, Engstrom PF, Enzinger PC, Fichera A, Grem JL, Grothey A, Hochster HS, Hoffe S, Hunt S, Kamel A, Kirilcuk N, Krishnamurthi S, Messersmith WA, Mulcahy MF, Murphy JD, Nurkin S, Saltz L, Sharma S, Shibata D, Skibber JM, Sofocleous CT, Stoffel EM, Stotsky-Himelfarb E, Willett CG, Wu CS, Gregory KM, Freedman-Cass D (2017) Colon cancer, version 1.2017, NCCN clinical practice guidelines in oncology. JNCCN 15(3):370–398
31. Sepulveda AR, Hamilton SR, Allegra CJ, Grody W, Cushman-Vokoun AM, Funkhouser WK, Kopetz SE, Lieu C, Lindor NM, Minsky BD, Monzon FA, Sargent DJ, Singh VM, Willis J, Clark J, Colasacco C, Rumble RB, Temple-Smolkin R, Ventura CB, Nowak JA (2017) Molecular biomarkers for the evaluation of colorectal cancer: guideline summary from the American Society for clinical pathology, College of American Pathologists, Association for Molecular Pathology, and American Society of Clinical Oncology. J Oncol Pract 19 (2):187–225
32. Sorich MJ, Wiese MD, Rowland A, Kichenadasse G, McKinnon RA, Karapetis CS (2015) Extended RAS mutations and anti-EGFR monoclonal antibody survival benefit in metastatic colorectal cancer: a meta-analysis of randomized, controlled trials. Ann Oncol 26 (1):13–21
33. Tran E, Robbins PF, Lu YC, Prickett TD, Gartner JJ, Jia L, Pasetto A, Zheng Z, Ray S, Groh EM, Kriley IR, Rosenberg SA (2016) T-Cell Transfer Therapy Targeting Mutant KRAS in Cancer. N Engl J Med 375(23):2255–2262
34. Rosenberg SA, Tran E, Robbins PF (2017) T-Cell Transfer Therapy Targeting Mutant KRAS. N Engl J Med 376(7):e11
35. Prenen H, De Schutter J, Jacobs B, De Roock W, Biesmans B, Claes B, Lambrechts D, Van Cutsem E, Tejpar S (2009) PIK3CA mutations are not a major determinant of resistance to the epidermal growth factor receptor inhibitor cetuximab in metastatic colorectal cancer. Clin Cancer Res 15(9):3184–3188
36. Sartore-Bianchi A, Martini M, Molinari F, Veronese S, Nichelatti M, Artale S, Di Nicolantonio F, Saletti P, De Dosso S, Mazzucchelli L, Frattini M, Siena S, Bardelli A (2009) PIK3CA mutations in colorectal cancer are associated with clinical resistance to EGFR-targeted monoclonal antibodies. Cancer Res 69(5):1851–1857

37. De Roock W, Claes B, Bernasconi D, De Schutter J, Biesmans B, Fountzilas G, Kalogeras KT, Kotoula V, Papamichael D, Laurent-Puig P, Penault-Llorca F, Rougier P, Vincenzi B, Santini D, Tonini G, Cappuzzo F, Frattini M, Molinari F, Saletti P, De Dosso S, Martini M, Bardelli A, Siena S, Sartore-Bianchi A, Tabernero J, Macarulla T, Di Fiore F, Gangloff AO, Ciardiello F, Pfeiffer P, Qvortrup C, Hansen TP, Van Cutsem E, Piessevaux H, Lambrechts D, Delorenzi M, Tejpar S (2010) Effects of KRAS, BRAF, NRAS, and PIK3CA mutations on the efficacy of cetuximab plus chemotherapy in chemotherapy-refractory metastatic colorectal cancer: a retrospective consortium analysis. Lancet Oncol 11(8):753–762
38. Karapetis CS, Jonker D, Daneshmand M, Hanson JE, O'Callaghan CJ, Marginean C, Zalcberg JR, Simes J, Moore MJ, Tebbutt NC, Price TJ, Shapiro JD, Pavlakis N, Gibbs P, Van Hazel GA, Lee U, Haq R, Virk S, Tu D, Lorimer IA, Group NCT, the Australasian Gastro-Intestinal Trials G (2014) PIK3CA, BRAF, and PTEN status and benefit from cetuximab in the treatment of advanced colorectal cancer—results from NCIC CTG/AGITG CO.17. Clin Cancer Res 20 (3):744–753
39. Chan AT, Giovannucci EL, Meyerhardt JA, Schernhammer ES, Wu K, Fuchs CS (2008) Aspirin dose and duration of use and risk of colorectal cancer in men. Gastroenterology 134(1):21–28
40. Flossmann E, Rothwell PM, British Doctors Aspirin T, the UKTIAAT (2007) Effect of aspirin on long-term risk of colorectal cancer: consistent evidence from randomised and observational studies. Lancet 369 (9573):1603–1613
41. Jacobs EJ, Thun MJ, Bain EB, Rodriguez C, Henley SJ, Calle EE (2007) A large cohort study of long-term daily use of adult-strength aspirin and cancer incidence. J Natl Cancer Inst 99(8):608–615
42. Domingo E, Church DN, Sieber O, Ramamoorthy R, Yanagisawa Y, Johnstone E, Davidson B, Kerr DJ, Tomlinson IP, Midgley R (2013) Evaluation of PIK3CA mutation as a predictor of benefit from nonsteroidal anti-inflammatory drug therapy in colorectal cancer. J Clin Oncol 31(34):4297–4305
43. Liao X, Lochhead P, Nishihara R, Morikawa T, Kuchiba A, Yamauchi M, Imamura Y, Qian ZR, Baba Y, Shima K, Sun R, Nosho K, Meyerhardt JA, Giovannucci E, Fuchs CS, Chan AT, Ogino S (2012) Aspirin use, tumor PIK3CA mutation, and colorectal-cancer survival. N Engl J Med 367(17):1596–1606
44. Kothari N, Kim R, Jorissen RN, Desai J, Tie J, Wong HL, Faragher I, Jones I, Day FL, Li S, Sakthinandeswaren A, Palmieri M, Lipton L, Schell M, Teer JK, Shibata D, Yeatman T, Sieber OM, Gibbs P, Tran B (2015) Impact of regular aspirin use on overall and cancer-specific survival in patients with colorectal cancer harboring a PIK3CA mutation. Acta Oncol 54(4):487–492
45. Saltz LB, Meropol NJ, Loehrer PJ Sr, Needle MN, Kopit J, Mayer RJ (2004) Phase II trial of cetuximab in patients with refractory colorectal cancer that expresses the epidermal growth factor receptor. J Clin Oncol 22(7):1201–1208
46. Cunningham D, Humblet Y, Siena S, Khayat D, Bleiberg H, Santoro A, Bets D, Mueser M, Harstrick A, Verslype C, Chau I, Van Cutsem E (2004) Cetuximab monotherapy and cetuximab plus irinotecan in irinotecan-refractory metastatic colorectal cancer. N Engl J Med 351(4):337–345
47. Chung KY, Shia J, Kemeny NE, Shah M, Schwartz GK, Tse A, Hamilton A, Pan D, Schrag D, Schwartz L, Klimstra DS, Fridman D, Kelsen DP, Saltz LB (2005) Cetuximab shows activity in colorectal cancer patients with tumors that do not express the epidermal growth factor receptor by immunohistochemistry. J Clin Oncol 23(9):1803–1810
48. Italiano A, Follana P, Caroli FX, Badetti JL, Benchimol D, Garnier G, Gugenheim J, Haudebourg J, Keslair F, Lesbats G, Lledo G, Roussel JF, Pedeutour F, Francois E (2008) Cetuximab shows activity in colorectal cancer patients with tumors for which FISH analysis does not detect an increase in EGFR gene copy number. Ann Surg Oncol 15(2):649–654
49. Scartozzi M, Bearzi I, Mandolesi A, Pierantoni C, Loupakis F, Zaniboni A, Negri F, Quadri A, Zorzi F, Galizia E, Berardi R, Biscotti T, Labianca R, Masi G, Falcone A, Cascinu S (2009) Epidermal Growth Factor Receptor (EGFR) gene copy number (GCN) correlates with clinical activity of irinotecan-cetuximab in K-RAS wild-type colorectal cancer: a fluorescence in situ (FISH) and chromogenic in situ hybridization (CISH) analysis. BMC Cancer 9:303
50. Bertotti A, Migliardi G, Galimi F, Sassi F, Torti D, Isella C, Cora D, Di Nicolantonio F, Buscarino M, Petti C, Ribero D, Russolillo N, Muratore A, Massucco P, Pisacane A, Molinaro L, Valtorta E, Sartore-Bianchi A, Risio M, Capussotti L, Gambacorta M, Siena S, Medico E, Sapino A, Marsoni S,

Comoglio PM, Bardelli A, Trusolino L (2011) A molecularly annotated platform of patient-derived xenografts ("xenopatients") identifies HER2 as an effective therapeutic target in cetuximab-resistant colorectal cancer. Cancer Discov 1(6):508–523

51. Leto SM, Sassi F, Catalano I, Torri V, Migliardi G, Zanella ER, Throsby M, Bertotti A, Trusolino L (2015) Sustained Inhibition of HER3 and EGFR Is Necessary to Induce Regression of HER2-Amplified Gastrointestinal Carcinomas. Clin Cancer Res 21 (24):5519–5531
52. Blackwell KL, Burstein HJ, Storniolo AM, Rugo H, Sledge G, Koehler M, Ellis C, Casey M, Vukelja S, Bischoff J, Baselga J, O'Shaughnessy J (2010) Randomized study of Lapatinib alone or in combination with trastuzumab in women with ErbB2-positive, trastuzumab-refractory metastatic breast cancer. J Clin Oncol 28(7):1124–1130
53. Li J, Qin S, Xu R, Yau TC, Ma B, Pan H, Xu J, Bai Y, Chi Y, Wang L, Yeh KH, Bi F, Cheng Y, Le AT, Lin JK, Liu T, Ma D, Kappeler C, Kalmus J, Kim TW, Investigators C (2015) Regorafenib plus best supportive care versus placebo plus best supportive care in Asian patients with previously treated metastatic colorectal cancer (CONCUR): a randomised, double-blind, placebo-controlled, phase 3 trial. Lancet Oncol 16(6):619–629
54. Xu Q, Xu AT, Zhu MM, Tong JL, Xu XT, Ran ZH (2013) Predictive and prognostic roles of BRAF mutation in patients with metastatic colorectal cancer treated with anti-epidermal growth factor receptor monoclonal antibodies: a meta-analysis. J Dig Dis 14(8):409–416
55. Yuan ZX, Wang XY, Qin QY, Chen DF, Zhong QH, Wang L, Wang JP (2013) The prognostic role of BRAF mutation in metastatic colorectal cancer receiving anti-EGFR monoclonal antibodies: a meta-analysis. PLoS One 8(6): e65995
56. Gavin PG, Colangelo LH, Fumagalli D, Tanaka N, Remillard MY, Yothers G, Kim C, Taniyama Y, Kim SI, Choi HJ, Blackmon NL, Lipchik C, Petrelli NJ, O'Connell MJ, Wolmark N, Paik S, Pogue-Geile KL (2012) Mutation profiling and microsatellite instability in stage II and III colon cancer: an assessment of their prognostic and oxaliplatin predictive value. Clin Cancer Res 18(23):6531–6541
57. Cremolini C, Loupakis F, Antoniotti C, Lupi C, Sensi E, Lonardi S, Mezi S, Tomasello G, Ronzoni M, Zaniboni A, Tonini G, Carlomagno C, Allegrini G, Chiara S, D'Amico M, Granetto C, Cazzaniga M, Boni L, Fontanini G, Falcone A (2015) FOLFOXIRI plus bevacizumab versus FOLFIRI plus bevacizumab as first-line treatment of patients with metastatic colorectal cancer: updated overall survival and molecular subgroup analyses of the open-label, phase 3 TRIBE study. Lancet Oncol 16 (13):1306–1315
58. Pietrantonio F, Petrelli F, Coinu A, Di Bartolomeo M, Borgonovo K, Maggi C, Cabiddu M, Iacovelli R, Bossi I, Lonati V, Ghilardi M, de Braud F, Barni S (2015) Predictive role of BRAF mutations in patients with advanced colorectal cancer receiving cetuximab and panitumumab: a meta-analysis. Eur J Cancer 51(5):587–594
59. Rowland A, Dias MM, Wiese MD, Kichenadasse G, McKinnon RA, Karapetis CS, Sorich MJ (2015) Meta-analysis of BRAF mutation as a predictive biomarker of benefit from anti-EGFR monoclonal antibody therapy for RAS wild-type metastatic colorectal cancer. Br J Cancer 112(12):1888–1894
60. Corcoran RB (2015) New therapeutic strategies for BRAF mutant colorectal cancers. J Gastrointest Oncol 6(6):650–659
61. Corcoran RB, Atreya CE, Falchook GS, Kwak EL, Ryan DP, Bendell JC, Hamid O, Messersmith WA, Daud A, Kurzrock R, Pierobon M, Sun P, Cunningham E, Little S, Orford K, Motwani M, Bai Y, Patel K, Venook AP, Kopetz S (2015) Combined BRAF and MEK Inhibition With Dabrafenib and Trametinib in BRAF V600-Mutant Colorectal Cancer. J Clin Oncol 33(34):4023–4031
62. Temraz S, Mukherji D, Shamseddine A (2015) Dual Inhibition of MEK and PI3K Pathway in KRAS and BRAF Mutated Colorectal Cancers. Int J Mol Sci 16(9):22976–22988
63. Corcoran R, Andre T, Yoshino T, Bendell J, Atreya C, Schellens J et al (2016) Efficacy and circulating tumor DNA (ctDNA) analysis of the BRAF inhibitor dabrafenib (D), MEK inhibitor trametinib (T), and anti-EGFR antibody panitumumab (P) in patients (pts) with BRAF V600E-mutated (BRAFm) metastatic colorectal cancer (mCRC). Ann Oncol 27 (suppl_6):455O
64. Kopetz S, McDonough S, Morris V, Lenz H-J, Magliocco T, Atreya C, Diaz LA, Allegra C, Wang S, Lieu C, Eckhardt SG, Semrad T, Kaberle K, Guthrie K, Hochster H (2017) Randomized trial of irinotecan and cetuximab with or without vemurafenib in BRAF-mutant metastatic colorectal cancer (SWOG 1406). J Clin Oncol 35(suppl 4S):abstract 520
65. Ahronian LG, Corcoran RB (2016) Effective MAPK Inhibition is critical for therapeutic

responses in colorectal cancer with BRAF mutations. Mol Cell Oncol 3(1):e1048405

66. Ahronian LG, Sennott EM, Van Allen EM, Wagle N, Kwak EL, Faris JE, Godfrey JT, Nishimura K, Lynch KD, Mermel CH, Lockerman EL, Kalsy A, Gurski JM Jr, Bahl S, Anderka K, Green LM, Lennon NJ, Huynh TG, Mino-Kenudson M, Getz G, Dias-Santagata D, Iafrate AJ, Engelman JA, Garraway LA, Corcoran RB (2015) Clinical acquired resistance to RAF inhibitor combinations in BRAF-Mutant colorectal cancer through MAPK pathway alterations. Cancer Discov 5(4):358–367
67. Oddo D, Sennott EM, Barault L, Valtorta E, Arena S, Cassingena A, Filiciotto G, Marzolla G, Elez E, van Geel RM, Bartolini A, Crisafulli G, Boscaro V, Godfrey JT, Buscarino M, Cancelliere C, Linnebacher M, Corti G, Truini M, Siravegna G, Grasselli J, Gallicchio M, Bernards R, Schellens JH, Tabernero J, Engelman JA, Sartore-Bianchi A, Bardelli A, Siena S, Corcoran RB, Di Nicolantonio F (2016) Molecular landscape of acquired resistance to targeted therapy combinations in BRAF-Mutant colorectal cancer. Cancer Res 76 (15):4504–4515
68. Jubb AM, Hurwitz HI, Bai W, Holmgren EB, Tobin P, Guerrero AS, Kabbinavar F, Holden SN, Novotny WF, Frantz GD, Hillan KJ, Koeppen H (2006) Impact of vascular endothelial growth factor-A expression, thrombospondin-2 expression, and microvessel density on the treatment effect of bevacizumab in metastatic colorectal cancer. J Clin Oncol 24(2):217–227
69. Foernzler D, Delmar P, Kockx M, Cassidy J, Saltz L, Scherer SJ (2010) Tumor tissue based biomarker analysis in NO16966: A randomized phase III study of first-line bevacizumab in combination with oxaliplatin-based chemotherapy in patients with mCRC. In: ASCO gastrointestinal cancers symposium, Orlando, FL, 22–24 January 2010, p Abstract 374
70. Gerger A, LaBonte M, Lenz HJ (2011) Molecular predictors of response to antiangiogenesis therapies. Cancer J 17(2):134–141
71. Hegde PS, Jubb AM, Chen D, Li NF, Meng YG, Bernaards C, Elliott R, Scherer SJ, Chen DS (2013) Predictive impact of circulating vascular endothelial growth factor in four phase III trials evaluating bevacizumab. Clin Cancer Res 19(4):929–937
72. Kopetz S, Hoff PM, Morris JS, Wolff RA, Eng C, Glover KY, Adinin R, Overman MJ, Valero V, Wen S, Lieu C, Yan S, Tran HT, Ellis LM, Abbruzzese JL, Heymach JV (2010) Phase II trial of infusional fluorouracil, irinotecan, and bevacizumab for metastatic colorectal cancer: efficacy and circulating angiogenic biomarkers associated with therapeutic resistance. J Clin Oncol 28(3):453–459
73. Semrad TJ, Kim EJ, Tanaka MS, Sands J, Roberts C, Burich RA, Li Y, Gandara DR, Lara P Jr, Mack PC (2017) Phase II study of dovitinib in patients progressing on anti-vascular endothelial growth factor therapy. Cancer Treat Res Commun 10:21–26
74. Parsons MT, Buchanan DD, Thompson B, Young JP, Spurdle AB (2012) Correlation of tumour BRAF mutations and MLH1 methylation with germline mismatch repair (MMR) gene mutation status: a literature review assessing utility of tumour features for MMR variant classification. J Med Genet 49(3):151–157
75. Sargent DJ, Marsoni S, Monges G, Thibodeau SN, Labianca R, Hamilton SR, French AJ, Kabat B, Foster NR, Torri V, Ribic C, Grothey A, Moore M, Zaniboni A, Seitz JF, Sinicrope F, Gallinger S (2010) Defective mismatch repair as a predictive marker for lack of efficacy of fluorouracil-based adjuvant therapy in colon cancer. J Clin Oncol 28 (20):3219–3226
76. Diaz LA Jr, Le DT (2015) PD-1 Blockade in Tumors with Mismatch-Repair Deficiency. N Engl J Med 373(20):1979
77. Hochster HS, Bendell JC, Cleary JM et al (2017) Efficacy and safety of atezolizumab (atezo) and bevacizumab (bev) in a phase 1b study of microsatellite instability (MSI)-high metastatic colorectal cancer (mCRC). J Clin Oncol 35(suppl 4S):abstract 673
78. Overman MJ, Lonardi S, Leone F et al (2017) Nivolumab in patients with DNA mismatch repair deficient/microsatellite instability high metastatic colorectal cancer: update from CheckMate 142. J Clin Oncol 35(suppl 4S): abstract 519
79. Bendell J, Kim TW, Goh BC, Wallin J, Oh D-Y, Han S-W, Lee C, Hellmann MD, Desai J, Lewin J, Solomon BJ, Chow LQ, Miller WH, Gainor J, Flaherty K, Infante J, Thakur MD, Foster P, Cha E, Bang Y-J (2016) Clinical activity and safety of cobimetinib and atezolizumab in colorectal cancer. J Clin Oncol 34 (suppl):abstr 3052
80. Budinska E, Popovici V, Tejpar S, D'Ario G, Lapique N, Sikora KO, Di Narzo AF, Yan P, Hodgson JG, Weinrich S, Bosman F, Roth A, Delorenzi M (2013) Gene expression patterns unveil a new level of molecular heterogeneity in colorectal cancer. J Pathol 231(1):63–76
81. Marisa L, de Reynies A, Duval A, Selves J, Gaub MP, Vescovo L, Etienne-Grimaldi MC,

Schiappa R, Guenot D, Ayadi M, Kirzin S, Chazal M, Flejou JF, Benchimol D, Berger A, Lagarde A, Pencreach E, Piard F, Elias D, Parc Y, Olschwang S, Milano G, Laurent-Puig P, Boige V (2013) Gene expression classification of colon cancer into molecular subtypes: characterization, validation, and prognostic value. PLoS Med 10(5):e1001453

82. Roepman P, Schlicker A, Tabernero J, Majewski I, Tian S, Moreno V, Snel MH, Chresta CM, Rosenberg R, Nitsche U, Macarulla T, Capella G, Salazar R, Orphanides G, Wessels LF, Bernards R, Simon IM (2014) Colorectal cancer intrinsic subtypes predict chemotherapy benefit, deficient mismatch repair and epithelial-to-mesenchymal transition. Int J Cancer 134 (3):552–562
83. Sadanandam A, Lyssiotis CA, Homicsko K, Collisson EA, Gibb WJ, Wullschleger S, Ostos LC, Lannon WA, Grotzinger C, Del Rio M, Lhermitte B, Olshen AB, Wiedenmann B, Cantley LC, Gray JW, Hanahan D (2013) A colorectal cancer classification system that associates cellular phenotype and responses to therapy. Nat Med 19(5):619–625
84. De Sousa EMF, Wang X, Jansen M, Fessler E, Trinh A, de Rooij LP, de Jong JH, de Boer OJ, van Leersum R, Bijlsma MF, Rodermond H, van der Heijden M, van Noesel CJ, Tuynman JB, Dekker E, Markowetz F, Medema JP, Vermeulen L (2013) Poor-prognosis colon cancer is defined by a molecularly distinct subtype and develops from serrated precursor lesions. Nat Med 19(5):614–618
85. Schlicker A, Beran G, Chresta CM, McWalter G, Pritchard A, Weston S, Runswick S, Davenport S, Heathcote K, Castro DA, Orphanides G, French T, Wessels LF (2012) Subtypes of primary colorectal tumors correlate with response to targeted treatment in colorectal cell lines. BMC Med Genet 5:66
86. Cancer Genome Atlas N (2012) Comprehensive molecular characterization of human colon and rectal cancer. Nature 487(7407):330–337
87. Dienstmann R, Vermeulen L, Guinney J, Kopetz S, Tejpar S, Tabernero J (2017) Consensus molecular subtypes and the evolution of precision medicine in colorectal cancer. Nat Rev Cancer 17(4):268
88. Guinney J, Dienstmann R, Wang X, de Reynies A, Schlicker A, Soneson C, Marisa L, Roepman P, Nyamundanda G, Angelino P, Bot BM, Morris JS, Simon IM, Gerster S, Fessler E, De Sousa EMF, Missiaglia E, Ramay H, Barras D, Homicsko K, Maru D, Manyam GC, Broom B, Boige V, Perez-Villamil B, Laderas T, Salazar R, Gray JW, Hanahan D, Tabernero J, Bernards R, Friend SH, Laurent-Puig P, Medema JP, Sadanandam A, Wessels L, Delorenzi M, Kopetz S, Vermeulen L, Tejpar S (2015) The consensus molecular subtypes of colorectal cancer. Nat Med 21(11):1350–1356
89. Marisa L, Ayadi M, Balogoun R, Pilati C, Le Malicot K, Lepage C, Emile JF, Salazar R, Aust DE, Duval A, Selves J, Guenot D, Milano G, Seitz JF, Taieb J, Boige V, de Reynies A, Laurent-Puig P (2017) Clinical utility of colon cancer molecular subtypes: validation of two main colorectal molecular classifications on the PETACC-8 phase III trial cohort. J Clin Oncol 35(suppl):abstract 3509
90. Lenz HJ, Ou FS, Venook AP, Hochster H, Niedzwiecki D, Goldberg RM, Mayer RJ, Bertagnolli MM, Blanke CD, Zemla T, Qu X, Innocenti F, Kabbarah O (2017) Impact of consensus molecular subtyping (CMS) on overall survival (OS) and progression free survival (PFS) in patients (pts) with metastatic colorectal cancer (mCRC): Analysis of CALGB/SWOG 80405 (Alliance). J Clin Oncol 35(suppl):abstract 3511
91. Stintzing S, Wirapati P, Lenz HJ, Neureiter D, von Weikersthal LF, Decker T, Kiani A, Vehling-Kaiser U, Al-Batran SE, Heintges T, Kahl C, Kullmann F, Moehler M, Scheithauer W, Held S, Modest DP, Jung A, Kirchner T, Tejpar S, Heinemann V, Investigators F (2017) Consensus molecular subgroups (CMS) of colorectal cancer (CRC) and first-line efficacy of FOLFIRI plus cetuximab or bevacizumab in the FIRE3 (AIO KRK-0306) trial. J Clin Oncol 35(suppl):abstract 3510

Check for updates

Chapter 19

Testing Cell-Based Immunotherapy for Colorectal Cancer

Jong Soon Kang, Yeo Dae Yoon, Myeong Youl Lee, Chang Woo Lee, Suk Jong Lee, and Sang-Bae Han

Abstract

Cell-based immunotherapy for cancer is emerging as an attractive alternative to conventional small-molecule or antibody-based treatment. Due to the characteristics of cell-based therapy, validation of test materials before in vivo administration is required. Here we describe general validation steps for preclinical evaluation of cell-based immunotherapy. We also describe a xenograft model of human colorectal cancer. This model can be used for applied to preclinical evaluation of various cell-based therapy regimens for colorectal cancer treatment.

Key words Immunotherapy, Immune cells, Colorectal cancer, Cell line, Human tumor xenograft model

1 Introduction

Cell-based immunotherapy, which aims at treating cancer patients by stimulating the response of their own immune system with autologous or allogeneic cells, is a promising tool for cancer treatment [1]. The major objective of cell-based cancer immunotherapy is the destruction of cancer cells by targeting tumor-specific or tumor-associated antigen(s) by means of boosting the antigen-specific immune response. Cell-based immunotherapy for cancer uses several types of immune cells, including T cells, dendritic cells, and natural killer cells [2–4]. Colorectal cancer (CRC) is one of the most prevalent cancers worldwide [1]. Although advances in treatment have improved the overall survival, further treatment options are required for efficient management of colorectal cancer patients. Among various therapeutic options, cell-based immunotherapy is considered promising for CRC treatment [1]. Clinical and preclinical development of cell-based immunotherapy using dendritic cells [5], T lymphocytes [6], and cytokine-induced killer cells [1] for CRC treatment has been reported, but currently there is no clinically approved cell-based immunotherapy for CRC. To use these

Jean-François Beaulieu (ed.), *Colorectal Cancer: Methods and Protocols*, Methods in Molecular Biology, vol. 1765, https://doi.org/10.1007/978-1-4939-7765-9_19,

cells as therapy regimens, they need to be collected, expanded, and characterized. However, due to their complexity, these cells cannot be fully characterized. Nevertheless, the biological activities and characteristics of these cells need to be determined and validated for their proper use in research or for clinical purposes.

Here, we describe several essential characteristics that need to be validated before preclinical evaluation of cell-based immunotherapy. We also describe general protocols for human tumor xenograft models that use various colorectal cancer cell lines.

2 Materials

2.1 Cell Viability Analysis and Phenotyping by Flow Cytometry

1. Phosphate-buffered saline (PBS): Dissolve 8 g of NaCl, 0.2 g of KCl, 1.44 g of Na_2HPO_4, and 0.24 g of KH_2PO_4 in 800 mL of H_2O. Adjust the pH to 7.4 with HCl, and then add H_2O to 1 L. Store at room temperature.
2. PBS containing 1% bovine serum albumin (PBS/BSA): Add 1 g of BSA to 100 mL of PBS. If desired, add 0.2 mL of 10% sodium azide. Store at 4 °C.
3. Propidium iodide (PI) staining solution: 10 μg/mL of propidium iodide in PBS (*see* **Note 1**). Store at 4 °C. Protect from light.
4. Fluorescein-conjugated antibodies.

2.2 In Vitro Cytotoxicity Assay

1. A U-bottomed 96-well plate.
2. 2% Triton X-100 in culture medium.
3. Scintillation vials.
4. Scintillation cocktail.
5. ^{51}Cr.
6. γ-counter.

2.3 Cell Culture and Preparation for Injection

1. Colon cancer cells lines: HCT-116 (ATCC® CCL-247™), HCT-15 (ATCC® CCL-225™), HT-29 (ATCC® HTB-38™), SW620 (ATCC® CCL-227™), COLO 205 (ATCC® CCL-222™), DLD-1 (ATCC® CCL-221™), SW480 (ATCC® CCL-228™), WiDr (ATCC® CCL-218™).
2. Cell culture media: RPMI-1640, McCoy's 5a, Eagle's Minimum Essential Medium (MEM), or Leibovitz's L-15, with or without 10% fetal bovine serum (FBS).
3. A cell culture incubator: a 37 °C incubator with a humidified atmosphere equilibrated with 5% CO_2 and 95% air.
4. Trypsin–EDTA solution: add 2.5 g trypsin and 0.2 g EDTA·4Na to 800 mL PBS and then add PBS to 1 L. Store in aliquots at −20 °C.

5. A Coulter counter or hemocytometer.
6. Basement membrane matrix proteins: Matrigel or CultrexBME.

2.4 Transplantation

1. Immunodeficient mice: nude mice, severe combined immunodeficiency (SCID) mice, or nonobese diabetic (NOD)/SCID mice.
2. 70% ethanol: mix 73.7 mL of 95% ethanol and 26.3 mL of distilled water. Store at room temperature.
3. A 1 cc syringe with a 21 G, 23 G, or 26 G needle.
4. Vernier calipers.

3 Methods

3.1 Cell Viability Analysis

1. Harvest and wash 1×10^6 cells once with 1 mL of PBS. Collect cells by centrifugation at $225 \times g$ and discard the supernatant. Resuspend cells in 100 μL of PBS and add 5–10 μL of PI staining solution just prior to analysis.
2. Analyze cells by flow cytometry (Fig. 1, *see* **Note 2**).

3.2 Phenotyping of Immune Cells

1. Harvest and wash 1×10^6 cells once with 1 mL of PBS/BSA. Collect cells by centrifugation and discard the supernatant. Resuspend cells in 100 μL of PBS/BSA.
2. Incubate cells with appropriate antibodies for 30 min at 4 °C. Wash twice with 1 mL of PBS/BSA, collect cells by centrifugation, and discard the supernatant. Resuspend cells in 400 μL of PBS/BSA.
3. Analyze cells by flow cytometry (Fig. 1, *see* **Note 3**).

3.3 Evaluation of Cytotoxicity In Vitro (see Note 4)

1. Label 2×10^6 target cancer cells with 100 μCi of ^{51}Cr for 4 h in a cell culture incubator at 37 °C. Wash cells three times with 10 mL of culture medium and resuspend them in 10 mL of culture medium.
2. Plate target cells (1×10^4 cells per well in 50 μL of culture medium) into U-bottomed 96-well plates and incubate them for 4 h with 100 μL of effector cells at various effector-to-target ratios (*see* **Note 5**).
3. Remove the cells by centrifugation and transfer 100 μL of the supernatant into a scintillation vial. Add scintillation cocktail and measure radioactivity using a γ-counter.
4. Calculate the percentage of specific lysis by using the following formula: (experimental release − target spontaneous release)/(target maximum release − target spontaneous release) × 100%.

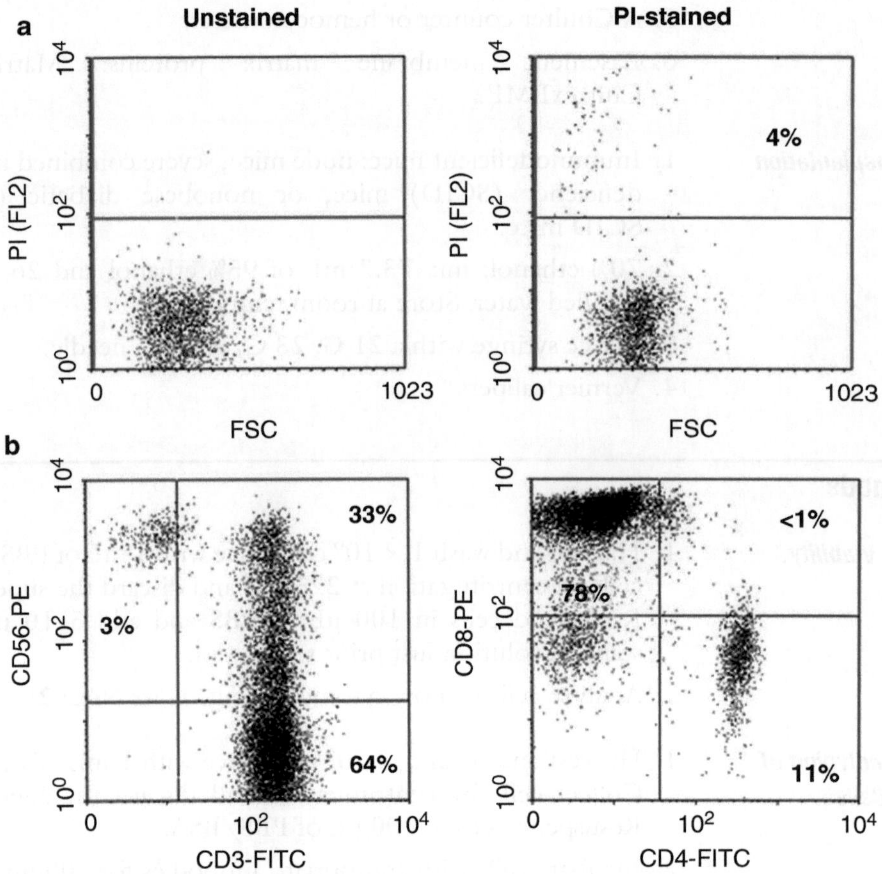

Fig. 1 Examples of the analysis of viability and phenotype of immune cells. (**a**) Viability of cytokine-induced killer cells was determined by PI staining and flow cytometry. (**b**) Phenotypes of cytokine-induced killer cells were analyzed before injection into mice

3.4 Cell Culture and Preparation for Injection

1. Thaw cells and culture them in appropriate medium (Table 1) at 37 °C in an incubator with a humidified atmosphere equilibrated with 5% CO_2 and 95% air (*see* **Notes 6** and **7**). Maintain cells in an exponential growth phase and passage before they reach confluence.

2. Harvest cells during exponential growth using trypsin–EDTA solution (*see* **Note 8**). Resuspend cells in medium containing FBS. Count cells in a Coulter counter or a hemocytometer. Centrifuge cells at 225 × *g* for 5 min. Remove the medium and resuspend cells in medium without FBS at an appropriate concentration (Table 1). Keep the suspension on ice until transplantation (*see* **Note 9**).

3. (Optional) Certain cancer cells, such as SW480, require basement membrane matrix proteins for tumor formation. Thaw basement membrane matrix proteins, such as Matrigel or CultrexBME, on ice (*see* **Note 10**). Add cold medium without FBS

Table 1
Commonly used CRC cell lines, recommended culture media, and cell numbers for transplantation

Cell line	Culture medium	Cell number for transplantation (per mouse)
HCT 116	McCoy's 5a	1.2×10^7
HCT-15	RPMI-1640	1.2×10^7
HT-29	McCoy's 5a	9×10^6
SW620	Leibovitz's L-15	9×10^6
COLO 205	RPMI-1640	9×10^6
DLD-1	RPMI-1640	9×10^6
SW480[a]	Leibovitz's L-15	9×10^6
WiDr	Eagle's MEM	9×10^6

[a]Transplantation requires the use of basement membrane matrix proteins

to the cell pellet (the volume depends on the desired final injection volume) and mix with an equal volume of basement membrane matrix proteins (*see* **Note 11**).

3.5 Transplantation

1. Clean the injection area with 70% ethanol. Agitate the cell suspension to disperse the cells homogeneously and withdraw it into a 1 cc syringe with the needle removed. Install a 26 G needle and inject 0.3 mL of the cell suspension into the flank of an appropriate immunodeficient mouse subcutaneously (*see* **Note 12**).
2. Monitor tumor growth and initiate treatment when tumor volumes reach an appropriate size (*see* **Note 13**). Measure tumor volume 2–3 times a week using vernier calipers. Calculate tumor volumes using the following equation (*see* **Note 14**).

$$\text{Tumor volume}\ (\text{mm}^3) = \pi/6 \times [\text{length (mm)} \times \text{width (mm)} \times \text{height (mm)}].$$

4 Notes

1. Although PI is not currently listed as a carcinogen by NTP (National Toxicology Program of the US Department of Health and Human Services), IARC (International Agency for Research on Cancer of the World Health Organization), or OSHA (Occupational Safety and Health Administration of the US Department of Labor), PI is a suspected carcinogen and should be handled with care.
2. Analyze cell viability every time after cell preparation before injection.

3. Select appropriate surface antigens for characterization of the cells to be injected and analyze the phenotype of these cells every time after cell preparation before injection.
4. Cytotoxicity can also be assayed by using other methods. For example, if you cannot use a radioisotope, you can label target cells with Calcein-AM and analyze cytotoxicity by measuring fluorescence in the culture supernatant.
5. Effector-to-target ratio can be set from 0.3:1 to 100:1 depending on the activity of effector cells.
6. When culturing cells in Leibovitz's L-15 medium, allow free gas exchange with atmospheric air. Leibovitz's L-15 medium is designed for use in CO_2-free systems, and culturing cells in this medium in a mixture of CO_2 and air is detrimental to cells.
7. Cells should be tested for possible contamination with mycoplasma or viruses, which might be harmful to immunodeficient mice.
8. Before detaching cells with trypsin–EDTA, rinse them with PBS to remove residual serum.
9. Inject collected cells as soon as possible. Certain cancer cells do not initiate tumor formation if they are kept in suspension for a long time before injection. We usually inject cancer cells within 30 min of collection. If the number of animals is large, collect only part of cancer cells at a time to reduce the time from cell collection to injection.
10. After thawing Matrigel or CultrexBME, keep it on ice at all times. Thawed Matrigel or CultrexBME should be inverted several times to ensure even mixing. Undiluted Matrigel or CultrexBME can be aliquoted and refrozen at −20 °C or −80 °C or stored at 4 °C for a few days [7].
11. Cell suspension should be cold when basement membrane matrix proteins are added. Use prechilled pipettes and syringes when handling basement membrane matrix proteins or cell suspensions.
12. Because cancer cells listed in Table 1 are small, a 26 G needle is adequate. If the cells are large, use a 23 G or 21 G needle to avoid cell damage.
13. We usually initiate treatment when the tumor volume reaches 50–150 mm^3. Initial tumor volume may vary depending on the purpose of the experiment.
14. Tumor volume can be calculated by using other formulas. The formulas that estimate tumor mass most accurately are $\pi/6 \times$ [length (mm) $\times$ width (mm) $\times$ height (mm)] or $1/2 \times$ [length (mm) $\times$ width (mm) $\times$ height (mm)]. However, many researchers use simplified formulas,

$1/2 \times$ [length (mm) $\times$ width (mm)^2] or $\pi/6 \times$ [length (mm) $\times$ width (mm)^2], for convenience. If tumors are multi-lobed, the volume of each lobe is calculated, and the final value is calculated by summation of the volumes of all lobes.

Acknowledgment

This work was supported by grants funded by the KRIBB Research Initiative Program and the Korean Government (NRF-2008-0062275).

References

1. Kim JS, Kim YG, Park EJ, Kim B, Lee HK, Hong JT et al (2016) Cell-based immunotherapy for colorectal cancer with cytokine-induced killer cells. Immune Netw 16(2):99–108
2. Houot R, Schultz LM, Marabelle A, kohrt H (2015) T-cell-based immunotherapy: adaptive cell transfer and checkpoint inhibition. Cancer Immunol Res 3(10):1115–1122
3. Sabado RL, Balan S, Bhardwaj N (2017) Dendritic cell-based immunotherapy. Cell Res 27 (1):74–95
4. Subrahmanyam PB, Sun W, East JE, Li J, Webb TJ (2012) Natural killer T cell based immunotherapy. J Vaccines Vaccin 3:144
5. Kajihara M, Takakura K, Kanai T, Ito Z, Saito K, Takami S et al (2016) Dendritic cell-based cancer immunotherapy for colorectal cancer. World J Gastroenterol 22(17):4275–4286
6. Zhen YH, Liu XH, Yang Y, Li B, Tang JL, Zeng QX et al (2015) Phase I/II study of adjuvant immunotherapy with sentinel lymph node T lymphocytes in patients with colorectal cancer. Cancer Immunol Immunother 64 (9):1083–1093
7. Fridman R, Benton B, Aranoutova I, Kleinman HK Bonfil RD (2012) Increased initiation and growth of tumor cell lines, cancer stem cells and biopsy materials in mice using basement membrane matrix protein (Cultrex or Matrigel) co-injection. Nat Protoc 7(6):1138–1144

Chapter 20

Patient-Derived Xenograft Models of Colorectal Cancer: Procedures for Engraftment and Propagation

Danielle M. Burgenske, David J. Monsma, and Jeffrey P. MacKeigan

Abstract

Preclinical compounds tested in animal models often demonstrate limited efficacy when transitioned into patients. As a result, individuals are assigned to treatment regimens that may be ineffective at treating their disease. The development of more clinically relevant models, such as patient-derived xenografts (PDXs), will (1) more completely mimic the human condition and (2) more accurately predict tumor responses to previously untested therapeutics.

PDX models are clinically relevant as tumor tissue is implanted directly from human donor to the mouse recipient. Therefore, these models prevent cell population selection, intentional or unintentional, as the human tissue adapts to an in vitro, two-dimensional environment prior to implantation into a three-dimensional in vivo murine host. Often, cell heterogeneity and tumor architecture can be maintained from human to the PDX model in the mouse. This protocol describes the engraftment and propagation processes for establishing colorectal (CRC) PDX models in mice, using tumor tissue from human subjects.

Key words Tumor heterogeneity, Preclinical in vivo efficacy, Drug screening, Colorectal cancer, Patient-derived xenograft, Tumorgraft

1 Introduction

Collaborations between oncology providers and biomedical research organizations provide opportunities to conduct science that can transform current clinical practices. The propagation of patient-derived tumor samples in immunocompromised mice allows laboratories to (1) replenish this valuable but limited resource and (2) generate relevant PDX models that accurately reflect cancer's inherent heterogeneity. Therefore, PDX models can aid researchers in investigating the pressing questions in the oncology field. PDX models are particularly valuable for preclinical drug testing, as simpler mouse models cannot accurately predict the antitumor efficacy of novel therapeutics [1–4].

Excluding skin cancers, CRC is the third most common cancer in the United States. The American Cancer Society (ACS) projects

Jean-François Beaulieu (ed.), *Colorectal Cancer: Methods and Protocols*, Methods in Molecular Biology, vol. 1765, https://doi.org/10.1007/978-1-4939-7765-9_20,

135,430 individuals will be diagnosed with CRC in 2017 with 50,260 succumbing to their disease [5]. While 5-year survival rates remain high for patients diagnosed in the early stages of disease, a stage IV diagnosis reduces survival to near 10%. This low survival rate highlights the lack of clinical advances for late stage colorectal cancer; many agents that show promise in early preclinical testing have ultimately failed in human clinical trials.

This high attrition rate demonstrates the inability of current preclinical CRC models to evaluate novel therapeutic regimens and identify proper patient populations for these targeted therapies [6]. While the factors that influence the utility of a given preclinical model are complex, evidence suggests that long term culturing of cancer cell lines promotes the loss of specific cell populations in conjunction with genomic alterations [7, 8]. To address this problem, CRC PDX models were established to better recapitulate the histological features of the disease, while also maintaining a high degree of genomic complexity [9–11]. These characteristics are uncommon in most other preclinical models [4, 12]. Given this high degree of fidelity to its human counterpart, PDX models are a valuable resource in the study of therapeutics, including chemotherapy, targeted therapy, and personalized medicine approaches.

Here we describe a method in which we isolate freshly resected tumor specimens from colorectal cancer patients for subcutaneous engraftment into athymic nude mice. This approach supports tissue viability and maintains sterility, and also creates stocks from which these PDX models can be established. The detailed instructions will provide a step-by-step protocol for colorectal PDX model generation. Moreover, this protocol uses consumables, equipment, and media components usually found within a general laboratory environment to facilitate initiation of PDX studies.

2 Materials

Note: All cell culture and tumor isolation work should be performed inside a tissue culture hood to maintain sterility.

2.1 Tissue

Surgically resected primary tissue (colon or rectal tumors) or patient-derived xenograft tissue.

2.2 Supplies

1. Sterile petri dishes (100 mm).
2. Sterile conical centrifuge tubes (50 mL).
3. Serological pipettes (25, 10, and 10 mL).
4. Sterile cryovials (2 mL).
5. Wet ice.
6. Dry ice pellets.

2.3 Surgical Tools

1. Sterilized scalpel, #10.
2. Sterilized dissecting straight scissors, 14/15 mm blade.
3. Sterilized dissecting forceps.
4. Surgical staples, 9 mm.
5. Hypodermic needle, 27 g.
6. Syringes, 1 cc.
7. Surgical gloves.

2.4 Equipment

1. Animal ear-tag punch.
2. Heating pad.
3. Calipers.
4. Rodent anesthesia machine (Parkland Scientific, USA).
5. CO_2 tank.
6. 37 °C water bath.
7. Mr. Frosty™ Freezing container (Nalgene, USA).

2.5 Media, Buffers, and Solutions

1. Sterile phosphate buffered saline, pH 7.2.
2. Ketoprofen (Ketofen®, Zoetis, USA).
3. Betadine or 70% ethanol.
4. Isoflurane (Abbot Labs, USA).
5. Isopropyl alcohol.

2.6 Transport Media

1. Sterile tissue culture media (RPMI-1640 medium with L-glutamine and 25 mM HEPES).
2. Fetal bovine serum.
3. Penicillin–streptomycin.
4. Heparin, 25,000 units.

2.7 Cryopreservation Media

1. Sterile tissue culture media (RPMI-1640 medium with L-glutamine and 25 mM HEPES).
2. Fetal bovine serum.
3. Penicillin–streptomycin.
4. Dimethyl sulfoxide (DMSO).

2.8 Animals

Most immunocompromised mice are acceptable for the experiment.

Six-to-ten-week-old immunocompromised [athymic nude (nu/nu), severe combined immune deficiency (SCID), or NOD *scid* gamma (NSG) mouse strains].

3 Methods

3.1 Implantation of Patient Tumor Samples into Mice (See Note 1)

1. Prepare transport media prior to tumor resection [RPMI 1640 media, 10% fetal bovine serum, 1% penicillin–streptomycin, and 50 units/mL heparin].
2. Using an ear punch or other IACUC approved method of animal identification, confirm that each experimental animal has been marked to allow for individual tumors to be tracked at engraftment. Mice should be gender-matched to the donor patient.
3. Resected tumor specimens are aseptically collected into 50 mL conical tubes containing 25 mL transport media. The corresponding sample log sheet should denote the location of specimen, diagnosis, and time of resection.
4. Specimens are transported to the lab on wet ice as rapidly as possible, 30–60 min post-surgery (*see* **Note 2**).
5. Aseptic techniques and appropriate personal protective equipment (PPE) are required. Upon receipt, move tumor specimens to individual 100 mm petri dishes containing 10 mL of sterile phosphate buffered saline.
6. Use scalpel and dissecting forceps to separate tumor into 3 mm × 3 mm × 3 mm fragments, removing any necrotic tissue as necessary. Healthy tumor tissue will appear pink or reddish in color with tumor vascularization and a range in texture from soft with firmer nodules to generally firm tissue. Necrotic tissue is typically abnormally colored, with either a gelatinous/liquid or a hard fibrotic consistency (*see* **Note 3**).
7. An ideal surgically resected tissue size would allow for five or more tumor fragments (3 mm × 3 mm × 3 mm). Implant three mice with fresh tumor fragments, while two tumor fragments are banked for future use. Snap-freeze one fragment for genomic analysis and formalin-fix the remaining fragment for histology. This exact number of tumor fragments will be dependent on the size and amount of viable tumor tissue that is received. Typically a maximum of five animals are implanted with fresh tumor fragments.
8. Weigh each mouse and administer an intraperitoneal dose of the analgesic Ketoprofen (5 mg/kg body weight) using a 27 g hypodermic needle.
9. Following induction of anesthesia using 2% isoflurane and induction chamber, confirm that the animal exhibits loss of pedal reflex.
10. Position animal in surgical station, under 2% isoflurane via nose cone, with right flank orientated up (*see* **Note 4**).

11. Clean right flank with Betadine or 70% ethanol at the surgical site.
12. Lifting the right flank with a forceps, use the dissection scissors to make a 1 cm incision.
13. While holding the incision open with forceps, make a pocket under the skin by blunt dissection with the scissors.
14. Using a second forceps, carefully insert the tumor fragment into the subcutaneous pocket, minimizing contact of the tumor fragment with the skin surface as much as possible (*see* **Note 5**).
15. Close the subcutaneous pocket using a single 9 mm surgical staple.
16. Following closure, return animals to their cage and place on a warmer until animals are fully recovered (*see* **Note 6**).
17. Return animals to their normal housing location.
18. Observe mice weekly collecting both body weight measurements and caliper-based tumor volumes during tumorgraft development (*see* **Note 7**).
19. Euthanize mice when tumors either reach 1500 mm^3 in size, exhibit no observable growth at 6 months following implantation, or animals meet any IACUC criteria for euthanasia.
20. Use aseptic techniques to harvest tumor for (1) further propagation, (2) cryopreservation, and (3) formalin fixation (*see* **Note 8**).

3.2 Serial Propagation of Flank Tumor Xenografts

1. Euthanize tumor-bearing mice using CO_2 and anesthesia machine.
2. Aseptically clean the site around the tumor with Betadine or 70% ethanol.
3. Using a forceps and scalpel, carefully separate the skin from the tumor below, minimizing contact with the tumor.
4. Using a sterile forceps, carefully lift tumor from muscle wall and place into a sterile petri dish containing 10 mL PBS (*see* **Note 5**).
5. Repeat **steps 3.1.6–3.1.16** above.

3.3 Cryopreservation of Xenograft Tumor Samples

1. Label cryovials with the lineage information of each tumor being frozen.
2. Prepare cryo media prior to tumor resection [RPMI 1640 media, 10% fetal bovine serum, 1% penicillin–streptomycin, and 10% DMSO].
3. Add 1.0 mL of cryopreservation media into each cryovial.
4. Repeat **steps 3.2.1–3.2.4** above.

5. Use scalpel and dissecting forceps to separate tumor into 3 mm × 3 mm × 3 mm fragments, removing any necrotic tissue as necessary.
6. Place tumor fragments each into a cryovial.
7. Slow freeze cryovials using a Mr. Frosty™ Freezing Container and isopropyl alcohol, or similar apparatus in a −80 °C freezer for 24 h, and then transfer the samples to long term storage in cryogenic liquid nitrogen storage.

3.4 Xenograft Restoration from Cryopreserved Samples

1. Remove cryovials from cryogenic liquid nitrogen storage and transport to surgical site on dry ice.
2. After the animal is prepped for surgery, rapidly thaw the vial by immersion in 37° C degree water bath and place tumor tissue and residual media into a 10 cm petri dish containing 10 mL PBS.
3. Repeat **steps 3.1.6–3.1.16** above.

4 Notes

1. Prior to initiating tumorgraft studies, the appropriate Institutional Review Board (IRB) and Institutional Animal Care and Use Committee (IACUC) approvals must be in place to use human tissue and animal models, respectively.
2. Time between resection and engraftment should be prompt as delayed engraftment can negatively impact tumor take rates. Therefore, time of shipment and receipt should be recorded for each sample.
3. The tumor tissue may not be viable if tissue is difficult to tease apart or separate into necessary tumor fragment sizes.
4. This protocol is a subcutaneous heterotopic PDX model. Examples of orthotopic CRC PDX models can be found in the literature [13–15].
5. Whenever possible, use separate sterile instruments when handling or manipulating the skin of the animal and when handling the tumor tissue. Goal is to minimize risk of introducing any foreign material or pathogen into the subcutaneous pocket.
6. While our group routinely uses warmers to facilitate animal recovery, others labs that create PDX models may or may not use warming pads.
7. Tumors could take up to 1 year to grow following implantation of a primary tumor. Most implantations will form palpable tumor within 6 months, but some may take longer.

8. It is also possible to establish short-lived explant cultures from isolated tumors as well. Tumors should be minced into fine pieces before being placed inside sterile dishes suitable for tissue culture, topping off with fresh.

References

1. Burgenske DM, Monsma DJ, Dylewski D, Scott SB, Sayfie AD, Kim DG, Luchtefeld M, Martin KR, Stephenson P, Hostetter G, Dujovny N, MacKeigan JP (2014) Establishment of genetically diverse patient-derived xenografts of colorectal cancer. Am J Cancer Res 4(6):824–837
2. Monsma DJ, Cherba DM, Richardson PJ, Vance S, Rangarajan S, Dylewski D, Eugster E, Scott SB, Beuschel NL, Davidson PJ, Axtell R, Mitchell D, Lester EP, Junewick JJ, Webb CP, Monks NR (2014) Using a rhabdomyosarcoma patient-derived xenograft to examine precision medicine approaches and model acquired resistance. Pediatr Blood Cancer 61(9):1570–1577
3. Monsma DJ, Cherba DM, Eugster EE, Dylewski DL, Davidson PT, Peterson CA, Borgman AS, Winn ME, Dykema KJ, Webb CP, MacKeigan JP, Duesbery NS, Nickoloff BJ, Monks NR (2015) Melanoma patient derived xenografts acquire distinct Vemurafenib resistance mechanisms. Am J Cancer Res 5 (4):1507–1518
4. Siolas D, Hannon GJ (2013) Patient-derived tumor xenografts: transforming clinical samples into mouse models. Cancer Res 73 (17):5315–5319
5. Society AC (2017) Cancer Facts & Figures 2017
6. Tentler JJ, Tan AC, Weekes CD, Jimeno A, Leong S, Pitts TM, Arcaroli JJ, Messersmith WA, Eckhardt SG (2012) Patient-derived tumour xenografts as models for oncology drug development. Nat Rev Clin Oncol 9 (6):338–350
7. Hidalgo M, Amant F, Biankin AV, Budinska E, Byrne AT, Caldas C, Clarke RB, de Jong S, Jonkers J, Maelandsmo GM, Roman-Roman S, Seoane J, Trusolino L, Villanueva A (2014) Patient-derived xenograft models: an emerging platform for translational cancer research. Cancer Discov 4(9):998–1013
8. Brown KM, Xue A, Mittal A, Samra JS, Smith R, Hugh TJ (2016) Patient-derived xenograft models of colorectal cancer in pre-clinical research: a systematic review. Oncotarget 7(40):66212–66225
9. Bertotti A, Migliardi G, Galimi F, Sassi F, Torti D, Isella C, Cora D, Di Nicolantonio F, Buscarino M, Petti C, Ribero D, Russolillo N, Muratore A, Massucco P, Pisacane A, Molinaro L, Valtorta E, Sartore-Bianchi A, Risio M, Capussotti L, Gambacorta M, Siena S, Medico E, Sapino A, Marsoni S, Comoglio PM, Bardelli A, Trusolino L (2011) A molecularly annotated platform of patient-derived xenografts ("xenopatients") identifies HER2 as an effective therapeutic target in cetuximab-resistant colorectal cancer. Cancer Discov 1(6):508–523
10. Julien S, Merino-Trigo A, Lacroix L, Pocard M, Goere D, Mariani P, Landron S, Bigot L, Nemati F, Dartigues P, Weiswald LB, Lantuas D, Morgand L, Pham E, Gonin P, Dangles-Marie V, Job B, Dessen P, Bruno A, Pierre A, De The H, Soliman H, Nunes M, Lardier G, Calvet L, Demers B, Prevost G, Vrignaud P, Roman-Roman S, Duchamp O, Berthet C (2012) Characterization of a large panel of patient-derived tumor xenografts representing the clinical heterogeneity of human colorectal cancer. Clin Cancer Res 18 (19):5314–5328
11. Migliardi G, Sassi F, Torti D, Galimi F, Zanella ER, Buscarino M, Ribero D, Muratore A, Massucco P, Pisacane A, Risio M, Capussotti L, Marsoni S, Di Nicolantonio F, Bardelli A, Comoglio PM, Trusolino L, Bertotti A (2012) Inhibition of MEK and PI3K/mTOR suppresses tumor growth but does not cause tumor regression in patient-derived xenografts of RAS-mutant colorectal carcinomas. Clin Cancer Res 18(9):2515–2525
12. Williams SA, Anderson WC, Santaguida MT, Dylla SJ (2013) Patient-derived xenografts, the cancer stem cell paradigm, and cancer pathobiology in the 21st century. Lab Investig 93 (9):970–982
13. Puig I, Chicote I, Tenbaum SP, Arques O, Herance JR, Gispert JD, Jimenez J, Landolfi S, Caci K, Allende H, Mendizabal L, Moreno D, Charco R, Espin E, Prat A, Elez ME, Argiles G, Vivancos A, Tabernero J, Rojas S, Palmer HG (2013) A personalized preclinical model to evaluate the metastatic potential of patient-derived colon cancer

initiating cells. Clin Cancer Res 19 (24):6787–6801
14. Furukawa T, Kubota T, Watanabe M, Kuo TH, Nishibori H, Kase S, Saikawa Y, Tanino H, Teramoto T, Ishibiki K et al (1993) A metastatic model of human colon cancer constructed using cecal implantation of cancer tissue in nude mice. Surg Today 23 (5):420–423
15. Fu X, Herrera H, Kubota T, Hoffman RM (1992) Extensive liver metastasis from human colon cancer in nude and scid mice after orthotopic onplantation of histologically-intact human colon carcinoma tissue. Anticancer Res 12(5):1395–1397

Check for updates

Chapter 21

Use of Organoids to Characterize Signaling Pathways in Cancer Initiation

Christina Oatway, Calley L. Hirsch, and Alex Gregorieff

Abstract

The development of intestinal organoid technology has greatly accelerated research in the field of colorectal cancer. Contrary to traditional cancer cell lines, organoids are composed of multiple cell types arranged in 3D structures highly reminiscent of their native tissues. Thus, organoids provide a near-physiological and readily accessible model to study tissue morphogenesis, adult stem cell behavior and tumorigenesis. Here, we provide protocols for establishing intestinal organoid cultures from genetically modified mouse lines and describe methods to overexpress and knockout genes of interest using lentiviral-based approaches.

Key words Organoid, Intestinal stem cells, Wnt, Apc, Yap, Lentiviral infection

1 Introduction

Colorectal cancer remains one of the major causes of cancer death in the Western world. Over the last 30 years, significant advances have been made regarding our understanding of the genetic and cellular lesions that drive transformation of normal colonic epithelium into adenomas and ultimately cancer. In the classical route, colorectal cancer is initiated by loss of function mutations in the tumor suppressor Apc, a key gatekeeper component of the Wnt signaling pathway [1, 2]. In normal colonic epithelium, intact Apc orchestrates proteosomal degradation of β-catenin and thereby restricts Wnt-driven cellular proliferation. In the absence of Apc, the β-catenin destruction complex is disassembled leading to accumulation of transcritpionally active β-catenin and induction of Wnt target genes. In addition to alterations in the Wnt pathway, tumor progression is also driven by mutations targeting KRAS, PI3K, TGFβ, and p53 signaling networks [3]. However, the precise mechanisms underpinning deregulation of these signaling modules in relation to tumor growth and dissemination remain incompletely understood.

Jean-François Beaulieu (ed.), *Colorectal Cancer: Methods and Protocols*, Methods in Molecular Biology, vol. 1765, https://doi.org/10.1007/978-1-4939-7765-9_21,

The development of Cre-lox technology has greatly facilitated the ability to model various human cancers. In the context of colorectal cancer, conditional deletion of *Apc* using gut specific Cre mouse lines has offered key insights into tumor initiation, as sporadic deletion of *Apc* causes the rapid development of benign adenomas; whereas deletion of *Apc* throughout the gut epithelium results in massive crypt expansion, hyperproliferation, and induction of Wnt target genes [4, 5]. These robust phenotypes have served as useful functional readouts to genetically test the role of numerous genes in cancer initiation and progression [6–10]. Furthermore, targeted deletion of *Apc* in specific populations of the gut epithelium has allowed researchers to track tumor initiating cells during adenoma formation and study clonal dynamics [11–13].

Beyond these in vivo models, the relatively recent development of organoid cultures [14, 15] offers another system to dissect the early events in tumorigenesis. When cultured ex vivo, *Apc* mutant organoids adopt a spheroid organization, which mimic in many respects the morphology of aberrant crypt foci or early adenomas observed in vivo (Fig. 1a). Furthermore, *Apc* mutant spheroids show high nuclear expression of the Hippo signaling effector Yap and induction of numerous genes associated with adenoma initiation [11]. Importantly, organoids are also highly amenable to pharmacological treatments and gene manipulations through lentiviral infections.

A common method to obtain *Apc* mutant organoids is to breed *Apc* floxed mice with a gut specific Cre deleter line such as *Villin-CreERT* mice or intestinal stem cell specific *Lgr5GFPCreERT* mice. Organoids are then derived from the crypt epithelium of uninduced $Apc^{fl/fl}$;*VillinCreErt* or $Apc^{fl/fl}$;*Lgr5CreERT* mice and *Apc* deletion is performed ex vivo in organoid cultures by tamoxifen addition. Alternatively, *Apc* mutant organoids are directly isolated from tamoxifen-induced *Apc* mutant mouse crypts. Additionally, researchers may bypass the need for genetic mouse models by directly inactivating *Apc* and other genes implicated in colorectal cancer using gene editting technology. Indeed, work from the Clevers and Sato labs have described methodologies for generating specific lesions using CRISPR/Cas9 to create precise colorectal cancer models from normal intestinal organoids [16, 17]. Here, we provide methods to generate intestinal $Apc^{-/-}$ organoids and describe lentiviral-based techniques to assess gene function in the context of *Apc* mutant organoids (Fig. 1b).

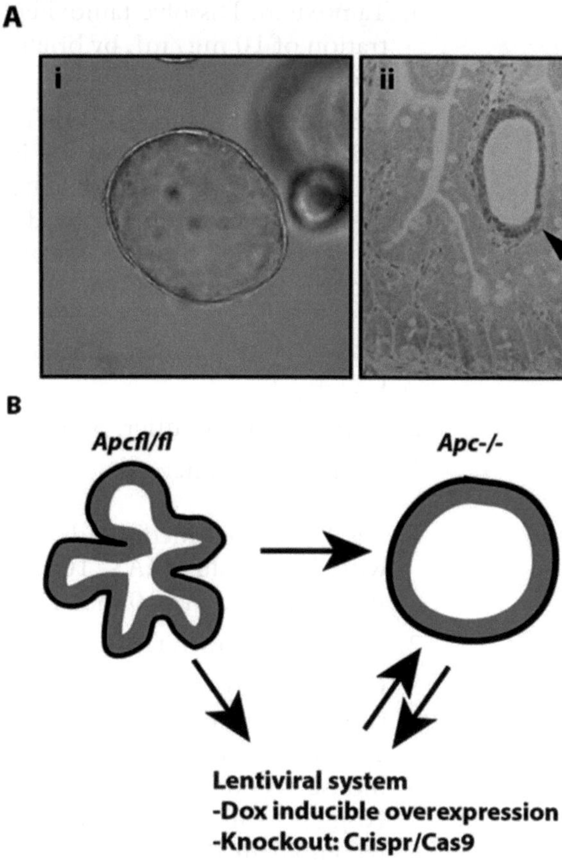

Fig. 1 Apc mutant organoids as a model of tumor initiation. (**a**) Bright field image of a Apc mutant spheroid in Matrigel (panel 1). Yap immunostaining of an early adenoma from *Lgr5GFPCreERT;Apc*$^{fl/fl}$ mice induced with tamoxifen (panel 2). Arrow indicates spherical morphology and strong Yap nuclear accumulation in early adenomas. (**b**) Schematic representation of general work-flow described in the Methods. Cre-mediated induction of *Apc*$^{fl/fl}$*;VilCreErt* organoids using 4-OHT leads to their conversion into *Apc* mutant spheroids. Gene function can be assessed in both noninduced and induced *Apc*$^{fl/fl}$*;VillinCreErt* organoids using a variety of lentiviral systems

2 Materials

2.1 Mouse Strains and Preparation of Tamoxifen

1. For a complete list of conditional floxed Apc alleles available refer to the MGI data base. The Jackson Laboratory distributes Apc^{tm1Tyj} and $Apc^{tm1Rsmi}$.
2. VillinCreErt mice (Obtained from Sylvie Robine, Institut Curie, France).
3. Lgr5GFPCreErt mice (Jackson Laboratory).

4. Tamoxifen. Dissolve tamoxifen freshly in corn oil at a concentration of 10 mg/mL by briefly heating between 65 and 90 °C and vortexing.
5. 4-hydroxytamoxifen (4-OHT). Prepare a stock solution of 0.25 mM 4-OHT in 100% ETOH. Briefly heat solution at 65 °C and vortex to facilitate dissolving 4-OHT. Prepare a 500× working solution by diluting stock solution 1/100 in 100% ETOH. Stock solution can be sored at −20 °C for months (*see* **Note 1**).

2.2 Crypt Isolation

1. PBS−/−: Phosphate Buffered Saline without Mg++ and Ca++.
2. Crypt isolation buffer: 5 mM EDTA in PBS−/−.
3. 70 μm cell strainer.

2.3 Culturing Organoids

1. Basal organoid media: Advanced DMEM/F12 supplemented with 2 mM GlutaMAX, 100 U mL^{-1} penicillin–100 μg mL^{-1} streptomycin, and 10 mM HEPES.
2. Matrigel (Growth factor reduced basement membrane matrix).
3. Organoid growth media: Basal organoid media plus 1× N2 supplement and 1× B-27 supplement (Life Technologies), 1.25 mM n-acetylcysteine, 10 mM nicotinamide, 50 ng/mL mouse recombinant EGF, 100 ng/mL mouse recombinant Noggin, 150 ng/mL human Rspo1. As a replacement for recombinant Rspo1, 1–2% of conditioned media derived from 293 T cells expressing Rspo1-Fc (Trevigen) can be added to basal organoid media.
4. Antibiotics: Puromycin, blasticidin, and doxycycline.
5. Additional supplements: Gsk3 inhibitor CHIR 99021 (Sigma) and ROCK inhibitor Y-27632 (Selleck Chemicals LLC).

2.4 Lentiviral Infections

1. 293 T cells.
2. Opti-MEM (Life Technologies).
3. Lipofectamine 2000 (Life Technologies).
4. Viral harvest media: DMEM supplemented with 10% fetal bovine serum, 0.2 g/mL BSA, and 100 U mL^{-1} penicillin–100 μg mL^{-1} streptomycin.
5. Polybrene (Hexadimethrine bromide). A 1000× stock solution of polybrene solution can be prepared by dissolving 4 mg of polybrene per mL of distilled water. Aliquot and store at −20 °C. Discard after single use.
6. Collagenase type IV 1 mg/mL (STEMCELL Technologies).
7. Lentiviral plasmids:
   (a) psPAX2 (Addgene, Depositor: Didier Trono),

(b) pMD2.G (Addgene, Depositor: Didier Trono),

(c) pCW57.1 (Addgene, Depositor: David Root)

All-in-one doxycycline inducible lentiviral vector harboring the rtTA and puromycin resistance gene. Multiple cloning site available to insert genes of interest.

(d) pCW57-GFP-2A-MCS (Addgene, Depositor: Adam Karpf)

All-in-one doxycycline inducible lentiviral vector harboring the rtTA and puromycin resistance gene. Gene of interest is expressed in bicistronic fashion with turboGFP using P2A self-cleaving peptide.

(e) lentiCRISPR v2 (Addgene, Depositor: Feng Zhang) Lentiviral vector which drives bicistronic expression of hSpCas9 and puromycin. Single gRNAs are inserted using a BsmBI sites.

8. Sequences used to knockout Apc were previously described by Doench et al. [18]:

(a) sgRNA_1_F—CACCGCCTTCTACACAGTACACCCG and sgRNA_1_R—AAACCGGGTGTACTGTGTAGAAGGC.

(b) sgRNA_2_F—CACCGATCACTACACCCCTATTGAG and sgRNA_2_R—AAACCTCAATAGGGGTGTAGTGATC.

(c) sgRNA_3_F—CACCGGGTTCCCCTTGACCTATATG and sgRNA_3_R—AAACCATATAGGTCAAGGGGAACCC.

(d) sgRNA_4_F—CACCGGTCTTAAAGTAACACTGTAG and sgRNA_4_R—AAACCTACAGTGTTACTTTAAGACC.

2.5 Protein Expression Analysis

1. Matrigel dissolving solution: PBS−/− containing 5 mM EDTA, 1 mM $NaVO_4$, 1.5 mM NaF, leupeptin, 1 mM PMSF, 2 μg/mL aprotinin, 8 μg/mL leupeptin, 1 μg/mL pepstatin A.
2. Protein lysis buffer: 50 mM Tris–HCl pH 7.6, 150 mM NaCl, 0.5% Triton X-100, 1 mM EDTA, 1 mM $NaVO_4$, 1.5 mM NaF, 1 mM PMSF, 2 μg/mL aprotinin, 8 μg/mL leupeptin, 1 μg/mL pepstatin A.
3. PBST: PBS−/− plus 0.1% Tween.
4. 10% Neutral buffered Formalin.
5. 4% paraformaldehyde (PFA): For 50 mL of PFA, dissolve 2 g of PFA powder into 50 mL of PBS−/− by heating in a 65 °C water bath.

6. O.C.T. Compound.
7. Sucrose solution (15%, 30%): Dissolve appropriate amount of sucrose in PBS−/−.
8. Cryomolds.
9. Mounting medium: 100 mM Tris (pH 8.5), 25% glycerol, 10% Mowiol 4-88 (Calbiochem), and 2.5% 1,4-diazabicyclo[2.2.2] octane (DABCO). To prepare, all components except for DABCO, are mixed in a 50 mL conical tube by rocking at room temperature (RT) overnight. The medium is then incubated at 55 °C for 30 min or longer to dissolve the Mowiol 4-88. After cooling, DABCO is added and the medium is spun at 5000 × *g* for 10 min to clear. The supernatant is aliquoted into microtubes and stored at −20 °C.

3 Methods

3.1 Generation of Apc Mutant Organoids from Genetic Mouse Models

Prior to preparing organoids, *Apc* floxed mice must be bred to mice harboring an inducible Cre recombinase expressed in the gut epithelium. For robust Cre-mediated deletion in the gut, we recommend the use of *VillinCreERT* mice. The *VillinCreERT* transgene drives expression of a tamoxifen-inducible Cre throughout the gut epithelium including the stem cell compartment. In the resulting $Apc^{fl/fl}$;*VillinCreERT* mice, Cre recombinase excises critical exons of the *Apc* gene by recognizing flanking LoxP sites. As an alternative, *Lgr5GFPCreERT* mice may also be utilized for deletion of *Apc* specifically in the intestinal stem cells.

1. Set aside a 500 mL bottle of cold PBS−/−, 40 mL of crypt isolation buffer, 25 mL of basal organoid media and 5–10 mL of organoid growth media. Prewarm a 24-well plate by placing it in the 37 °C incubator.
2. Sacrifice $Apc^{fl/fl}$;*VillinCreERT* mice and harvest small intestine using standard surgical procedures.
3. Cut small intestine into three sections (proximal, middle, and distal). Flush luminal contents from each part with cold PBS−/− using a syringe and 22 gauge needle. For this purpose, apply needle into the luminal side of intestinal segment and gently apply pressure to syringe to slowly release PBS−/− (*see* **Note 2**).
4. Cut intestinal pieces lengthwise with surgical scissors to expose the epithelial cells. By holding the gut tube with fine tweezers insert one sharp end of the scissors into luminal side and start cutting until entire piece is opened.
5. Wash fecal material at least five times in 15 mL PBS−/− in 50 mL conical tubes. All subsequent steps are performed in conical tubes.

6. Following last wash, replace PBS−/− with 40 mL of Crypt isolation buffer. Gently rock intestines for 30–45 min at 4 °C.
7. Remove crypt dissociation buffer and replace with 15 mL of PBS−/−.
8. Shake tubes with intestinal pieces vigorously for 2–3 s to dissociate epithelium from basement membrane. Solution should appear cloudy due to release of epithelial cells.
9. Collect epithelial cells in suspension in a second conical tube. Intestinal pieces are then placed in original tube containing 15 mL of fresh PBS−/−.
10. Repeat **steps 8** and **9** until 45–50 mL of epithelial cell suspension is collected.
11. Apply 8–10 mL of epithelial cell suspension through a 70 μm cell strainer to separate villous fraction from crypts and collect flow through in a new prerinsed 50 mL conical tube (*see* **Note 3**).
12. Repeat **step 11** until entire cell suspension has been filtered.
13. Centrifuge filtered suspension from **steps 11** to **12** at 200 × *g* to precipitate crypt fraction.
14. Resuspend crypt fraction in 10 mL of basal organoid media and place crypt suspension on ice.
15. Remove 10 μL from crypt suspension and count the number of crypts per 10 μL drops from the crypt suspension. Take the corresponding volume out of the crypt suspension to plate 100–500 crypts per well (24-well plate), and transfer to 4 mL of basal growth media in a new 15 mL conical tube (*see* **Note 4**).
16. Centrifuge at 200 × *g* for 5 min.
17. Aspirate supernatant and resuspend crypts in appropriate volume of Matrigel to obtain 100–500 crypts per 30 μL of Matrigel. *Typically 25–30* μL *of organoid–Matrigel suspension is plated per well (24-well plate)*.
18. Apply crypt–Matrigel suspension on prewarmed 24-well plates so that a dome is formed in the center of each well (*see* **Note 5**).
19. Allow Matrigel to harden by placing plates in the incubator 37 °C for 10 min.
20. Overlay Matrigel with 500 μL of organoid growth media and culture at 37 °C, 5% CO_2.

3.2 Passaging of Organoids and Cre-Mediated Deletion

1. Passage organoids on day 4–5 post-seeding or when confluent by mechanically breaking down organoids by repeatedly pipetting up and down (approximately 20 times) the culture media using p1000 tips and pipettor. This will cause organoids to breakdown into smaller aggregates of cells.

2. Transfer suspension to a 15 mL conical tube containing 4 mL of basal organoid media.
3. Centrifuge at 185 × *g* for 5 min and resuspend in appropriate volume of Matrigel. Typically, each well can be split into 3–4 wells (30 μL of Matrigel/well) for routine passaging. Overlay Matrigel with 500 μL of organoid growth media and culture at 37 °C, 5% CO_2.
4. At day 3–4 post passaging, replace media with fresh organoid growth media containing 5 μM 4-OHT and grow organoids for an additional 16–24 h (*see* **Notes 6** and 7).
5. Passage organoids as in **step 1** and **3**.
6. Centrifuge at 185 × *g* for 5 min and resuspend in appropriate volume of Matrigel. Typically organoids from each well induced with 4-OHT can be split into three wells. Overlay Matrigel with 500 μL of organoid growth media lacking Rspo1 to select for Apc−/− organoids (*see* **Note 8**). Culture organoids at 37 °C, 5% CO_2.
7. Maintain Apc−/− organoids indefinitely in organoid growth media minus Rspo1 and passage every 3–5 days as described in **steps 1–3**.

3.3 Preparation of Lentiviral Particles

1. Thaw and grow low passage 293 T cells in DMEM including 10% FBS and 100 U mL^{-1} penicillin–100 μg mL^{-1} streptomycin.
2. Plate 4 × 10^5 293 T cells per well in a six-well plate into DMEM/10% FBS media and incubate overnight at 37 °C.
3. The next day, carefully replace media with 1.2 mL of fresh DMEM (without penicillin–streptomycin) including 10% FBS media 1 h before transfections.
4. Combine plasmids as indicated below into a microtube containing 150 μL of Opti-MEM (at room temperature). Amounts needed for transfection of a single well in a six-well plate: 0.7 μg psPAX2, 0.3 μg pMD2.G, and 1 μg of lentiviral plasmid in 150 μL of Opti-MEM.
5. In a separate microtube add 5 μL of Lipofectamine 2000 to 145 μL of Opti-MEM and incubate for 5 min at room temperature.
6. Add the Lipofectamine–Opti-MEM mixture to the DNA–Opti-MEM mix and incubate for 20 min at room temperature.
7. Gently add the 300 μL of transfection mix dropwise to each well.
8. Incubate cells overnight at 37 °C, 5%CO_2.

9. The following day (approximately 16 h later) remove media and add 1.8 mL of viral harvest media.
10. Incubate cells overnight at 37 °C, 5%CO_2.
11. Collect the viral media at least 24 h after the last media change and store at 4 °C (*see* **Note 9**).
12. Centrifuge viral media at 300 × *g* for 5 min.
13. Remove only the supernatant and pass through a 0.45 μm filter.

Viral particles are stored at 4 °C for a week or aliquoted and stored at −80 °C for longer periods (3–4 months) (*see* **Note 10**).

3.4 Infection of Organoids by Spinoculation

Lentiviral infection of $Apc^{fl/fl}$;*VillinCreERT* organoids can be performed before or after Cre induction, depending on the experimental purpose. To improve infection efficiency of organoids, pretreatment with the GSK3 inhibitor (CHIR 99021) and ROCK inhibitor (Y-27632) is recommended to promote robust proliferation prior to viral infection. The protocol below was originally described by Koo et al. [19] with a few modifications.

1. For each infection prepare 2–3 wells (from 24-well plate) of $Apc^{fl/fl}$;*VillinCreERT* organoids.
2. Grow organoids at 37 °C, 5% CO_2 for 3 days in organoid growth media supplemented with 10 μM CHIR 99021 and 10 μM Y-27632 (*see* **Note 11**).
3. Remove growth media and add 200 μL of collagenase type IV per 24-well plate. Incubate at 37 °C, 5% CO_2 for 5 min. Add 1 mL of basal media to collect organoids and transfer into a 50 mL conical tube containing 5 mL of cold basal growth media.
4. Pass cells 10–15 times through a 22 gauge blunt ended needle using a 10 mL syringe. Typically this treatment will reduce spheroids to single cells or small cellular aggregates. A small aliquot can be removed and observed under the microscope to monitor cells.
5. Cell suspensions are transferred to 15 mL conical tube containing 5 mL of basal growth media and centrifuged at 185 × *g* for 5 min.
6. Aspirate supernatant and resuspend cell pellet in 1 mL of viral media (*see* **Note 12**). Supplement viral media with 1× N2 supplement, 1× B27 supplement, 1.25 mM N-Acetylcysteine, 10 mM Nicotinamide, 50 ng/mL Egf, 100 ng/mL Noggin, 150 ng/mL Rspo1,10 μM CHIR 9902, 10 μM Y-27632 and 4 μg/mL of polybrene.
7. Place tubes in centrifuge and spin at 600 × *g* for 1 h at 37 °C.

8. Remove tubes and place directly at 37 °C, 5% CO_2 for 5–6 h.
9. After this time, pipette the infected cell pellet to resuspend and add 10 mL of basal media.
10. Spin at 185 g for 5 min.
11. Aspirate media and resuspend pellet in 90 μL of Matrigel. Seed Matrigel–cell suspension in three wells (24-well plate) as described above (Subheading 3.1, **step 18**).
12. Allow Matrigel to solidify and overlay with organoid growth media supplemented with 10 μM CHIR 99021 and 10 μM Y-27632.
13. After 48 h replace organoid growth media 10 μM CHIR 99021 and 10 μM Y-27632. Begin selecting organoids by addition of the appropriate antibiotic (*see* **Note 13**). For mouse organoids use a final concentration of 2–4 μg/mL of puromycin and 10 μg/mL of blasticidin.
14. Grow organoids for 3–7 days at 37 °C, 5% CO_2 in selection media. Passage organoids when wells appear confluent as described in Subheading 3.2.
15. After first passage organoids can be grown in regular organoid growth media lacking CHIR 99021 and Y-27632.

3.5 Loss and Gain of Function Studies in Apc Mutant Organoids

For gain of function studies, tetracycline-based lentiviral vectors offer a reliable method for inducible expression of genes of interest. In one scenario, organoids can be infected with lentiviral constructs that carry the reverse tetracyclin transactivator (rtTA) gene cassette, as well as a tetracycline responsive element to drive gene expression. Following a brief selection period for stable integration of the lentiviral construct, gene expression can be induced at high levels by treating organoids with doxycycline (dox). Similarly, lentiviral gene delivery systems also offer efficient means to perform loss of function experiments using short harpin RNAs (shRNAs) or CRISPR/Cas9 technology. In both cases a wide range of lentiviral systems exist, many of which are distributed by Addgene (see Materials). Below we describe a basic method for production of lentiviral particles and infection of organoids. In addition, we provide details of specific lentiviral systems to perform dox-inducible gene expression and generate Apc null organoids using a CRISPR/Cas9.

3.5.1 Dox-inducuble Gene Expression in Organoids

1. Clone gene of interest in lentiviral vector of choice. See Materials for examples of "all-in-one" lentiviral vectors, which harbor both cloning sites and doxycycline-responsive transactivator (rtTA).
2. Proceed with viral particle preparation and infection as per Subheadings 3.3 and 3.4.

3. Following selection with appropriate antibiotics, passage surviving polyclonal population of organoids as outlined in section into multiple wells in a 24-well plate. Induce transgene expression in one well by adding 1.5 μg/mL of doxycycline in organoid growth media.
4. Incubate doxycycline-treated organoids for 12–72 h at 37 °C, 5% CO_2.
5. Monitor expression levels of induced gene of interest by performing immunostaining as indicated in Subheadings 3.6.1 and 3.6.2 (*see* **Note 14**). Protein expression can also be visualized by western blot analysis as per Subheading 3.6.3. If immunostaining shows evidence of variable gene induction, the polyclonal population can be subcloned (continue below to **step 6**).
6. Culture polyclonal organoids in organoid growth media containing 10 μM CHIR 99021 and 10 μM Y-27632 for 2–3 days prior to passaging.
7. Break down spheroids from a single well by transferring organoids into a 50 mL conical tube containing 5 mL of cold basal growth media. Pass cells 10 times through a 22 gauge blunt ended needle using a 10 mL syringe. Transfer broken down organoids into a 15 mL conical containing 5 mL of basal organoid media.
8. Spin down cells at 185 g for 4 min. Remove supernatant and resuspend in appropriate volume of Matrigel to seed six wells (*see* **Note 15**).
9. Grow organoids in organoid growth media containing 10 μM CHIR 99021 and 10 μM Y-27632 at 37 °C, 5% CO_2.
10. Once organoids are visible to the naked eye (3–5 days post seeding), aspirate isolated organoids directly out of the Matrigel using yellow tips and a pipettor (*see* **Note 16**). To assist in picking individual organoids, a dissecting microscope can be used.
11. Picked organoids are then placed in round bottom or v-bottom well of a 96-well plate containing 10 μL of basal organoid media. Keep plate on ice.
12. Mechanically break down organoids into smaller pieces by pipetting basal organoid media up and down for 5–10 times in each well.
13. Resuspend organoids by adding 20 μL of Matrigel to each well and immediately seed organoid–Matrigel suspension in a new 24-well plate. Place plate at 37 °C to allow Matrigel to set.

14. Grow subcloned organoids to confluency in organoid growth media containing 10 μM CHIR 99021 and 10 μM Y-27632 (*see* **Note 17**). Passage organoids when needed.
15. Once sufficient number of organoids is obtained repeat doxycycline treatment as in **steps 3** and **4** and monitor gene induction by immunofluorescence. Select positive organoids for further study. Discard negative organoids.

3.5.2 Generation of Apc Mutant Organoids using CRISPR/Cas9

1. Specific guide RNAs targeting murine *Apc* are listed in the Materials section. For details on cloning sgRNAs into the lentiCRISPRv2 vector refer to the following link https://www.addgene.org/static/data/plasmids/52/52961/52961-attachment_B3xTwla0bkYD.pdf (see original references [20, 21]). Briefly, digest the vector using Esp3I or BsmBI, with the addition of FastAP. Run the digest on a gel and purify the larger band (approximately 12 kb). In parallel phosphorylate and anneal oligo pairs, and ligate with purified vector backbone. Transform ligation mix into competent bacteria.
2. Proceed with viral particle preparation and infection as per Subheadings 3.3 and 3.4. For CRISPR-mediated knockout of *Apc*, prepare organoids from wild-type mice.
3. Following infection, select for *Apc* null mutants using 3 μg/mL of puromycin in organoid growth media. Split organoids as required, with a total of 3–5 days in puromycin.
4. Once puromycin is removed, the organoids can be cultured in organoid growth media minus Rspo1. Following Rspo1 removal viable organoids will adopt a spheroid morphology.

3.6 Imaging and Protein Expression Analysis of Organoids

3.6.1 Whole-Mount Immunofluorescence

1. Sterilize glass circular coverslips by rinsing them in 70% ETOH and allow them to dry in a tissue culture hood. Place dried coverslips in appropriate number of wells of a 24-well plate.
2. Seed organoids in Matrigel in the center of the coverslips. Allow Matrigel to set and overlay with organoid growth media. Grow organoids at 37 °C, 5% CO_2.
3. Remove growth media and wash organoids twice in 1 mL of PBS−/−.
4. Add 2 mL of 10% neutral buffered formalin in each well. Fix organoids for 20–30 min (*see* **Note 18**).
5. Remove formalin and wash wells three times using 1 mL of PBST.
6. Add 1 mL of PBST including 0.5% Triton per well and allow solution to permeabilize organoids for 20 min.
7. Wash wells twice in PBST and block organoids in 500 μL of 2% BSA in PBS−/− for 30 min.

8. Prepare appropriate primary antibody dilution in PBST containing 1% BSA. Add 300 μL of antibody dilution per well and incubate overnight at 4 °C.
9. Wash wells 6× in PBST for 5 min each.
10. Prepare appropriate fluorescent secondary antibody dilution in PBST containing 1% BSA and 1 μg/mL of DAPI. Add 300 μL of antibody dilution per well and incubate for 2 h at room temperature or overnight at 4 °C.
11. Wash wells 6× in PBST for 5 min each.
12. Take out cover slips using fine forceps and dry excess PBST on a tissue.
13. Place coverslips with organoids facing down on top of a drop of mounting media on a glass microscopy slide. Visualize samples using fluorescent microscope.

3.6.2 Cryo-sectioning of Organoids

1. Disrupt Matrigel with organoids using a P1000 pipette and collect. Remove excess media and add 4% PFA (*see* **Note 19**), leave at 4 °C for 30 min.
2. Take the organoids and place them in 15% sucrose solution at 4 °C. The organoids can be removed from the solution once they have sunk to the bottom of the tube.
3. Place the organoids in 30% sucrose solution at 4 °C. They can be transferred to OCT compound once they have sunk to the bottom of the tube, or they can be kept at 4 °C for a couple of days.
4. Transfer the organoids to a plastic cryomold. Add OCT compound to submerge the organoids and place the mold on dry ice until the compound has solidified. The samples can then be sectioned or kept at −80 °C.
5. Section the samples using a cryostat. The samples can then be placed on prewarmed glass slides. Sample slides can be stored at −80 °C, if required.
6. Samples can be stained in the same manner as Subheading 3.6.1.

3.6.3 Preparing Protein Lysates from Organoids

1. Grow 2–3 wells of organoids (per lysate) to confluency in the appropriate growth media.
2. Aspirate growth media from each well and wash well twice in 1 mL of cold PBS−/−.
3. Add 500 μl of cold Matrigel dissolving solution in each well and collect organoids by breaking up Matrigel dome using a p1000 tip. Transfer Matrigel–organoids suspension into a 1.5 mL microtube.

4. Rock tubes at 4 °C for 20–30 min to dissolve Matrigel (*see* **Note 20**).
5. If pieces of Matrigel are no longer visible place microtubes in a tabletop centrifuge and spin at 200 × *g* for 2 min.
6. Remove as much of the supernatant as possible with yellow tip and pipettor.
7. Resuspend organoids in 80 μL of freshly prepared protein lysis buffer including standard proteinase inhibitors and allow lysis to continue for 15–30 min on ice. Spin down tubes at 16,000 × *g* for 5 min at 4 °C.
8. Remove supernatant and place into new microtube and proceed to analyse lysates by SDS-PAGE using standard procedures.

4 Notes

1. Stock solution will precipitate when frozen. Thus before use, stock solution should be reheated briefly to dissolve crystals.
2. It is not necessary to wash out completely all fecal material. The primary aim of this step is to fill the gut lumen with PBS−/− to facilitate opening of intestinal tube with scissors.
3. To avoid clogging of cell strainer wash away villous fraction remaining in the strainer with distilled water after each round of filtering. The 50 mL conical tube used for collection of crypt fraction should be briefly rinsed in 5 mL of basal organoid media. This step will prevent crypts from sticking to tube wall during centrifugation.
4. In most cases removal of 200 μL out of 10 mL of crypt suspension will be sufficient to plate 4–6 wells in 24-well plate.
5. Typically organoid growth will not be adversely affected if Matrigel spreads during plating and does not form a dome.
6. Cre activation by 4-OHT treatment may cause toxicity in organoids. To minimize these effects, 4-OHT should not be added to organoids harboring the *VillinCreERT* transgene immediately after passaging or during crypt seeding.
7. Apc deletion can also be performed in vivo by performing a single intraperitoneal injection of tamoxifen (dissolved in corn oil at 10 mg/Kg body weight,) in *Apc*$^{fl/fl}$;*VillinCreERT* mice aged at least 6 weeks. At 2–4 days post injection crypts can be isolated as described above and cultured in organoid growth media lacking Rspo1.

8. *Apc$^{fl/fl}$* organoids adopt a spheroid morphology after 2 days post 4-OHT treatment and no longer require addition of Rspo1.
9. The first collection will generally have a higher titer, so if a higher titer is needed only perform the first viral collection and collect 32 h after the last media change rather than 24 h and proceed with centrifugation and filtering of supernatant. Alternatively, two viral collections can be performed at 24–48 h following last media change. If performing a second viral collection, add 1.8 mL of additional viral harvest media to transfected 293 T cells and incubate cells overnight at 37 °C, 5% CO_2.
10. Viral particles can be concentrated by ultracentrifugation of supernatants at 50,400 × *g* for 2–3 h. Pellets are then resuspended in 250 μL organoid growth media.
11. Noninduced *Apc$^{fl/fl}$;VillinCreERT* organoids are grown 2–3 days prior to infection in organoid growth media supplemented with CHIR 99021 and Y-27632. When performing infections on Apc mutant organoids the use of CHIR 99021 can be omitted.
12. When working with concentrated viral particles, resuspend cell pellet in 250 μL of organoid growth media and add 250 μL of concentrated viral suspension (*see* **Note 10**). Next, viral–cell suspension is supplemented with 10 μM CHIR 99021 and 10 μM Y-27632 and 4 μg/mL of polybrene.
13. When performing CRISPR/Cas9-mediated deletions, organoids can also be functionally selected for the correct mutational event.
14. In polyclonal populations induction of gene of interest upon doxycycline addition may vary from individual organoid to organoid or even vary within a given organoid. To control for variable expression it is preferable to perform immunostainings rather than western blot analysis. To facilitate visualization of proteins an epitope tag can be added to the gene of interest. Bicistronic lentiviral vectors co-expressing a fluorescent protein (e.g., pCW57-GFP-2A-MCS) are also useful to monitor expression of gene of interest within organoid population.
15. The object of this step is to passage organoids sparsely to facilitate picking of individual organoids in **step 10**. Thus exact dilution may vary depending on confluence of original well.
16. The number of individual organoids to be picked may vary depending on experiment. As a starting point researchers can pick 10–15 organoids.

17. When subcloned cultures have fully recovered, supplements (i.e., 10 μM CHIR 99021 and 10 μM Y-27632) can be omitted from growth media.

18. During fixation period organoids attach directly to the glass coverslips, while Matrigel will typically dissolve into the formalin solution.

19. PFA will disintegrate leftover Matrigel, there is no need to separate the organoids from the Matrigel.

20. Typically after 30 min Matrigel pieces will disappear and free organoids will settle to the bottom of the tube. If after 30 min pieces of Matrigel remain intact, allow organoids to settle to the bottom of the tube and remove supernatant. Add 1.2 mL of fresh Matrigel dissolving solution as in **step 3** and continue rocking tubes for an additional 20 min.

References

1. Holland JD, Klaus A, Garratt AN, Birchmeier W (2013) Wnt signaling in stem and cancer stem cells. Curr Opin Cell Biol 25 (2):254–264. https://doi.org/10.1016/j.ceb.2013.01.004
2. Krausova M, Korinek V (2014) Wnt signaling in adult intestinal stem cells and cancer. Cell Signal 26(3):570–579. https://doi.org/10.1016/j.cellsig.2013.11.032
3. Fearon ER (2011) Molecular genetics of colorectal cancer. Annu Rev Pathol 6:479–507. https://doi.org/10.1146/annurev-pathol-011110-130235
4. Jackstadt R, Sansom OJ (2016) Mouse models of intestinal cancer. J Pathol 238(2):141–151. https://doi.org/10.1002/path.4645
5. Sansom OJ, Griffiths DF, Reed KR, Winton DJ, Clarke AR (2005) Apc deficiency predisposes to renal carcinoma in the mouse. Oncogene 24(55):8205–8210. https://doi.org/10.1038/sj.onc.1208956
6. Ashton GH, Morton JP, Myant K, Phesse TJ, Ridgway RA, Marsh V, Wilkins JA, Athineos D, Muncan V, Kemp R, Neufeld K, Clevers H, Brunton V, Winton DJ, Wang X, Sears RC, Clarke AR, Frame MC, Sansom OJ (2010) Focal adhesion kinase is required for intestinal regeneration and tumorigenesis downstream of Wnt/c-Myc signaling. Dev Cell 19 (2):259–269. https://doi.org/10.1016/j.devcel.2010.07.015
7. Buller NV, Rosekrans SL, Metcalfe C, Heijmans J, van Dop WA, Fessler E, Jansen M, Ahn C, Vermeulen JL, Westendorp BF, Robanus-Maandag EC, Offerhaus GJ, Medema JP, D'Haens GR, Wildenberg ME, de Sauvage FJ, Muncan V, van den Brink GR (2015) Stromal Indian hedgehog signaling is required for intestinal adenoma formation in mice. Gastroenterology 148(1):170–180 e176. https://doi.org/10.1053/j.gastro.2014.10.006
8. Cordero JB, Ridgway RA, Valeri N, Nixon C, Frame MC, Muller WJ, Vidal M, Sansom OJ (2014) c-Src drives intestinal regeneration and transformation. EMBO J 33(13):1474–1491. https://doi.org/10.1002/embj.201387454
9. Marsh V, Winton DJ, Williams GT, Dubois N, Trumpp A, Sansom OJ, Clarke AR (2008) Epithelial Pten is dispensable for intestinal homeostasis but suppresses adenoma development and progression after Apc mutation. Nat Genet 40(12):1436–1444. https://doi.org/10.1038/ng.256
10. Sansom OJ, Meniel VS, Muncan V, Phesse TJ, Wilkins JA, Reed KR, Vass JK, Athineos D, Clevers H, Clarke AR (2007) Myc deletion rescues Apc deficiency in the small intestine. Nature 446(7136):676–679. https://doi.org/10.1038/nature05674
11. Gregorieff A, Liu Y, Inanlou MR, Khomchuk Y, Wrana JL (2015) Yap-dependent reprogramming of Lgr5(+) stem cells drives intestinal regeneration and cancer. Nature 526(7575):715–718. https://doi.org/10.1038/nature15382
12. Schepers AG, Snippert HJ, Stange DE, van den Born M, van Es JH, van de Wetering M, Clevers H (2012) Lineage tracing reveals Lgr5+ stem cell activity in mouse intestinal adenomas. Science 337(6095):730–735. https://doi.org/10.1126/science.1224676

13. Vermeulen L, Morrissey E, van der Heijden M, Nicholson AM, Sottoriva A, Buczacki S, Kemp R, Tavare S, Winton DJ (2013) Defining stem cell dynamics in models of intestinal tumor initiation. Science 342 (6161):995–998. https://doi.org/10.1126/science.1243148
14. Date S, Sato T (2015) Mini-gut organoids: reconstitution of the stem cell niche. Annu Rev Cell Dev Biol 31:269–289. https://doi.org/10.1146/annurev-cellbio-100814-125218
15. Leushacke M, Barker N (2014) Ex vivo culture of the intestinal epithelium: strategies and applications. Gut 63(8):1345–1354. https://doi.org/10.1136/gutjnl-2014-307204
16. Drost J, van Jaarsveld RH, Ponsioen B, Zimberlin C, van Boxtel R, Buijs A, Sachs N, Overmeer RM, Offerhaus GJ, Begthel H, Korving J, van de Wetering M, Schwank G, Logtenberg M, Cuppen E, Snippert HJ, Medema JP, Kops GJ, Clevers H (2015) Sequential cancer mutations in cultured human intestinal stem cells. Nature 521 (7550):43–47. https://doi.org/10.1038/nature14415
17. Matano M, Date S, Shimokawa M, Takano A, Fujii M, Ohta Y, Watanabe T, Kanai T, Sato T (2015) Modeling colorectal cancer using CRISPR-Cas9-mediated engineering of human intestinal organoids. Nat Med 21 (3):256–262. https://doi.org/10.1038/nm.3802
18. Doench JG, Fusi N, Sullender M, Hegde M, Vaimberg EW, Donovan KF, Smith I, Tothova Z, Wilen C, Orchard R, Virgin HW, Listgarten J, Root DE (2016) Optimized sgRNA design to maximize activity and minimize off-target effects of CRISPR-Cas9. Nat Biotechnol 34(2):184–191. https://doi.org/10.1038/nbt.3437
19. Koo BK, Stange DE, Sato T, Karthaus W, Farin HF, Huch M, van Es JH, Clevers H (2011) Controlled gene expression in primary Lgr5 organoid cultures. Nat Methods 9(1):81–83. https://doi.org/10.1038/nmeth.1802
20. Sanjana NE, Shalem O, Zhang F (2014) Improved vectors and genome-wide libraries for CRISPR screening. Nat Methods 11 (8):783–784. https://doi.org/10.1038/nmeth.3047
21. Shalem O, Sanjana NE, Hartenian E, Shi X, Scott DA, Mikkelsen TS, Heckl D, Ebert BL, Root DE, Doench JG, Zhang F (2014) Genome-scale CRISPR-Cas9 knockout screening in human cells. Science 343(6166):84–87. https://doi.org/10.1126/science.1247005

Chapter 22

Identification of Novel Molecules Targeting Cancer Stem Cells

Yannick D. Benoit

Abstract

Multiple studies focused on tumor heterogeneity and cellular hierarchies have demonstrated the role of cancer stem cells (CSC) in tumor initiation and recurrence. Colorectal cancer is one of the leading causes of cancer-related death and is hierarchically organized, with the majority of tumor cells descending from a small population of colon cancer stem cells (CCSCs). Such a rare self-renewing population is marked by the acquisition of distinct chromatin regulation and transcriptional programs. Fundamental molecular deviations between CCSCs and bulk tumor cells as well as normal tissues represent a unique therapeutic access to develop novel, selective anticancer therapies.

In this chapter, we describe a methodological pipeline to identify novel molecules to selectively target human CCSC. We present a point-by-point description of a typical phenotypic molecular screening experiment, aiming to identify selective modulators of human CCSCs vs. normal intestinal progenitor cells.

Key words Cancer stem cells, Colon cancer, Small molecules, Phenotypic screening, Drug discovery

1 Introduction

Multiple studies focused on tumor heterogeneity and cellular hierarchies demonstrate continued support for the concept of cancer stem cells (CSC), which harbor self-renewal and tumor initiation capacities [1–3]. Numerous reports have highlighted the role of CSCs in tumor initiation and recurrence through the acquisition of chemoresistance/radioresistance properties, and the ability to form metastases at distant sites [2]. Investigations of this rare subset of malignant cells have emphasized the importance of understanding CSC biology in order to develop novel, selective anticancer therapies [2]. Colorectal cancer, which is one of the leading causes of cancer-related death in North America [4], is among the types of malignancies shown to be hierarchically organized and to contain such a small population of self-renewing and highly tumorigenic colon cancer stem cells (CCSCs) [5]. As in several other types of human tumors, CCSCs are marked by the acquisition of distinct

Jean-François Beaulieu (ed.), *Colorectal Cancer: Methods and Protocols*, Methods in Molecular Biology, vol. 1765, https://doi.org/10.1007/978-1-4939-7765-9_22,

chromatin regulation and transcriptional programs compared to normal mucosa or bulk tumor population, conferring them with unique oncogenic properties [6–8]. Such fundamental differences result in aberrant gene expression, protein stability or enzymatic activation that is CSC-specific. Therefore, this opens new perspectives toward identifying CCSC vulnerabilities, creating unique opportunities to develop novel therapeutics.

High-throughput chemical screening (HTS) was shown as an efficient strategy to identify new anticancer compounds, which directly or indirectly target essential molecular features of CSC maintenance and development. The basics of HTS in drug discovery are generally characterized by the miniaturization of a chemical or biological assay, allowing a time and cost-efficient identification of active compounds from a molecular library. Compound libraries exist in diverse sizes and generally consist of collections of natural products, FDA-approved or other experimental drugs, as well as uncharacterized chemicals. One of the current debates in drug discovery is to determine whether a phenotypic or a target-based approach is most appropriate to design and perform a HTS project. While target-based strategies measure the effects of molecules from a library on an isolated macromolecular target, phenotypic approaches instead involve complete biological systems, such as mammalian cells or microorganisms, to identify drugs capable of modifying a specific cellular phenotype (Fig. 1). Although target-based chemical screening has been the mainstream approach in the pharmaceutical industry over several decades, phenotypic screening is currently gaining popularity and could represent the future of anticancer drug development. This could be mainly due to the high rate of failure observed in Phase-III clinical trials using drugs identified from target-based screening endeavors in [9]. A possible explanation could reside in the fact that complex heterogeneous diseases such as cancer are not likely to converge toward a single target or pathway [10]. Moreover, phenotypic screening is more likely to identify drug candidates with pathologically relevant molecular mechanism of action [11], conferring more chances of success to a lead compound when tested for its antitumor efficacy at the later stages of drug development. In this regard, a recent study reported that a majority (56%) of the 50 first-in-class new molecular entities used in cancer drug development were originally discovered using a phenotypic molecular screening approach, while target-based approaches accounted for less than 35% of the discoveries from this same category [12]. From the perspective of fundamental innovation, target-based HTS is usually more hypothesis-driven than phenotypic approaches, which leaves less room for authentic discovery of novel therapeutic targets. Despite these advantages, phenotypic screening also involves important drawbacks in the drug discovery field. These mainly relate to the considerable investment in time and resources required to identify the target(s) of a

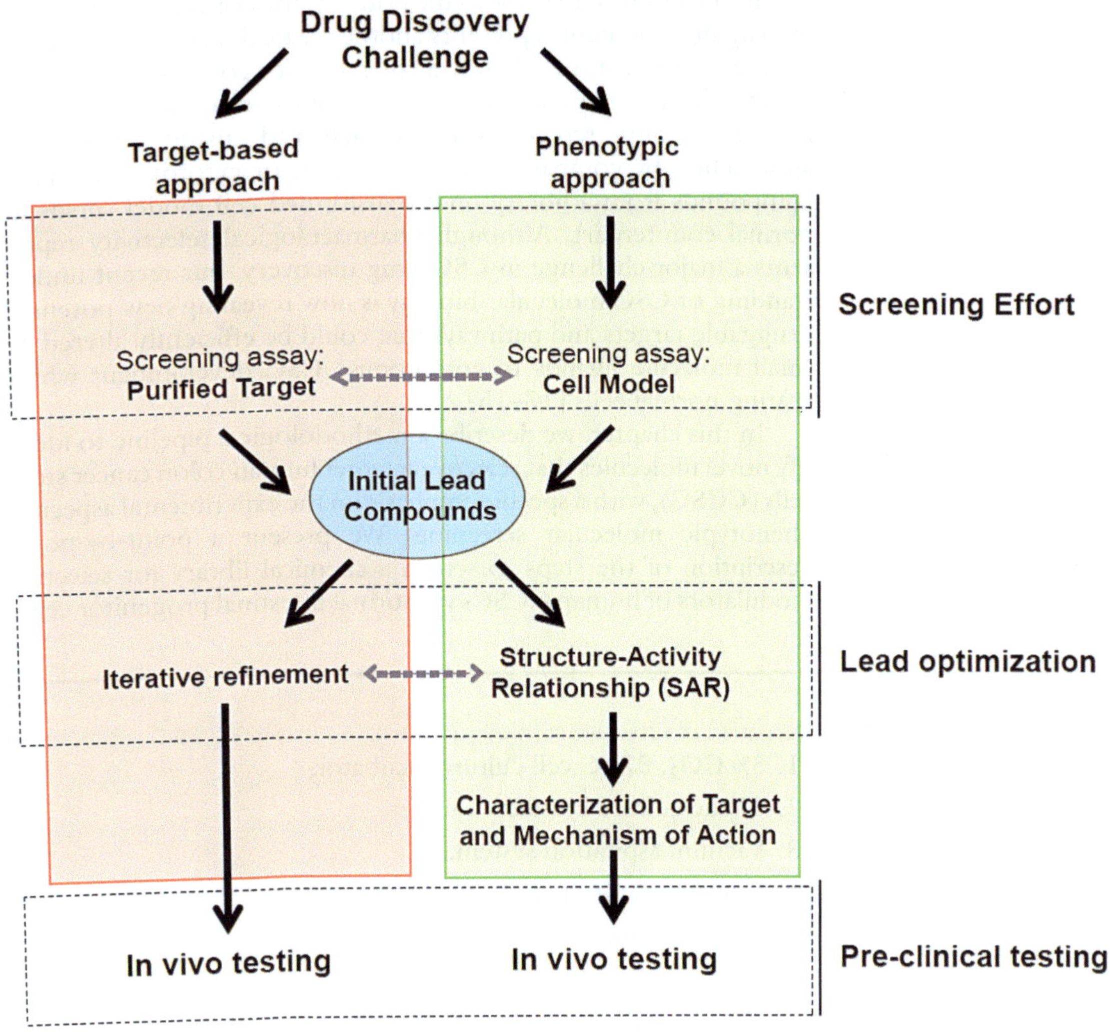

Fig. 1 Target-based and phenotypic molecular screening approaches. Flowchart of a drug discovery project, depending on the choice of molecular screening approach. Both, target-based (red) and phenotypic (green) screening strategies are aiming at the identification and optimization of lead compounds. However, the phenotypic screening approach often requires considerable time and rescources investment to identify the target(s) and characterize the molecular mechanism of action of drug candidate(s) prior to preclinical in vivo efficacy testing. Gray arrows represent possible interconnections between the two strategies: (1) A phenotypic assay can be used as a secondary screen to an initial target-based screening effort. (2) A target-based screening step can be used as a secondary assay following an initial target-informed phenotypic screen. (3) SAR and iterative refinement can complement each other to optimize potency of identified lead compounds

lead compound and to characterize its molecular mechanism of action [10]. However, the emergence of new technologies in molecular biology is now helping to overcome these hurdles, including advances in small molecule labeling, proteomics, and next-generation sequencing.

In addition to small molecule potency, the concept of selectivity in drug development represents another critical layer of complexity in the optimization of novel therapeutic compounds, where selected lead candidates will not compromise normal tissue integrity. Selectivity screens can be achieved using phenotypic approaches, by comparing antiproliferative or cytotoxic effects of compounds from a library on a transformed cell model versus its normal counterpart. Although pharmacological selectivity represents a major challenge in CSC drug discovery, our recent understanding of CSC molecular biology is now revealing new potential druggable targets and pathways that could be efficiently altered by small molecule ligands to compromise CSC development whilst sparing normal cells [13–15].

In this chapter, we describe a methodological pipeline to identify novel molecules that selectively target human colon cancer stem cells (CCSC), with a specific emphasis on the experimental aspect of phenotypic molecular screening. We present a point-by-point description of the steps to screen a chemical library for selective modulators of human CCSCs vs. normal intestinal progenitor cells.

2 Materials

2.1 Equipment

1. 5% CO_2, 37 °C cell culture incubator.
2. Tissue culture biosafety cabinet.
3. Vacuum aspiration system.
4. 4 °C laboratory fridge.
5. −20 °C laboratory freezer.
6. −80 °C laboratory freezer.
7. 37 °C water bath.
8. Benchtop centrifuge with versatile swinging bucket rotor.
9. Countess Automated Cell Counter + chamber slides.
10. Motorized pipette.
11. 300 μL multichannel pipette.
12. P2, P20, P200, and P1000 single channel pipettes.
13. Handheld multichannel aspirator system.
14. Microlab NIMBUS automated liquid handling system (Hamilton Robotics) (Optional, *see* **Note 1**).
15. Fluorescence microscope system with microplate stage (Leica DMi8 or equivalent).
16. Operetta High-Content Imaging system (PerkinElmer) (Optional, *see* **Note 2**).

2.2 Consumables

1. Disposable pipetting reservoirs.
2. Disposable P2, P20, P200, and P1000 filtered tips.
3. 5 mL, 10 mL, 25 mL sterile serological pipettes.
4. Disposable 15–50 mL conical tubes.
5. T-25 (25 cm^2) tissue culture-treated flasks.
6. Ultralow attachment T-25 (25 cm^2) flasks.
7. 96-well flat clear bottom black polystyrene tissue culture-treated optical micro plates.
8. 96-well deep V-bottom, 0.5 mL sterile plates with lids.
9. Aluminum foil.
10. Cling-wrap or Parafilm.

2.3 Cell Culture Reagents and Molecular Biology Supplies

1. HIEC-6 cells (ATCC, CRL-3266) and culture medium (Table 1).
2. Primary tumor derived CCSCs (derived from surgical resection) and culture medium (Table 2).
3. 18Co cells (ATCC, CRL-1459) and culture medium (Table 3).
4. Sterile 1× Phosphate buffered saline (PBS).
5. 16% stock Paraformaldehyde (w/v) (ThermoFisher). Use a 1:8 dilution (2%) in 1× PBS as a working solution.
6. 10× Perm/Wash buffer (BD Biosciences). Use a 1× dilution in PBS as a working solution.
7. KnockOut D-MEM (ThermoFisher).
8. Matrigel® Basement membrane matrix. Add 10 mL of cold KnockOut D-MEM to a 10 mL bottle of Matrigel to get 15× stock solution. Store at −20 °C as 1 mL aliquots in 15 mL conical tubes.
9. TrypLE Express cell dissociation reagent (ThermoFisher).
10. Dimethyl Sulfoxide (DMSO).

Table 1
Human Intestine Epithelial Crypt (HIEC) cell culture media composition

Reagent	Final volume/concentration
Opti-MEM (*see* **Note 3**)	470 mL
1 M HEPES	5 mL/10 mM
GlutaMAX supplement (100×)	5 mL
Fetal bovine serum (FBS) (*see* **Note 4**)	4% (20 mL)
Epithelial growth factor (EGF)	10 ng/mL

Table 2
Human patient-derived Colorectal Cancer Stem Cell (CCSC) culture media composition

Reagent	Final volume/ concentration
DMEM/F-12 (*see* **Note 5**)	480 mL
Nonessential amino acids supplement (100×)	5 mL
N2 supplement (100×) (*see* **Note 6**)	5 mL
B-27 supplement (50×) (*see* **Note 6**)	10 mL
Basic fibroblast growth factor (b-FGF)	20 ng/mL
Epithelial growth factor (EGF)	40 ng/mL
Heparin	4 μg/mL

Table 3
Culture media to grow 18Co human myofibroblasts

Reagent	Supplier	Final volume/concentration
MEM	ThermoFisher	450 mL
Fetal bovine serum (FBS)	Wisent	10% (50 mL)
L-Glutamine (*see* **Note 7**)	ThermoFisher	2 mM

11. Compound library (*see* **Note 3**), distributed in 96-well plate format, at 1 mM or 10 mM for each compound.
12. 3-deazaneplanocin A Hydrochloride (DZNep).
13. Hoechst 33,342, 1000× stock solution 10 mg/mL.

3 Methods

Typically, drug discovery projects require a logical stepwise progression through a specific experimental pipeline before reaching clinical trial phases (Fig. 2) [16]. Upon the identification of a specific clinical challenge, the optimization of an accurate cellular readout assay, and subsequent phenotypic HTS represent cornerstone steps of such a pipeline. Suitability of a screening assay is defined by its Z-factor (or Z-prime), meaning the statistical coefficient of signal dynamics and data variation within the assay [16, 17]. The inclusion of pharmacological negative (Lo) and positive (Hi) controls in a cellular assay is critical to assess its quality by calculating its Z-factor, and essential for appropriate hit identification [16]. In addition to HTS, there are other important steps that

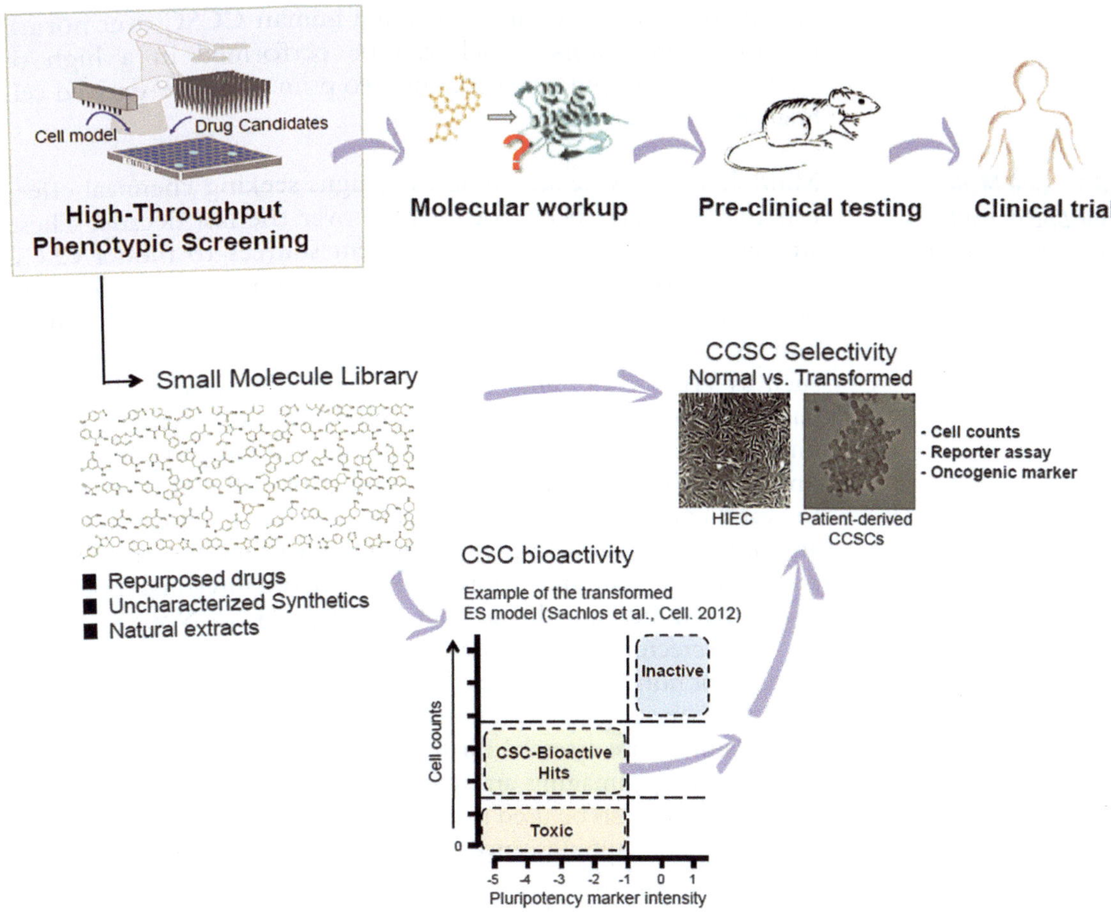

Fig. 2 Stepwise illustration of a typical drug discovery pipeline designed around phenotypic molecular screening effort. Upon identification of a drug discovery challenge, molecular high-throughput screening represents the first critical step, before molecular workup (hit validation, target identification, characterization of the mechanism of action, lead optimization) and preclinical in vivo efficacy testing, in order to move novel compounds toward clinical trial phases. Small molecule libraries from different sources are screened for selective disruptors of human CCSC biology. Chemical screening can be directly performed on normal vs. CCSCs primary tissue derived assay or, alternatively, a high-throughput primary screening step (e.g., CSC-bioactivity screen, Sachlos et al., 2012) can be used to scale down the number of compounds to be tested in the selectivity assay

constitute a phenotypic-based drug discovery effort, which are illustrated in (Fig. 2). These include molecular workup to identify drug candidate target(s) and mechanism of action, as well as evaluation of drug in vivo efficacy [16]. Important parameters have to be considered in the design of a phenotypic HTS experiment, such as the choice of a chemical library, the type of cellular model to be used, the type of readout and detection method(s), as well as the possibility of performing sequential primary and secondary assays (Fig. 2) or even counterscreen steps [18]. The following section will focus on the methodological aspect of a phenotypic screen to identify selective compounds affecting human CCSC over normal intestinal progenitors, which can be performed in a high or medium-throughput fashion using two primary tissue-derived cellular models (Fig. 2).

3.1 Cell Models for CSC-Based Screening Assays

Multiple phenotypic screening campaigns seeking chemical effectors of CSCs have been documented over the last decade. These studies have used a variety of different sources to model CSCs, including common cancer lines, embryonic stem cells, and patient-derived primary tissues [15, 19, 20]. Unlike common human cancer cell lines or ES cells, primary tissue-derived models such as HIEC [21] and CCSC [22] are highly relevant to the pathophysiology of colorectal cancers but may present technical limitations like costly maintenance and limited lifespan. Depending on the size of the library and the number of different doses tested for each compound, it may be most practical to filter down the amounts of unique compounds through a primary screen before proceeding with human primary tissue-derived intestinal models in a secondary, medium-throughput step (Fig. 2) (*see* **Note 8**).

The screening method herein described is applied to adherent cultures of normal HIEC [21] and primary tumor derived CCSCs derived from surgical resections [22], where unique compounds from a library are assessed for impacts on cell growth/viability by nuclei staining, imaging and counts. Alternatively, human CCSC and HIEC can also be used in a similar screening setup, by using an ATP detection luminescence assay as the experimental output to measure cell viability.

3.2 CCSC-selective Compound Screening Assays

A general and simplified workflow of a phenotypic screening project is illustrated in (Fig. 3). Briefly, selected cell models are initially seeded in Matrigel-coated multiwell optical plates. Concomitantly, stock compounds, stored in "master plates," are appropriately diluted into "daughter plates" to be used for subsequent drug treatments. Upon incubation with library and control compounds, cells are fixed and imaged. Plate imaging and data analysis will lead to the identification of compounds with the capacity to selectively affect neoplastic stem cells, with limited biological impact on normal counterpart models.

3.2.1 Optical Plates

1. Prepare a 1:15 solution of Matrigel from 1 mL stock aliquots using KnockOut D-MEM. Plan a final volume of 6 mL of 1:15 Matrigel per experimental plate.
2. Mix all tubes well with a 25 mL pipette and transfer contents to a pipetting reservoir.
3. Dispense 50 μL/well to each optical plate (*see* **Note 9**).

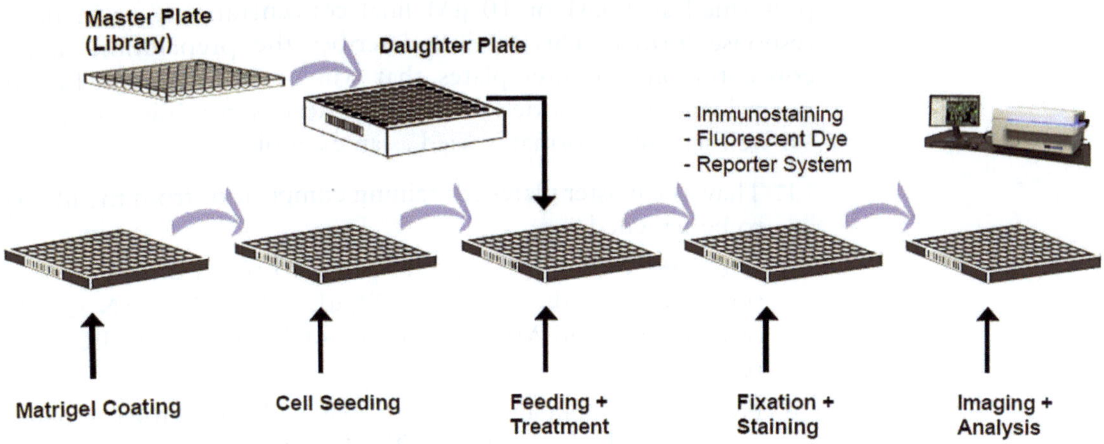

Fig. 3 Step-by-step representation of the human CCSC-selective compound screening assays. Subheading 3.2.1: Preparation the optical plates (Matrigel coating). Subheading 3.2.2: Seeding cells on Matrigel-coated optical plates. Subheading 3.2.3: Preparation of small molecule dilutions (Daughter plates) from the chemical library (Master plates). Subheading 3.2.4: Feeding and small molecule treatments of human HIEC and CCSC models. Subheadings 3.2.5 and 3.2.6: Cell fixation and designated cellular staining for cell count, oncogenic marker, differentiation marker and/or reporter assessment

4. Wrap plates tightly in plastic cling-wrap and incubate at 4 °C (minimum of 2 h) before placing them at room temperature ½ h before the seeding step.

3.2.2 Seeding Cells

HIEC maintained as monolayer in TC-treated plastics, while CCSCs are grown as suspension aggregates in ultralow adhesion flasks, as previously described [21–25] using culture media prepared as described above. To preserve human CCSC in an undifferentiated, self-renewing state while maintained in adherent conditions, myofibroblast conditioned medium (MFCM) must be used throughout the screening process (*see* **Note 10**).

1. Prepare HIEC and CCSC cell suspensions in Opti-MEM and MFCM respectively. Both cell type suspensions are obtained from TrypLE enzymatic dissociation (5 min at 37 °C).
2. While preparing cell suspensions, carefully aspirate Matrigel from the optical plates using a multichannel aspirator system.
3. Seed the cells at a predetermined density, avoiding CCSC and HIEC cells to reach confluence within 84 h (*see* **Note 11**).
4. Put the plates in a tissue culture incubator, as stacks of three plates maximum to ensure proper gas exchange.

3.2.3 Preparation of Small Molecule Dilutions

Small molecule libraries can generally be purchased and stored as 96- or 384-well plate formats at 1 mM or 10 mM concentrations (*see* **Note 12** for examples of available chemical libraries). Depending on the user's experimental design, screening experiments can be performed at 1 μM or 10 μM final concentrations, or in dose-response format. This section describes the preparation of 5× concentration daughter plates that will be used to test human normal and CSC models in a single-dose screening assay. The 96-well screening format is used as an example.

1. Thaw the master plates containing compounds from the library to be screened.
2. Use deep V-bottom Daughter plates to prepare the 5× dilutions and prefill the wells with 200 μL of MFCM (*see* **Note 11**) or complete Opti-MEM (Table 1) for CCSC and HIEC cells, respectively.
3. For each 96-well daughter plate, plan eight wells for Lo (negative) control (5× = 0.5% DMSO) and eight wells for Hi (positive) control (*see* **Note 13**).
4. Depending of the working dilution, transfer the appropriate volume of stock compounds from the master plate to the daughter plate. For instance, if the master plate is at 10 mM and the screening is performed at 10 μM, a 1:200 dilution will give a 5× concentration in the daughter plate (*see* **Note 14**).
5. Relid the daughter plates and replace cap mats (if applicable) on the master plates. Daughter plates can be wrapped plastic cling-wrap or Parafilm and stored at 4 °C until the cells are ready to be treated. The recapped master plates can be stored at −80 °C.

3.2.4 Feeding and Small Molecule Treatments

To prevent CCSC differentiation in adherent culture conditions, CCSCs must be both fed and drug-treated in MFCM (*see* **Note 11**). HIEC are fed and treated in complete Opti-MEM (Table 1). Small molecule treatments start 48 hours post seeding.

1. In advance, allow the daughter plates to reach room temperature and incubate the media bottles in a 37 °C water bath.
2. From the CCSC and HIEC culture plates, carefully remove the culture media using a multichannel aspirator system (*see* **Note 1**).
3. Add 160 μL per well of MFCM and complete Opti-MEM media to CCSC and HIEC plates respectively.
4. From the daughter plates, pipet 40 μL of the 5× compound preparations and dispense it to the culture plates according to your experimental design for a final 1× compound concentration into 200 μL). Generally, each compound should be tested at least in duplicate on both CCSCs and HIECs in two independent plates. Therefore, a total of 160 μL (4 × 40 μL) of drug preparation will be used from each well of a daughter plate.
5. Place the culture plates back in the incubator for 48 h.

3.2.5 Cell Counts

In order to determine the effect of individual tested compounds on CCSC and HIEC cells, proceed to quantification of cell number in each well, based on nuclear staining and microscopy imaging.

1. Take the plates out of the incubator and carefully remove the culture media using a multichannel aspirator system (*see* **Note 1**).
2. Using a multichannel pipet, distribute 80 μL of 2% PFA/1× PBS per well and incubate the plates for 10 min at room temperature.
3. Discard PFA and proceed to three successive washes with 100 μL of 1× Perm/wash buffer per well. For the third wash, keep the buffer in the wells for 10 min.
4. In each well, dispense 100 μL of a 1:1000 solution of Hoechst 33,342 (*see* **Note 15**) prepared in 1× Perm/wash. Incubate the plates for 10 min at room temperature.
5. Perform two quick washes of the plates using 1× PBS (100 μL per well) followed by a final wash with 100 μL of 1× PBS per well.
6. Relid plates and wrap them as stacks in tinfoil to protect them from light exposure. Plates can be stored in the fridge for up to 7 days until imaging.
7. Proceed to plate imaging using the method of your choice, in order to obtain cell (nuclei) count values for each tested compound, as well as positive and negative controls (*see* **Note 2**).

3.2.6 Reporter or Differentiation/Oncogenic Marker-Based Assays

Depending on screening goals, multiple phenotypic parameters other than cell count can be assessed, including variation in oncogenic or differentiation marker expression, modulation of a given morphological feature such as actin cytoskeleton organization, or tracking of specific fluorescent reporter systems. For the case of fluorescent reporter systems, apply the steps described in Subheading 3.2.5 combined to the appropriate imaging method in order to quantify the signal from the reporter in each compound-treated and control wells. However, for specific marker quantification, immunostaining may be required as described below.

1. Prepare a preestablished dilution of the primary antibody to be used to detect the marker(s) of interest, in 1× Perm/Wash buffer.
2. Execute the **steps 1–3** as described in subheading 3.2.5.
3. Discard Perm/Wash buffer from the last washing step, add 100 μL/well of the primary antibody suspension and incubate the plates at 4 °C for 12–18 h.
4. Discard the antibody solution and proceed to three successive washes with 100 μL/well of 1× Perm/wash buffer.

5. Prepare a preestablished dilution of the secondary antibody (ies) (in 1× Perm/Wash buffer) to detect the isotype(s) of the primary antibody(ies) of interest.
6. Add 100 μL/well of the secondary antibody suspension and incubate the plates, wrapped in tinfoil at room temperature for 1 h. Minimize light exposure for all subsequent steps.
7. Discard the secondary antibody solution and proceed to three successive washes with 100 μL of 1× Perm/wash buffer per well.
8. Execute the **steps 4–6** as described in subheading 3.2.5 and proceed to plate imaging in order to accurately measure signals from the immunostaining (*see* **Notes 16** and **17**).

4 Notes

1. This is not an issue if using an automated liquid handling platform like a Microlab Nimbus. If using a multichannel aspirator system, make sure not to remove cells from the monolayers as it may affect final cell counts.
2. It is recommended to use an automated high-content imaging system (e.g., PerkinElmer Operetta or equivalent) to perform unbiased plate imaging, and subsequently obtain cell count data. Such an imaging method suits all sizes of screening experiments, although for smaller-scale endeavor, standard fluorescence microscopy imaging equipment can be used.
3. Opti-MEM medium can be purchased presupplemented with GlutaMAX.
4. Use premium quality serum such as Wisent Premium.
5. DMEM/F-12 media can be purchased presupplemented with nonessential amino acids such as Advanced DMEM/F-12 (ThermoFisher).
6. N2 and B-27 supplements are available from ThermoFisher
7. MEM media can be purchased without L-glutamine, as Advanced MEM (ThermoFisher).
8. Using a primary HTS step involving models like transformed human ES cells [15] or embryonic carcinoma cells [26] may represent a practical option to filter CSC-bioactive molecular entities from a large-scale chemical library before proceeding to a focused screen for CCSC-selective compounds.
9. If performing a cell viability assay using an ATP quantification luminescent method [19] such as CellTiter-Glo (Promega), use opaque wall luminescence plates. Also, plan a full column

(eight wells) per plate as a "no cell" control to assess the background from the luminescent reagent.

10. MFCM is obtained by culturing 18Co myofibroblasts (initially maintained using medium described in Table 3) with EGF/b-FGF-free CCSC medium for 24 h, as previously described by Vermeulen et al. [27].
11. Predetermining seeding density for cell models used in a cellular assay is critical before proceeding to molecular screening. As an example, previous screening experiments using human transformed ES cells [15, 28] and primary human breast cancer stem cells [19] seeded 5000 cells/well and 1000 cells/well, respectively, in 96-well plates, 24 h prior to drug treatment. This step can be achieved with superior consistency using an automated liquid handling platform, e.g., Microlab NIMBUS (Hamilton Robotics).
12. The following links provide information on standard, commercially available chemical libraries:
    (a) http://www.prestwickchemical.com/prestwick-chemical-library.html
    (b) http://www.selleckchem.com/screening-libraries.html
    (c) https://www.chromadex.com/natural-product-libraries/
    (d) http://www.chemdiv.com/products/screening-libraries/complete-list/
13. Generally, classic anticancer compounds such as Etoposide can be used as a Hi control at a 1× concentration of 10 μM. However, in this specific case, 3-deazaneplanocin A (DZNep) was previously shown to have a robust selective apoptosis-inducing effect against CCSCs (≥10-fold) over HIECs when used at a 5 μM final concentration [29] (5× = 50 μM DZNep). If using t-hESCs as a CSC model for a primary HTS assay as described by Sachlos et al., BMP4 (5× = 0.5% DMSO +100 ng/mL) represents a suitable Hi control [15].
14. Although this section describes preparation of daughter plates for a single-dose screening assay, it is possible to apply the same procedure for 8–10 point dose-response screening assays by purchasing or preparing master plates in order to preserve a common dilution factor to achieve 5× concentrated daughter plates.
15. Other DNA staining dye such as 4′,6-diamidine-2′-phenylindole dihydrochloride (DAPI) can also be used.
16. Unlike most nuclear dyes, plates stained with fluorescence-conjugated antibodies should not usually stay for prolonged periods of time at 4 °C due to possible fluorescence signal

fading. Thus, plate imaging might have to be performed with minimal delay following antibody staining.

17. Calculation methods and data interpretation will differ across assays and users based on multiple experimental factors, including size of the assay (compound library), specific output parameter(s), imaging methods and equipment, as well as Hi and Lo controls and assay-specific Z-factor.

References

1. Bonnet D, Dick JE (1997) Human acute myeloid leukemia is organized as a hierarchy that originates from a primitive hematopoietic cell. Nat Med 3(7):730–737
2. Visvader JE, Lindeman GJ (2012) Cancer stem cells: current status and evolving complexities. Cell Stem Cell 10(6):717–728. https://doi.org/10.1016/j.stem.2012.05.007
3. Kreso A, Dick JE (2014) Evolution of the cancer stem cell model. Cell Stem Cell 14 (3):275–291. https://doi.org/10.1016/j.stem.2014.02.006
4. Siegel RL, Miller KD, Jemal A (2016) Cancer statistics, 2016. CA Cancer J Clin 66(1):7–30. https://doi.org/10.3322/caac.21332
5. O'Brien CA, Pollett A, Gallinger S, Dick JE (2007) A human colon cancer cell capable of initiating tumour growth in immunodeficient mice. Nature 445(7123):106–110. https://doi.org/10.1038/nature05372
6. Widschwendter M, Fiegl H, Egle D, Mueller-Holzner E, Spizzo G, Marth C, Weisenberger DJ, Campan M, Young J, Jacobs I, Laird PW (2007) Epigenetic stem cell signature in cancer. Nat Genet 39(2):157–158. https://doi.org/10.1038/ng1941
7. Suva ML, Riggi N, Bernstein BE (2013) Epigenetic reprogramming in cancer. Science 339 (6127):1567–1570. https://doi.org/10.1126/science.1230184
8. Merlos-Suárez A, Barriga FM, Jung P, Iglesias M, Céspedes MV, Rossell D, Sevillano M, Hernando-Momblona X, da Silva-Diz V, Muñoz P, Clevers H, Sancho E, Mangues R, Batlle E (2011) The intestinal stem cell signature identifies colorectal cancer stem cells and predicts disease relapse. Cell Stem Cell 8(5):511–524. https://doi.org/10.1016/j.stem.2011.02.020
9. Williams R (2013) Discontinued drugs in 2012: oncology drugs. Expert Opin Investig Drugs 22(12):1627–1644. https://doi.org/10.1517/13543784.2013.847088
10. Kotz J (2012) Phenotypic screening, take two. Sci BX 5(15). https://doi.org/10.1038/scibx.2012.380
11. Swinney DC (2013) Phenotypic vs. target-based drug discovery for first-in-class medicines. Clin Pharmacol Ther 93(4):299–301. https://doi.org/10.1038/clpt.2012.236
12. Swinney DC, Anthony J (2011) How were new medicines discovered? Nat Rev Drug Discov 10(7):507–519. https://doi.org/10.1038/nrd3480
13. Benoit YD, Guezguez B, Boyd AL, Bhatia M (2014) Molecular pathways: epigenetic modulation of Wnt-glycogen synthase kinase-3 signaling to target human cancer stem cells. Clin Cancer Res 20(21):5372–5378. https://doi.org/10.1158/1078-0432.CCR-13-2491
14. Kahn M (2014) Can we safely target the WNT pathway? Nat Rev Drug Discov 13 (7):513–532. https://doi.org/10.1038/nrd4233
15. Sachlos E, Risueño RM, Laronde S, Shapovalova Z, Lee JH, Russell J, Malig M, McNicol JD, Fiebig-Comyn A, Graham M, Levadoux-Martin M, Lee JB, Giacomelli AO, Hassell JA, Fischer-Russell D, Trus MR, Foley R, Leber B, Xenocostas A, Brown ED, Collins TJ, Bhatia M (2012) Identification of drugs including a dopamine receptor antagonist that selectively target cancer stem cells. Cell 149(6):1284–1297. https://doi.org/10.1016/j.cell.2012.03.049
16. Hughes JP, Rees S, Kalindjian SB, Philpott KL (2011) Principles of early drug discovery. Br J Pharmacol 162(6):1239–1249. https://doi.org/10.1111/j.1476-5381.2010.01127.x
17. Zhang JH, Chung TD, Oldenburg KR (1999) A simple statistical parameter for use in evaluation and validation of high throughput screening assays. J Biomol Screen 4(2):67–73. https://doi.org/10.1177/108705719900400206

18. Thorne N, Auld DS, Inglese J (2010) Apparent activity in high-throughput screening: origins of compound-dependent assay interference. Curr Opin Chem Biol 14(3):315–324. https://doi.org/10.1016/j.cbpa.2010.03.020
19. Gupta PB, Onder TT, Jiang G, Tao K, Kuperwasser C, Weinberg RA, Lander ES (2009) Identification of selective inhibitors of cancer stem cells by high-throughput screening. Cell 138(4):645–659. https://doi.org/10.1016/j.cell.2009.06.034
20. Yasgar A, Titus SA, Wang Y, Danchik C, Yang SM, Vasiliou V, Jadhav A, Maloney DJ, Simeonov A, Martinez NJ (2017) A high-content assay enables the automated screening and identification of small molecules with specific ALDH1A1-inhibitory activity. PLoS One 12(1):e0170937. https://doi.org/10.1371/journal.pone.0170937
21. Perreault N, Beaulieu JF (1996) Use of the dissociating enzyme thermolysin to generate viable human normal intestinal epithelial cell cultures. Exp Cell Res 224(2):354–364
22. Prasetyanti PR, Zimberlin C, De Sousa E, Melo F, Medema JP (2013) Isolation and propagation of colon cancer stem cells. Methods Mol Biol 1035:247–259. https://doi.org/10.1007/978-1-62703-508-8_21
23. Benoit YD, Lussier C, Ducharme PA, Sivret S, Schnapp LM, Basora N, Beaulieu JF (2009) Integrin alpha8beta1 regulates adhesion, migration and proliferation of human intestinal crypt cells via a predominant RhoA/ROCK-dependent mechanism. Biol Cell 101 (12):695–708. https://doi.org/10.1042/BC20090060
24. Benoit YD, Pare F, Francoeur C, Jean D, Tremblay E, Boudreau F, Escaffit F, Beaulieu JF (2010) Cooperation between HNF-1alpha, Cdx2, and GATA-4 in initiating an enterocytic differentiation program in a normal human intestinal epithelial progenitor cell line. Am J Physiol Gastrointest Liver Physiol 298(4): G504–G517. https://doi.org/10.1152/ajpgi.00265.2009
25. Sikandar SS, Pate KT, Anderson S, Dizon D, Edwards RA, Waterman ML, Lipkin SM (2010) NOTCH signaling is required for formation and self-renewal of tumor-initiating cells and for repression of secretory cell differentiation in colon cancer. Cancer Res 70 (4):1469–1478. https://doi.org/10.1158/0008-5472.CAN-09-2557
26. Barbaric I, Jones M, Harley DJ, Gokhale PJ, Andrews PW (2011) High-content screening for chemical modulators of embryonal carcinoma cell differentiation and survival. J Biomol Screen 16(6):603–617. https://doi.org/10.1177/1087057111406547
27. Vermeulen L, De Sousa E, Melo F, van der Heijden M, Cameron K, de Jong JH, Borovski T, Tuynman JB, Todaro M, Merz C, Rodermond H, Sprick MR, Kemper K, Richel DJ, Stassi G, Medema JP (2010) Wnt activity defines colon cancer stem cells and is regulated by the microenvironment. Nat Cell Biol 12 (5):468–476. https://doi.org/10.1038/ncb2048
28. Werbowetski-Ogilvie TE, Bhatia M (2008) Pluripotent human stem cell lines: what we can learn about cancer initiation. Trends Mol Med 14(8):323–332. https://doi.org/10.1016/j.molmed.2008.06.005
29. Benoit YD, Witherspoon MS, Laursen KB, Guezguez A, Beausejour M, Beaulieu JF, Lipkin SM, Gudas LJ (2013) Pharmacological inhibition of polycomb repressive complex-2-activity induces apoptosis in human colon cancer stem cells. Exp Cell Res 319 (10):1463–1470. https://doi.org/10.1016/j.yexcr.2013.04.006

Index

A

Aberrant crypt foci (ACF) 27, 79–84, 316
Adenomas .... vii, 27, 79, 81, 193–195, 197–201, 204, 217, 218, 242, 244, 315–317
Alkylation 158, 160, 262
Amphotericin B 88
Anchorage independent growth 34, 35
Angiogenesis 28, 37, 180, 288
Annexin V 103, 105, 109, 112–114, 117, 132, 273–276
Anoikis 34, 35, 100
Antibody 6, 14, 18, 32, 33, 51–54, 104–107, 110, 117, 119, 131, 133, 156, 159, 160, 169, 181–184, 188, 206, 207, 249, 259, 260, 262, 263, 268, 274–276, 282–288, 300, 301, 327, 343, 346
APC 58, 180, 194, 274, 315–317, 319, 320, 322–325, 328, 329
Apoptosis 34, 99–135, 173, 205, 271, 345
Area under ROC curve 210, 223, 235
Autophagy 99, 117, 167–174
Azoxymethane (AOM) 80–84

B

Bacteria 8, 47, 54, 59, 139–141, 150, 325
Bafilomycin A1 .... 168, 170, 172, 173
Bioinformatics 8, 24, 58, 60–61, 63, 140, 159, 163
Biomarker 28, 193, 204, 205, 230, 236, 237, 241–269, 282, 284, 285, 288, 291
Biopsy 143–145, 148–149
Bisulfite 6, 15, 17, 22
Blasticidin 318, 324
Blood samples 244, 272, 274, 275
Bradford assay 245, 252, 265
BRAF 180, 283, 284, 287–289

C

CA19-9 .... 272, 275
Cancer stem cells 333–346
Carcinogen 29, 79–82, 139, 189, 261, 303
Caspase 99, 101, 104–106, 112, 114–119, 121–129, 133–135
CDX2 .... 57, 58, 61, 63, 66, 70, 74, 75, 181, 182, 184, 186, 188
CEA 272–275
Cell counter 9, 30, 33, 336
Cell culture 5, 9, 31, 45, 59, 64, 102, 107, 111, 112, 114, 115, 132, 133, 155, 156, 159, 170, 300–302, 308, 336, 337
Cell growth 33, 35, 340
Cell invasion 35, 36
Cell line 3–22, 24, 29, 30, 32, 39, 45, 50, 54, 58, 59, 61, 63, 64, 70, 75, 101, 128, 134, 156, 159, 165, 168, 172, 173, 303, 308, 340
Cell lysate 32, 71–73, 120, 124, 170
Cell lysis 45, 48, 50, 103, 250, 263
Cell migration 35
Cell survival 99
CH_3CN (acetonitrile) 156, 158, 161, 164, 165, 231, 232, 248, 257
Chemical library 336, 339, 341, 344
Chemically-induced carcinogenesis 79
Chemotherapy 58, 282–284, 290, 308
Chemotherapy agent
  5-fluorouracil 282
  irinotecan 282
  leucovorin 284
  oxaliplatin 282
  trifluridine/tipiracil 282
Chemotherapy agent combination
  FOLFIRI 283
  FOLFIRINOX 287
  FOLFOX 288
Chromatin 43, 47–50, 53, 63, 79–85, 333
Chromatin immunoprecipitation 43, 47–50, 53
Chromosomal instability (CIN) 3, 88, 180
Colon cancer cell classification 53, 57
Colonocyte exfoliation 193
Colorectal cancer cell line
  Caco-2 .... 58, 59, 61, 75, 101
  Caco-2/15 .... 101, 123, 126, 132, 134, 156
  Colo-201 9
  Colo-205 .... 9, 300, 303

Jean-François Beaulieu (ed.), *Colorectal Cancer: Methods and Protocols*, Methods in Molecular Biology, vol. 1765,
https://doi.org/10.1007/978-1-4939-7765-9,

Colorectal cancer cell line (*cont.*)
Colo-320 ... 9
DLD-1 ... 156, 300, 303
HCT15 ... 23, 303
HCT116 ... 9, 23, 172, 300, 303
HT-29 ... 6, 101, 123, 126, 134, 156, 300, 303
LoVo ... 172
SNU175 ... 9, 23
SNUCI ... 9, 24
SW480 ... 8, 9, 24, 75, 101, 123, 134, 172, 300, 303
SW620 ... 24, 101, 123, 126, 134, 172, 300, 303
SW948 ... 9, 24
SW1116 ... 9, 24
T84 ... 24, 172
WiDr ... 6, 24, 300, 303
Colorectal cancer cells (CRC) ... 3, 4, 6, 8, 9, 12, 14, 15, 19, 20, 22, 27–29, 39, 87–94, 96, 101, 121, 123, 126, 131, 132, 134, 139, 155, 167, 179–189, 193–195, 197–201, 229–239, 241–269, 271–276, 281–291, 299–305
Confocal microscopy ... 36
Consensus molecular subtyping (CMS) ... 4, 179–181, 183, 189, 283, 290, 291
Construct ... 44, 58, 61, 64, 68, 69, 75, 211, 246, 324
CpG island methylator phenotype (CIMP) ... 3, 4, 6, 7, 15, 22
Cre-lox ... 316
CRISPR/Cas9 ... 316, 324, 325, 329
Cryo-embedding ... 102, 128, 131
Cytokeratin ... 156, 160, 181, 182, 184, 188
Cytotoxicity ... 300, 301, 304

D

3-Deazaneplanocin A hydrochloride (DZNep) ... 338, 345
Denaturing gradient gel electrophoresis (DGGE) ... 150
Dextran sodium sulfate (DSS) ... 80, 81, 83
DNA amplification ... 65, 197, 198
DNA extraction ... 114, 143–146, 194–197, 199, 201
DNA isolation ... 8, 21, 103
DNA laddering ... 103, 114, 115, 117, 121, 132–134
DNA profiling ... 3
DNA purification ... 46, 52, 55
DNA staining
4′,6-diamidine-2′-phenylindole dihydrochloride (DAPI) ... 345
Hoechst 33, 342 ... 338, 343
propidium iodine ... 300
Doxycycline ... 318, 319, 324–326, 329
Drug discovery ... 334–336, 338, 339
Drug screening ... 307
Dysbiosis ... 139

E

EGF receptor (EGFR) ... 4, 28, 40, 181, 282–288, 291
Electrophoresis
isoelectrofocusing ... 241, 247, 251, 253–254, 261, 266
SDS PAGE ... 104–105, 120–122, 241, 246
silver staining ... 256
two-dimensional ... 241
ELISA immunoassay ... 249, 250, 259–261
Enhancer ... 47, 58, 60, 61, 63–70, 72, 74, 75
Epidermal growth factor (EGF) ... 102, 156, 282, 284, 318, 337, 338, 345
Epithelial-mesenchymal transition (EMT) ... 101, 180, 181, 291
Epithelial-to-mesenchymal transformation ... 27
Explants ... 102, 107, 108, 112
Extracellular vesicles ... 88

F

Fecal immunochemical testing (FIT) ... 217, 218, 223, 230
Fecal occult blood test (FOBT) ... 204
Feces, *see* Stool
Fetal colon ... 107, 108
Fetal intestine ... 106–107, 337
Fibrin ... 272–275
Fibroblast ... 40, 87–97, 156, 159, 338
FL-DNA, *see* Fluorescence long DNA
Fluorogenic assay ... 105, 121–123
Formalin-fixed ... 5, 12, 18, 181
Fungi ... 140, 150, 261
Fungizone ... 88

G

Gas chromatography (GC) ... 66, 209, 224, 230
Gel electrophoresis ... 4, 59, 67, 104, 114, 133, 150, 158, 161, 241, 246, 254, 261
Genetic alteration ... 3, 27
Genistein ... 102, 107–109, 111, 112, 115, 119, 122, 124, 128, 133
Gentamicin ... 30, 102
GSK3 inhibitor ... 318, 323

H

Haemocytometer 9
Hematoxylin 37, 182, 184, 188, 189
Hepatocyte growth factor (HGF) 28, 288
HER2 .... 282, 283, 287
Hereditary non-polyposis colorectal cancer 289
HIEC cells 163, 341–343
High-performance liquid chromatography (HPLC) 159, 162
High-throughput chemical screening (HTS) 334, 338, 339, 344, 345
Human tumor xenograft models 300

I

Immune cells 299, 301, 302
Immunoblot (IB) 32, 33, 168, 171–173
Immunodeficient mice 13, 301, 304
Immunofluorescence 106–109, 111, 112, 114, 133, 173, 325, 326
Immunohistochemistry (IHC) 6, 14, 84, 179–189
Immunotherapy 282, 285, 289, 290, 299–305
Immunotherapy agent
  bevacizumab 282
  cetuximab 282
  panitumumab 282
In-gel trypsin digestion 158, 161
Integrin 100
Internal transcribed spacer (ITS) 140, 141, 150
Intestinal cell line HIEC 101, 123, 156, 337
Intestinal epithelial cells (IEC) 27, 123, 181
Intestinal stem cells 316, 320
ITGA6 .... 218, 223

K

KRAS 4, 28, 180, 230, 284–287, 290, 315

L

Laser capture microdissection 89, 91
LC3 .... 168, 169, 171–174
Lentiviral infections 316, 318, 323
Lgr5 .... 316, 317, 320
Liquid chromatography coupled to mass spectrometry (LC-MS) 159, 162, 230
Luciferase 44, 49, 54, 60, 61, 64–67, 71–73, 75, 77
Luciferase reporter assay 44
Lysosome 168

M

Magnetic beads 206, 208
MAP kinase signaling 287
Mass spectrometry (MS) 155, 156, 159, 162, 230, 241, 248, 255, 257, 258
Matrigel 5, 13, 20, 31, 37, 38, 40, 89, 92, 94, 95, 301, 302, 304, 317–319, 321, 322, 324, 325, 327, 328, 330, 337, 340, 341
MET receptor 28
Metabolite biomarker 237
Metabolomics profiling 229–239
Metabolomics 230
Metastasis .... vii, 28, 34, 35, 37, 39, 87, 95, 96, 101, 205, 272
Metastatic activity 37, 39
Methylation 3, 6, 15, 17, 18, 22, 46, 289
Microbial diversity 140–141, 150
Microbiome 139–151
Microparticle 271–276
Microparticulosome 272, 273
MicroRNA stools 230
MicroRNA tissues 211
Microsatellite instability (MSI) 3, 14–16, 20, 179, 180, 283, 289
Microsatellite testing 14, 20
Mismatch repair (MMR) 3, 14, 181, 289
Molecular subtype 3, 7, 9–11, 15, 17, 18, 22, 24
Molecular subtypes 179–189, 290
Mouse models 36, 272, 287, 307, 316, 320
Mucin 1 .... 272, 274, 275
MYC 44, 49, 53, 55, 180, 218, 223, 290
Mycoplasma 4, 5, 8–11, 19, 304

N

Neomycin 30, 32
Next-generation sequencing (NGS) 141, 335
Nucleoside diphosphate kinase A (NDKA) 241, 249

O

Online classification tool 179
Organ culture 102, 107
Organoids 315–330
Organotypic culture 89, 93, 94, 108, 128
Orthotopic location 95–96

P

Paraffin-embedded 5, 12, 18, 181
Patient derived xenograft (PDX) 4, 307–313
Penicillin 5, 59, 88, 97, 156, 309–311, 318, 322
Peptide purification 158, 162
Phenotypic screening 334, 335, 340
Phosphatidylserine (PS) 109–113, 272, 276
Phosphoinositide-3-kinase (PI3K) 3, 283, 285, 286, 315
Plasmid 30, 31, 44, 46–48, 54, 58–61, 64, 65, 67–71, 74–77, 194, 318, 322
Podoplanin 272, 274, 275
Polybrene 30, 32, 40, 318, 323, 329
PolyHEMA 30, 34, 102, 115, 117, 118, 120, 125, 126, 128, 133, 134
Polymerase chain reaction (PCR) 181, 193, 195
  cDNA preamplification step 211, 212
  droplet digital PCR (ddPCR) 218
  inhibitors 204
  multiplex 15, 222
  quantitative PCR (qPCR) 211, 213, 218
  reaction 9, 17, 21, 45–47, 52, 66, 140, 141, 209, 211, 213, 220–222, 225
  real-time 141, 207, 212–214, 221, 222
  reverse transcriptase (RT) 47, 208, 209, 211, 213
  TaqMan probes 207, 213, 224
Polyp 193, 204, 231, 232, 235–237
Primary tumor 35, 37, 272, 312, 337, 340
Profiling 4, 6, 8, 9, 58, 88, 89, 181, 230, 237, 241–269, 290
Promoter 3, 29, 43, 47–50, 53, 58, 60, 61, 63–66, 68–72, 74–76, 289
Promoter reporting assay 43, 47, 48, 58, 60, 61, 64, 68, 69, 74
Protein dosage 156, 160
Proteinase K 46, 52, 55, 103, 116, 133, 143–146, 151, 194–197
Proteomics 155–166, 204, 241–269, 335
PTGS2 218
Puromycin 318, 319, 324, 325

R

RAS 179, 181, 283–287
Receiver operating characteristic (ROC) curve 210, 223, 235, 237
Receptor 28, 29, 40, 181, 282, 284, 289
Reduction 79, 158, 160, 187, 210, 229
Regulated cell death (RCD) 99, 106, 109
Response element 43–55
RNA preservation solution 206
RNA-Seq 58
ROCK inhibitor 318, 323

S

Severe combined immune deficiency (SCID) 90, 95, 301, 309
Signaling pathway 28, 29, 35, 79, 82, 83, 284, 285, 287, 288, 315–330
Site directed mutagenesis 43, 47–50, 53
Sonication 50, 54, 250, 263
16S ribosomal RNA 140
18S ribosomal RNA 209
Stable isotope labeling 155, 231, 233, 234
Stable isotope labeling with amino acids in culture (SILAC) 155, 156, 159, 160, 164
Statistics analysis 207, 210, 223, 231, 235
Stool 143–146, 150, 193–195, 197–201, 204–208, 211, 212, 217–225, 230
Stool DNA 143, 144, 146–147, 193–195, 197–201, 230
Stool mRNA 205, 212, 217–225
Streptomycin 5, 88, 97, 156, 309–311, 318, 322
Stroma 4, 36, 88–91, 94, 180, 181, 184, 288
Subcellular fractionation 156, 159, 160
Surgically resected primary tissue 308, 310

T

Tamoxifen 316, 317, 320, 328
Tissue factor (TF) 272–275
Tissue sections OCT compound embedded for cryosections 128
Tissue sections paraffin-embedded 181, 188
TNM classification 211
Transcription factor (TF) 43, 46, 48, 51, 52, 59–61, 64, 69–71, 75–77
Transfection 30, 31, 44, 47, 49, 54, 61, 64, 69–76, 322, 329
Transwell 30, 35
Trypsin 5, 9, 30, 33, 36, 37, 59, 69, 70, 76, 88, 102, 112, 117, 119, 126, 158, 161, 162, 164, 248, 257, 267, 300, 302, 304
Tumor-derived microvesicle 271
Tumor heterogeneity 333–346
Tumorgraft 311, 312
Tumorigenesis 36, 79, 316
Tumour microenvironment (TME) 87, 88
TUNEL 103
Tyrosine kinase 28, 128, 284, 287

U

Uridine diphosphate glucuronosyltransferase (UGT) 283

V

Vascular endothelia growth factor (VEGF)................282, 283, 288, 291
Viral infection.. 40, 323

W

Western blot 119, 242, 243, 253
Western blotting...................................92, 104, 117–122, 134, 169, 248, 249, 257, 259, 262, 265
Whole-mount immunofluorescence 325
WNT 3, 4, 58, 80, 82, 83, 180, 290, 315, 316

X

Xenograft..........4, 5, 13, 14, 18, 21, 287, 300, 307–313

Y

Yap 316, 317

V

Vascular endothelial growth factor (VEGF) 262, 283, 285, 291
Viral infection 49, 326

W

Western blot 119, 282, 284, 285
Western blotting 95, 104, 117–122, 184, 185, 218, 240, 247, 258, 263, 265
Whole mount immunofluorescence 325
WNT 3, 4, 8, 79, 82, 83, 180, 290, 315, 324

X

Xenograft 3, 6, 13, 14, 15, 27, 282, 300, 307, 312

Y

Yap 310, 317

MIX
Papier aus verantwortungsvollen Quellen
Paper from responsible sources
FSC® C105338

If you have any concerns about our products,
you can contact us on
ProductSafety@springernature.com

In case Publisher is established outside the EU,
the EU authorized representative is:
Springer Nature Customer Service Center GmbH
Europaplatz 3, 69115 Heidelberg, Germany

Printed by Libri Plureos GmbH
in Hamburg, Germany